Title ... related interest

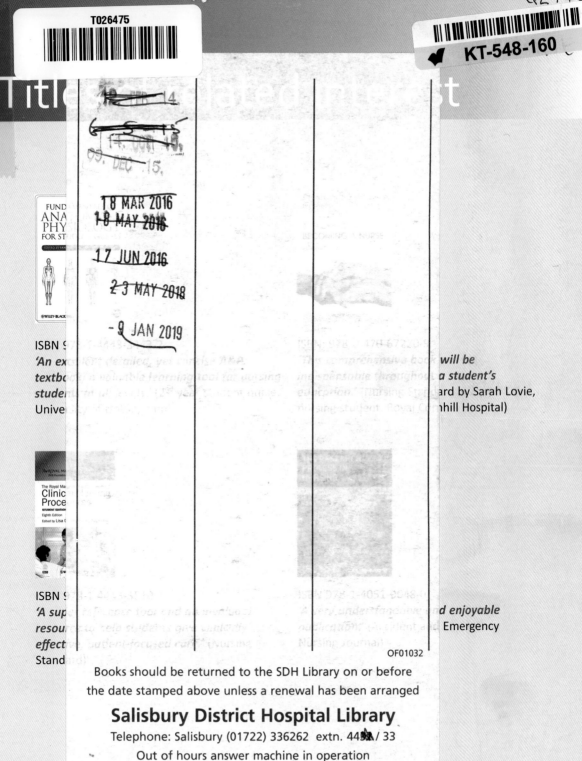

FUND...
ANA...
PHY...
FOR ST...

@WILEY-BLACK...

ISBN 9...
'An ex...lent detailed, yet concise textbook...a valuable learning tool for nursing student...' (*...* 1st year student nurse, University of...)

Clinic
Proce
Eighth Edition
Edited by Lisa ...

ISBN 9...
'A supe...reference tool and assessment resour...to help students give patient effectiv...' student-focused care' (*Nursing Standard*)

...BECOMING A NURSE...

ISBN 978 ... 17H-67220-...
'This comprehensive book will be indispensable throughout a student's education' (*Nursing Standard* by Sarah Lovie, nursing tutor, Royal Cornhill Hospital)

ISBN 978 1-4051 6048-...
A very understanding and enjoyable education' (*Student ...* Emergency *Nursing Journal*)

OF01032

Fundamentals of

Applied Pathophysiology

*For all the students we have had the pleasure of working with,
helping them to develop their knowledge and skills.*

SECOND EDITION

Fundamentals of
Applied
Pathophysiology

An essential guide for
nursing and healthcare students

EDITED BY

MURALITHARAN NAIR

Senior Lecturer, University of Hertfordshire

AND

IAN PEATE

Visiting Professor of Nursing, University of West London
Independent Consultant and *Editor in Chief* British Journal of Nursing

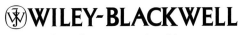

A John Wiley & Sons, Ltd., Publication

Library of Congress Cataloging-in-Publication Data
Fundamentals of applied pathophysiology : an essential guide for nursing and healthcare students / edited by Muralitharan Nair and Ian Peate. – 2nd ed.
     p.   cm.
   Includes bibliographical references and index.
   ISBN 978-0-470-67062-0 (pbk. : alk. paper)   1. Physiology, Pathological.   2. Nursing.   I. Nair, Muralitharan.
II. Peate, Ian.
   RB113.F86 2013
   616.07–dc23
                                                2012028351

A catalogue record for this book is available from the British Library.

Contents

About the series

Wiley's *Fundamentals* series are a wide-ranging selection of textbooks written to support pre-registration nursing and other healthcare students throughout their course. Packed full of useful features such as learning objectives, activities to test knowledge and understanding, and clinical scenarios, the titles are also highly illustrated and fully supported by interactive MCQs, and each one includes access to a Wiley E-Text powered by VitalSource – an interactive digital version of the book including downloadable text and images and highlighting and note-taking facilities. Accessible on your laptop, mobile phone or tablet device, the *Fundamentals* series is *the* most flexible, supportive textbook series available for nursing and healthcare students today.

Contributors

Carl Clare RN DipN BSc (Hons) MSc (Lond) PGDE (Lond)
Senior Lecturer, Department of Adult Nursing and Primary Care, School of Health and Social Work, University of Hertfordshire, Hatfield, Hertfordshire, UK

Carl began his nursing career as a Nursing Auxiliary in 1990. He later undertook a 3-year student nurse training at Selly Oak Hospital (Birmingham). He moved to the Royal Devon and Exeter Hospitals, then to the Northwick Park Hospital and finally to the Royal Brompton and Harefield NHS Trust as a Resuscitation Officer and Honorary Teaching Fellow of Imperial College (London). He has worked in nurse education since 2001. His key areas of interest are physiology, sociology, cardiac care and resuscitation. Carl has previously published work in the field of cardiac care and resuscitation.

Louise McErlean RGN MA BSc (Hons)
Senior Lecturer, Department of Adult Nursing and Primary Care, School of Health and Social Work, University of Hertfordshire, Hatfield, Hertfordshire, UK

Louise began her nursing career in 1986 in Glasgow, becoming a Registered General Nurse. She later completed the intensive care course for RGNs while working in Belfast as a staff nurse. Louise moved to London in 1997 and worked towards a Junior Sister's role in Intensive Care. She moved to the University of Hertfordshire in 2005 where she is currently employed as a senior lecturer. Her key areas of interest are learning and teaching pre-registration nursing and intensive care nursing.

Janet G. Migliozzi RGN BSc (Hons) MSc (London) PGD Ed. FHEA
Senior Lecturer, Department of Adult Nursing and Primary Care, School of Health and Social Work, University of Hertfordshire, Hatfield, Hertfordshire, UK

Janet commenced her nursing career in London, becoming a Staff Nurse in 1988. She has worked at a variety of hospitals across London, predominately in vascular, orthopaedic and high-dependency surgery before specialising in infection prevention and control. She has worked in nurse education since 1999. Her key interests include microbiology, particularly in relation to healthcare-associated infection, vascular/surgical nursing, health informatics and nurse education. Janet has previously published work in the field of minimising risk in relation to healthcare-associated infection and is a member of the Infection Prevention Society.

Muralitharan Nair SRN RMN DipN (Lond) RNT Cert Ed. Cert in Counselling BSc (Hons) MSc (Surrey) FHEA
Senior Lecturer, Department of Adult Nursing and Primary Care, School of Health and Social Work, University of Hertfordshire, Hatfield, Hertfordshire, UK

Muralitharan commenced his nursing career in 1971 at Edgware General Hospital, becoming a Staff Nurse. In 1975, he commenced his mental health nurse training at Springfield Hospital and worked as a Staff Nurse for approximately 1 year. He has worked at St Mary's Hospital, Paddington and Northwick Park Hospital, returning to Edgware General Hospital to take up the post of Senior Staff Nurse and then Charge Nurse. He has worked in nurse education since 1989. His key interests include physiology, diabetes, surgical nursing and nurse education. Muralitharan has published in journals and co-edited and written textbooks, and he is an experienced nurse educator.

Ian Peate EN(G), RGN, DipN (Lond), RNT, BEd (Hons), MA(Lond), LLM
Visiting Professor of Nursing, School of Nursing, Midwifery and Healthcare, Faculty of Health and Human Sciences, University of West London, Brentford, Middlesex, UK; Independent Consultant and Editor-in-Chief British Journal of Nursing

Ian began his nursing career in 1981 at the Central Middlesex Hospital, becoming an Enrolled Nurse working in an intensive care unit. He later undertook a 3-year student nurse training at Central Middlesex and Northwick Park Hospitals, becoming a Staff Nurse and then a Charge Nurse. He has worked in healthcare education since 1989. He is currently Professor of Nursing. His key areas of expertise focus on nursing theory and practice, sexual health, HIV and men's health. He is widely published and an experienced healthcare educator.

Anthony Wheeldon RN Dip HE BSc (Hons) MSc (Lond) PGDE
Senior Lecturer, Department of Adult Nursing and Primary Care, School of Health and Social Work, University of Hertfordshire, Hatfield, Hertfordshire, UK

After qualification in 1995, Anthony worked as a Staff Nurse and a Senior Staff Nurse in the Respiratory Directorate at the Royal Brompton and Harefield NHS Trust. He began teaching on postregistration courses in 2000 before moving into full-time nurse education at Thames Valley University in 2002. Anthony has a wide range of nursing interests, including cardiorespiratory nursing, anatomy and physiology, respiratory assessment and nurse education. He is currently a Senior Lecturer at the University of Hertfordshire.

Acknowledgements

We would like to thank all of our colleagues for their help, support, comments and suggestions.

Muralitharan would like to thank his wife, Evangeline, and his daughters, Samantha and Jennifer, for their continued support and patience.

Ian would like to thank his partner Jussi Lahtinen for all of his continued support and encouragement.

Copyright information

Several Wiley publications have contributed artwork to this book. We are grateful for permission to use and adapt the artwork.

Bulstrode and Swales (2007) The Musculoskeletal System at a Glance, Blackwell Publishing, Oxford

Graham-Brown and Burns (2002) Lecture Notes on Dermatalogy, 8th edition, Blackwell Publishing, Oxford

Grobowski and Tortora (2003) Principles of Anatomy and Physiology, 10th edition, John Wiley & Sons, Hoboken

Tortora and Derrickson (2011) Principles of Anatomy and Physiology, 13th edition, John Wiley & Sons, Hoboken

Tortora and Derrickson (2009) Principles of Anatomy and Physiology, 12th edition, John Wiley & Sons, Hoboken

Tortora and Derrickson (2007) Principles of Anatomy and Physiology, 11th edition, John Wiley & Sons, Hoboken

Artwork reproduced with permission from third-parties is credited at the end of the appropriate caption.

Preface

This second edition of the hugely popular *Fundamentals of Applied Pathophysiology* provides you with an up to date overview of pathophysiology and related care. This edition supplements a nursing focus by broadening the professional base to include all healthcare students; hence the title change to *Fundamentals of Applied Pathophysiology: An Essential Guide for Nursing and Healthcare Students*.

An integrated, multidisciplinary approach to the provision of health and social care is high up on the agendas of those who provide health and social care. This edition goes some way to ensuring that healthcare students work as a part of an interdisciplinary team. This text will help you develop critical thinking, innovation and creativity in relation to the health and well-being of the people you have the privilege to care for.

There are a number of new features that have been added in order to enhance learning and to encourage application of the theoretical principles to care provision – wherever this may be. Each chapter now incorporates two case studies related to the chapter content; there are questions at the end of each case study that provoke reflection and further thought. Word searches, fill in the blanks and label the diagram activities are provided at the end of each chapter, with answers given on the accompanying website; and on the website are 10 multiple choice questions for each chapter Each chapter offers a list of further resources that the reader may wish to use to enhance and develop learning. A glossary of terms is included at the end of each chapter.

How to get the best out of your textbook

Welcome to the new edition of *Fundamentals of Applied Pathophysiology: An Essential Guide for Nursing and Healthcare Students*. Over the next few pages you will be shown how to make the most of the learning features included in the textbook.

The Anytime, Anywhere Textbook ▶

For the first time, your textbook comes with free access to a **Wiley E-Text Edition** – a digital, interactive version of this textbook which you own as soon as you download it.

Your Wiley E-Text Edition allows you to:

Search: Save time by finding terms and topics instantly in your book, your notes, even your whole library (once you've downloaded more textbooks)

Note and Highlight: Colour code, highlight and make digital notes right in the text so you can find them quickly and easily

Organize: Keep books, notes and class materials organized in folders inside the application

Share: Exchange notes and highlights with friends, classmates and study groups

Upgrade: Your textbook can be transferred when you need to change or upgrade computers

Link: Link directly from the page of your interactive textbook to all of the material contained on the companion website

Copy and paste: Photographs and illustration can be placed into assignments, presentations and your own notes.

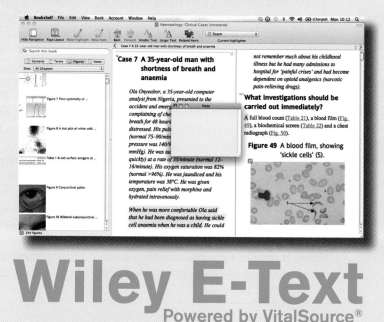

Wiley E-Text
Powered by VitalSource®

To access your Wiley E-Text Edition:

- Find the redemption code on the inside front cover of this book and carefully scratch away the top coating of the label. Visit **www.vitalsource.com/software/bookshelf/downloads** to download the Bookshelf application to your computer, laptop or mobile device.
- If you have purchased this title as an e-book, access to your Wiley E-Text Edition is available with proof of purchase within 90 days. Visit **http://support.wiley.com** to request a redemption code via the 'Live Chat' or 'Ask A Question' tabs.
- Open the Bookshelf application on your computer and register for an account.
- Follow the registration process and enter your redemption code to download your digital book.
- For full access instructions, visit **www.wiley.com/go/ fundamentalsofappliedpathophysiology**

CourseSmart gives you instant access (via computer or mobile device) to this Wiley-Blackwell eTextbook and its extra electronic functionality, at 40% off the recommended retail print price. See all the benefits at **www.coursesmart.com/students**

Instructors . . . receive your own digital desk copies!
It also offers instructors an immediate, efficient, and environmentally-friendly way to review this textbook for your course.

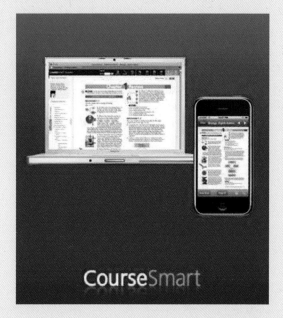

For more information visit **www.coursesmart.com/instructors**.
With CourseSmart, you can create lecture notes quickly with copy and paste, and share pages and notes with your students. Access your Wiley CourseSmart digital textbook from your computer or mobile device instantly for evaluation, class preparation, and as a teaching tool in the classroom.

Simply sign in at **http://instructors.coursesmart.com/bookshelf** to download your Bookshelf and get started. To request your desk copy, hit 'Request Online Copy' on your search results or book product page.

How to get the best out of your textbook

Features contained within your textbook

Every chapter begins with a contents list, some quick questions to test your knowledge, and the learning outcomes you should have achieved by the end of the chapter.

Case studies place the topics you read about into a real-life clinical context.

Case study

Mr Suresh Patel is a 46-year-old married man who works as a bus driver. This morning, while he was having breakfast, Mr Patel felt unwell and collapsed but regained consciousness. His wife called for an ambulance. He is admitted to A&E complaining of chest pain spreading to the shoulders, neck and arms. His wife states that he complained of not feeling well when he got up that morning and that he vomited a couple of times in the toilet. His wife indicates that generally he is a fit man but does suffer from hypertension for which he takes medications to control his blood pressure. She informs you that Mr Patel has a family history of diabetes and hypertension and that he is under stress as he fears he will lose his job as a result of cuts and that they are behind in their mortgage payments.

Your textbook is full of useful illustrations, photographs and tables.

Every chapter ends with a conclusion summing up what you've learnt, a glossary, references and a range of activities to test your understanding of what you've been studying.

Activities

Here are some activities and exercises to help test your learning. For the answers to these exercises, as well as further self-testing activities, visit our website at www.wiley.com/go/fundamentalsofappliedpathophysiology

We hope you enjoy your new textbook. Good luck with your studies!

4

Shock

Janet G. Migliozzi

Senior Lecturer, Department of Adult Nursing and Primary Care, School of Health and Social Work, University of Hertfordshire, Hatfield, Hertfordshire, UK

Contents

Key words

- Anaphylactic shock
- Anaerobic metabolism
- Cardiac output
- Distributive shock
- Homeostasis
- Hypovolaemic shock
- Hypoperfusion
- Neurogenic shock
- Obstructive shock
- Peripheral vasodilatation
- Septic shock
- Toxic shock syndrome

Test your prior knowledge

- What does the cardiovascular system consist of?
- What is homeostasis?
- How is blood pressure maintained at a constant level?
- List the different types of shock.

Learning outcomes

On completion of this chapter the reader will be able to:

- Describe the different types of shock and their causative factors.
- Describe the clinical presentation of the different types of shock.
- Describe the pathophysiology and three stages of shock.
- Understand the care of the patient in shock.

Table 8.1.   Summary of the solutes of the kidney.

Inorganic solutes	Organic solutes
Sodium	Urea
Potassium	Creatinine
Calcium	Uric acid
Magnesium	
Iron	
Chloride	
Sulphate	
Phosphate	
Bicarbonate	
Ammonia	

Adapted from Mader (2011).

Figure 8.6   Nephron with capillaries.

How to use the website

Don't forget to visit the companion website for this book:

www.wiley.com/go/fundamentalsofappliedpathophysiology

There you will find valuable instructor and student material designed to enhance your learning, including:

- instructor image bank
- interactive multiple choice questions
- interactive true/false exercises
- word searches
- label the diagram activities
- searchable glossary
- further reading and resources

Introduction

Ian Peate[1] and Muralitharan Nair[2]

[1]*Visiting Professor of Nursing, School of Nursing, Midwifery and Healthcare, Faculty of Health and Human Sciences, University of West London, Brentford, Middlesex; Independent Consultant and Editor in Chief British Journal of Nursing.*
[2]*Senior Lecturer, Department of Adult Nursing and Primary Care, School of Health and Social Work, University of Hertfordshire, Hatfield, Hertfordshire, UK.*

Pathophysiology

Pathophysiology is concerned with the disturbance of normal mechanical, physical and biochemical functions. The disturbance is either caused by disease, an abnormal syndrome or a condition. Porth (2009) looks at the word 'pathophysiology' – it is a combined word, from the Greek *pathos*, meaning disease, and physiology, meaning related to the various normal functions of the human body. Pathophysiology addresses both the cellular and the organ changes that occur with disease, as well as the effects these changes have on body function. When something impacts upon the normal physiological functioning of the body (i.e. disease), this then becomes a pathophysiological issue. It must, however, be remembered that normal health is not and cannot be exactly the same in any two individuals; therefore, the term 'normal' must be treated with caution.

This text has been written with the intention of making the sometimes complex subject of pathophysiology accessible and exciting. The human body has an extraordinary ability to respond to disease in a number of physiological and psychological ways; it is able to compensate for the changes that occur as a result of the disease process. This text considers those changes (the pathophysiological processes) and the effect they can have on a person.

Healthcare provision

The provision of healthcare is in a constant state of flux, not least because it should aim to respond to the global shift in the burden of disease; a larger number of people affected by long-term conditions is now seen. An integrated approach to health and social care is essential if the needs of people accessing services are to be met safely and effectively.

People who are affected by long-term conditions (patients and families) can often experience physical and mental health problems at the same time either as a consequence of their illness or independent of it, and they are entitled to receive care from healthcare professionals who are knowledgeable, kind, caring and compassionate.

There are a number of factors that impinge on the provision of healthcare, the maintenance of health and the prevention of disease, e.g.:

- health inequalities
- technological advances
- public expectation
- the role and function of the healthcare professional
- the role and function of other healthcare providers
- personal, social and cultural factors.

To be able to care for people, safely and effectively, the healthcare professional must have the appropriate knowledge and skills to meet needs:

- in a complex and diverse society where social inequality exists
- inside and outside hospital and across health and social care
- across public, private and voluntary health provider organisations
- of an increasing older population
- of those with long-term conditions
- across the patient care pathway
- in supporting lifestyle changes
- using disease prevention and health promotional interventions
- by treating patients as partners in healthcare and maximising choice
- through the use of technological advances
- in new and emerging roles that cross professional boundaries
- as leaders and members of multidisciplinary and interdisciplinary teams
- as lifelong learners in an ever-evolving healthcare environment.

In order for the healthcare student to aspire to and provide care that takes the above points into account, there must be a sound understanding of pathophysiological principles.

Fundamentals of Applied Pathophysiology

This is a foundation text that will enable the reader to grow personally and professionally in relation to the provision of healthcare. This textbook is primarily intended for healthcare students who will come into contact with patients who may have a variety of physically-related healthcare problems, such as pneumonia, diabetes mellitus and Alzheimer's disease, in both the hospital and community settings. The focus of the text is on the adult person. Illness and disease are discussed explicitly, emphasising the fact that individuals do become ill and experience disease.

It is the intention of this text to develop knowledge and skills both in theory and practice, and to apply this knowledge in order to provide safe and effective high-quality care. The overriding aim is to relate normal body function to pathological changes that may lead to disease processes, preventing the individual from leading a 'normal' life.

The level at which the text has been written will provide readers with a straightforward understanding of applied pathophysiology, providing healthcare students with an essential/fundamental understanding of applied pathophysiology in order to deliver high-quality care in any setting.

Fundamentals of Applied Pathophysiology is not only intended as a valuable textbook for students during their lectures, but also as a reference resource to be used in the practice setting (wherever this may be). It is not our intention that this text be read from cover to cover – the reader is encouraged to delve in and out of it; we aim to entice and encourage the reader to read further and in so doing instil a sense of curiosity. The book is written with healthcare students in mind and provides an approach to pathophysiological issues in a more user-friendly manner. Illustrations are used in abundance to assist the reader in understanding and appreciating the complex disease patterns that are being discussed.

Using a fundamental approach will provide readers with an essential understanding of applied pathophysiology. A result of working in a variety of healthcare settings is that students may find themselves assisting and working with other healthcare professionals in the care and management of the patient, e.g. assisting in radiology departments in the safe preparation of patients for special investigations, such as a barium meal, or re-enforcing the dietary advice given to patients by a dietician. An understanding of 'normal' and 'abnormal' pathophysiology can help the student and the patient.

A note about the terms used

There are a plethora of terms used to describe people who are the recipients of healthcare and choosing the correct term, one that will be appreciated by all readers, is challenging.

The term 'patient' can refer to all groups and individuals who have direct or indirect contact with all health and social care workers. Patient is the expression that is commonly used within the National Health Service (NHS) and it is a term that has been used throughout this text. It is recognised and respected that not everyone supports the use of the passive concept that can be associated with this term, but it is used here in the knowledge that it is widely understood; it may apply to those who are recipients of health and social care in hospitals, in the person's own home, in the primary care setting and in the independent and voluntary sector. We could have used other expressions, e.g. service user, client or consumer; however, for the sake of brevity the phrase patient has been used.

The chapters

The format of this text allows the reader to use it either as a quick reference guide to pathophysiology or in a more in-depth manner; this is an easy-to-use textbook providing the fundamental concepts associated with pathophysiological processes. The processes of specific diseases are introduced; treatments and care are provided in a clear and concise manner.

The text uses a sound evidence base throughout, drawing on contemporary literature to support discussion. The use of standards/frameworks produced by voluntary and statutory organisations is also included, e.g. patient safety and risk assessment. Government policy, in the guise of the National Service Frameworks, is referred to and readers are encouraged to probe deeper to inform their practice with the overriding aim of the provision of safe and effective care. However, the reader should always make reference to local guidance when necessary.

Each chapter begins with a list of key words, introducing the reader at an early stage to terms that will be discussed within the chapter. To assess current knowledge, the reader is invited to test this at the start of each chapter and again at the end. The intended learning outcomes outline what the chapters will cover. Illustrations have been included in order to ease and facilitate learning. There are two case studies in each chapter that bring to life the pathophysiology being discussed and at the end of each case study, a number of questions that encourage you to dig deeper and to give more thought to the issues being discussed.

At the end of each chapter, there are also another set of questions provided for you to test your knowledge; this can help you determine how far you have progressed after reading and assimilating the contents of the chapter. Other features that aim to enhance learning and aid retention of facts are various exercises for you to complete, a word search, fill in the blanks and a diagram that you are asked to label – the intention is to test yourself and to broaden your learning. In each chapter there are further resources related to the topics covered in the chapter to further enhance learning. A glossary of terms is available at the end of each chapter, providing you with the opportunity to develop your vocabulary further in relation to the terminology being used.

This interactive approach is provided in an attempt to prompt thinking and to encourage you to investigate and explore a field further in relation to the pathophysiological issues discussed or even those that have not been discussed.

Our overriding objective is to encourage and motivate you, as well as to instil confidence and competence to become a proficient provider of care. Providing care with a sound knowledge base and the desire to care with compassion and understanding is a hallmark of a healthcare professional. We believe that understanding and applying this understanding is the key to the provision of high-quality, safe and effective care, as well developing critical thinking, innovation and creativity.

The contributors have enjoyed the challenges of writing this second edition, and we hope that you find the chapters stimulating and thought provoking; above all, we hope that those you care for benefit as a result of your learning.

Reference

Porth, C.M. (2009). *Pathophysiology Concepts of Altered States*, 8th edn. Philadelphia: Lippincott.

1

Cell and body tissue physiology

Anthony Wheeldon

Senior Lecturer, Department of Adult Nursing and Primary Care, School of Health and Social Work, University of Hertfordshire, Hatfield, Hertfordshire, UK

Contents

Fundamentals of Applied Pathophysiology: An Essential Guide for Nursing and Healthcare Students, Second Edition. Edited by Muralitharan Nair and Ian Peate.
© 2013 John Wiley & Sons, Ltd. Published 2013 by John Wiley & Sons, Ltd.

1

Key words

- Plasma membrane
- Organelles
- Connective tissue
- Passive transport
- Nucleus
- Cell cycle
- Muscle tissue
- Active transport
- Cytoplasm
- Epithelial tissue
- Nervous tissue
- Bulk transport

Test your prior knowledge

- What are the three main parts of a human cell?
- Describe the structure and function of a human cell.
- Describe the phases of a cell cycle.

Learning outcomes

On completion of this chapter the reader will be able to:

- Outline the structure and function of a human cell.
- List and describe the functions of the organelles.
- Explain the phases of a cell cycle.
- Explain the cellular transport system.
- Describe the structure and function of epithelial tissue, connective tissue, muscle tissue and nervous tissue.
- Explain the process of tissue repair (inflammation).

Don't forget to visit to the companion website for this book (www.wiley.com/go/ fundamentalsofappliedpathophysiology) where you can find self-assessment tests to check your progress, as well as lots of activities to practise your learning.

Introduction

To understand the human body and how it works (and also how it fails to work properly), it is important to understand the anatomy and physiology of the cell. Living organisms show a wide diversity as regards their size, shape, colour, behaviour and habitat. In spite of this, however, there are many similarities between organisms, and this fundamental similarity is known as the 'cell theory'. This cell theory states that all living organisms are composed of one or more cells and the products of cells. Despite the fact that the cells belong to different organisms, and cells within the same organism may have different functions, there are many similarities between them. For example, there are similarities in their chemical composition, their chemical and biochemical behaviour and in their detailed structure.

All cells have many characteristics, but these characteristics can differ from cell to cell, such as:

- Cells are able to carry out certain specific functions, i.e. they are active.
- Cells need to consume food to live and to carry out their functions. Although they do not have mouths, they are still able to 'catch' and digest their food and use it for growth and reproduction. The correct term for this is endocytosis – they surround and engulf organisms such as bacteria and digest them.
- Cells can grow and repair.
- Similarly, cells can reproduce themselves. They do this by a process known as simple fission. This means that they reproduce themselves by dividing into two, and then each new cell grows to full size before it divides by simple fission and so on. In other words, cells replicate themselves.
- Like humans, cells can become irritable if something upsets or stimulates them.
- The nutrition that cells taken in is also used for the storage and release of energy (just like humans), thus enabling them to grow and repair themselves.
- Similarly, just as humans do not utilise all the food they eat – some of it cannot be used and so is excreted, cells excrete what they do not need or cannot use.
- Just as all humans will eventually die, so will cells. Some have a short life, whilst others survive many years – but eventually they will die.

So, cells are not all that different from humans in many respects. They do what humans do – albeit in different ways.

Anatomy of the cell

Each cell has a structure that is almost as complex as the human body (Figure 1.1). For example, each cell contains as many molecules as the body has cells. There is no such thing as a typical cell. However, each cell is surrounded by a membrane and contains protoplasm. This protoplasm consists of a nucleus, which is kept separate from the rest of the cell by a nuclear membrane (although the nuclear membrane disappears during the process of cell division), and an opaque substance called cytoplasm (Watson, 2005). The cells themselves consist of water, proteins, lipids,

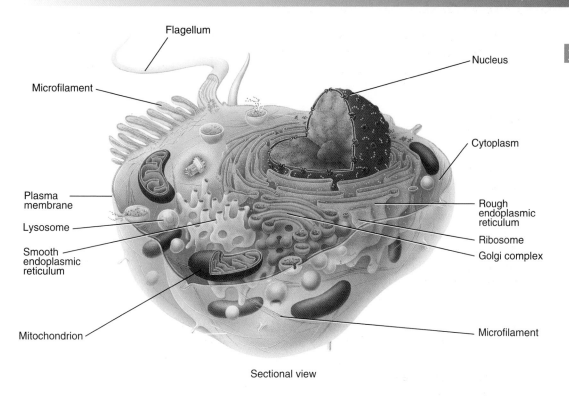

Flagellum

Nucleus

Microfilament

Cytoplasm

Plasma
membrane

Rough
endoplasmic
reticulum

Lysosome

Ribosome

Smooth
endoplasmic
reticulum

Golgi complex

Mitochondrion

Microfilament

Sectional view

Figure 1.1   Simplified structure of a cell.

carbohydrates and various ions such as potassium (K^+) and magnesium (Mg^{2+}). Within the cytoplasm there are also many complex protein structures called organelles.

Cells vary in size from 2 to 20 μm. For example, a lymphocyte (a type of blood cell) is about
8–10 μm in diameter.

All the cells in the body, apart from those on the surface of the body, are surrounded by a fluid
that is known as extracellular fluid (i.e. fluid outside of the cell).

The cell membrane

The cell membrane can vary from 7.5 to 10 nm in thickness. It acts just like a 'skin' that protects
the cell from the outside environment. In addition, it regulates the movement of water, nutrients
and waste products into and out of the cell.

The cell membrane is made up of a double layer (bilayer) of phospholipid (fatty) molecules with
protein molecules interspersed between them (Figure 1.2). A phospholipid molecule consists of
a polar 'head' which is hydrophilic (water loving) and 'tails' which are hydrophobic (water hating).
The hydrophilic 'heads' are attracted to water and are found on the inner and outer surfaces
of the cell (water is the main component of both extracellular and intracellular environments),
whilst the hydrophobic 'tails' are found in the middle of the cell membrane where they can avoid

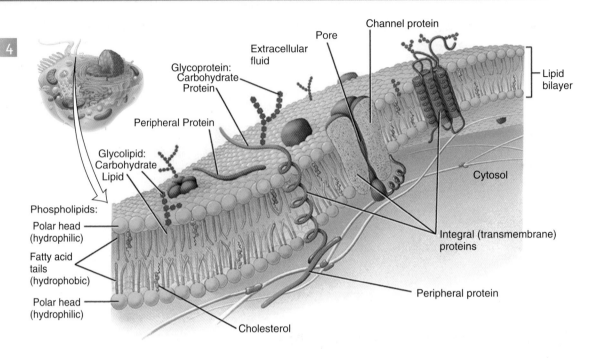

Phospholipids:

Polar head (hydrophilic)

Fatty acid tails (hydrophobic)

Polar head (hydrophilic)

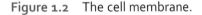

Figure 1.2   The cell membrane.

water. These phospholipid molecules are arranged as a bilayer with the heads facing outwards. This means that the bilayer is self-sealing. It is the central part of the plasma membrane, consisting of the hydrophobic 'tails', that makes the cell membrane impermeable to water-soluble molecules, and so prevents the passage of these molecules into and out of the cell (Marieb, 2010). However, if the membrane just consisted of these phospholipid molecules, then cells would not be able to function – within the cell membrane there are also plasma membrane proteins (PMPs), which can be either integral or peripheral.

Some of the integral PMPs are embedded amongst the tails of the phospholipid molecules, whilst others penetrate the membrane completely (Figure 1.2). Subunits of some of these integral proteins can form channels which allow for the transportation of materials into and out of the cell. Other subunits are able to bind to carbohydrates to form receptor sites. These receptor sites are important, as will be discussed in Chapter 3 – inflammation, immune response and healing.

Peripheral PMPs bind loosely to the surface of the cell membrane and so can easily be separated from it. Some of them function as enzymes to catalyse cellular reactions, whilst others are receptors for hormones and other chemicals, or function as binding sites for attachment to other structures (Marieb, 2010).

Functions

- Endocytosis and exocytosis – the transport of fluids and other matter into and out of the cell.

- Endocytosis is the intake of extracellular fluid and particulate material (small particles) ranging in size from macromolecules to whole cells (e.g. the bacteria engulfed and destroyed by macrophage cells).
- Exocytosis is the bulk transport of material out of the cells.

There are three types of endocytosis:

- Phagocytosis – involves the ingestion of large particles, even whole microbial cells.
- Pinocytosis – involves the ingestion of small particles and fluids.
- Receptor-mediated endocytosis – involves large particles, notably proteins, but also has the important feature of being highly selective.

Endocytosis involves part of the cell membrane being drawn into the cell along with the particles or fluid to be ingested (Figure 1.3). This membrane is then pinched off to form a membrane-bound vesicle within the cell, while at the same time the cell membrane as a whole reseals itself. Inside the cell, the fate of this vesicle depends upon the type of endocytosis involved as well as the material it contains. In some cases, the endocytic vesicle ultimately fuses with an organelle called a lysosome, after which processing of the ingested material can occur. Endocytosis is also the means by which many simple organisms obtain their nutrients.

Transport across the cell membrane

One of the key properties of the cell membrane with regards to transport is its selective permeability. This refers to its ability to let certain materials pass through, whilst preventing others from doing so. This selective permeability is based on the hydrophobicity (water hatred) of its component molecules. Because the phospholipid tails in the centre of the bilayer are composed entirely of hydrophobic fatty acid chains (lipids are fats), it is very difficult for water-soluble (hydrophilic) molecules to penetrate to the membrane interior. The result is a very effective permeability barrier.

However, this barrier can be penetrated, but only by way of specific transport systems. These control what goes into and out of the cell, or what crosses from one subcellular compartment to another. Cell membranes control metabolism by restricting the flow of glucose and other water-soluble metabolites in and out of cells and between subcellular compartments. This is known as compartmentation. The cells store energy in the form of transmembrane ion gradients by allowing high concentrations of particular ions to accumulate on one side of the membrane.

Ions pass from inside to outside of the cell (or the other way round) so that there are more supplies of these ions just outside the cell or inside it and the membrane controls the speed/rate at which these ions pass through the membrane. The controlled release of such ion gradients can be used to:

- extract nutrients from surrounding fluids
- pass electrical messages (known as nerve excitability)
- control cell volume and stop cells bursting from excess fluid.

To return to the cell membrane itself, there are four factors that decide the degree of permeability of a membrane:

- Size of molecules – large molecules cannot pass through the integral membrane proteins, but small ones such as water and amino acids can.

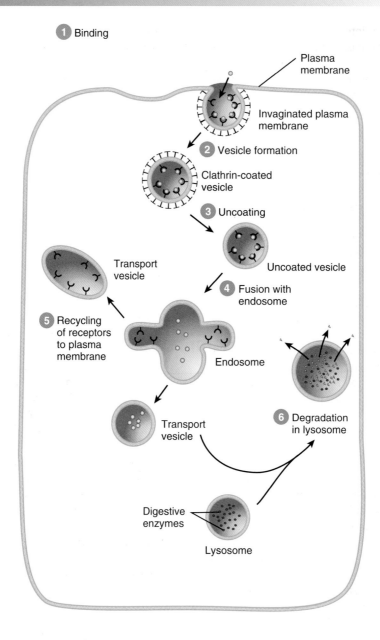

Figure 1.3   Endocytosis.

- Solubility in lipids (fats) – substances that easily dissolve in lipids can pass through the membrane more easily than non–lipid-soluble substances. Lipid-soluble substances include oxygen, carbon dioxide and steroid hormones.
- If an ion has an electrical charge opposite to that of the membrane, then it is attracted to the membrane and can more easily pass through it.

- Carrier integral proteins can carry substances across the membrane, regardless of their size, ability to dissolve in lipids or membrane electrical charge.

There are two ways in which substances can move across the membrane: passive or active. Passive processes are:

- diffusion
- facilitated diffusion
- osmosis
- filtration.

Active processes are:

- active transport pumps
- endocytosis
- exocytosis.

A passive process is one in which the substances move on their own down a concentration gradient from an area of higher to one of lower concentration. The cell does not expend any energy on the process. Think of it as rolling down a hill from an area of high altitude to one of lower altitude. Little energy is expended just rolling down a hill.

Diffusion is the most common form of passive transport in which a substance of higher concentration moves to an area where there is a lower concentration of that substance (Colbert *et al.*, 2011). This difference between the areas of high concentration and of low concentration is known as a concentration gradient. This process of diffusion is essential for respiration. It is through diffusion that oxygen is transported from the lungs to the blood and carbon dioxide makes the opposite journey from the blood to the lungs (Colbert *et al.*, 2011).

Facilitated diffusion is similar to diffusion, but with one exception. For this process to take place, there needs to be a substance that helps – a facilitator. Glucose is moved using this process. Although glucose can move part of the way through the membrane on its own, it needs something else (a carrier/transport protein) to give it that extra push to get it completely through the membrane (Colbert *et al.*, 2011; McCance *et al.*, 2010).

Osmosis is the process in which water travels through a selectively permeable membrane so that concentrations of a substance that is soluble in water (known as a solute) are the same on both sides of that membrane. This is known as osmotic pressure (Figures 1.4 and 1.5). The higher the concentration of the solute on one side of the membrane, the higher the osmotic pressure available for the movement of the water (Colbert *et al.*, 2011).

Filtration is similar to osmosis, except that pressure is applied in order to 'push' water and solutes across that membrane. The heart is a major supplier of the force that can lead to one type of filtration (renal filtration) as it pushes blood into the kidneys where filtration of the blood can take place (Colbert *et al.*, 2011).

An active process is one in which substances move against a concentration gradient from an area of lower to one of higher concentration. To do this, the cell must expend energy; this is released by splitting adenosine triphosphate (ATP) into adenosine diphosphate (ADP) and phosphate. ATP is a compound of a base, a sugar and three phosphate groups (triphosphate). These phosphate groups are held together by high-energy bonds, which when broken release a high level of energy. Once one of these phosphate bonds has been broken and a phosphate group has been released, that compound now has only two phosphate groups (diphosphate).

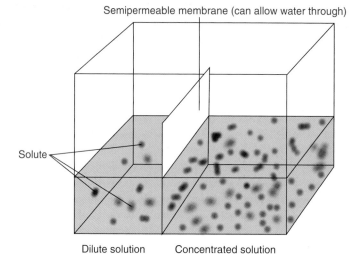

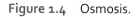

Figure 1.4   Osmosis.

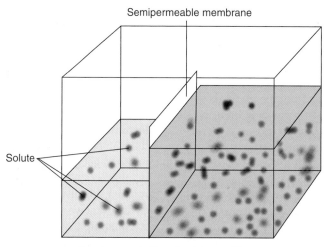

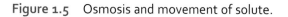

Figure 1.5   Osmosis and movement of solute.

The released phosphate group in turn joins up with another ADP group, so forming another molecule of ATP (with energy stored in the phosphate bonds), and the whole process continues to recur.

The energy is required because the cell is attempting to move a substance to an area that already has a high concentration of that substance. Think again of a hill. When walking up a hill, a lot of energy is expended. Obviously, the higher the concentration already present, the more energy required to move further molecules of the particular substance into that area – the steeper the hill, the more energy is used. For example, cells contain a lot of potassium (K^+); therefore, energy is required to transport more potassium through the membrane and into the cell.

Now, to turn to what is inside the cell membrane, starting with the cytoplasm.

Cytoplasm

Cytoplasm is a ground substance (also known as a matrix) in which various cellular components are found. 'Cyto' means cell, so any word that has 'cyto' in it is to do with cells.

Cytoplasm, itself, is a thick, semitransparent, elastic fluid containing suspended particles and the cytoskeleton. The cytoskeleton provides support and shape to the cell. In addition, it is involved in the movement of structures in the cytoplasm because some cells can change shape, e.g. phagocytic cells (see Figure 1.3).

Role of cytoplasm

- Chemically, cytoplasm is 75–90% water plus solid compounds – mainly carbohydrates, lipids and inorganic substances, and it is the substance in which chemical reactions occur.
- The cytoplasm receives raw materials from the external environment (such as from digested food) and converts them into usable energy by decomposition reactions.
- As well as the breakdown of raw materials to make energy, the cytoplasm is also the site where new substances are synthesised (produced) for the use of the cell.
- It is the place where various chemicals are packaged for transport to other parts of the cell, or to other cells in the body.
- It is in the cytoplasm that various chemicals facilitate the excretion of waste materials.

Nucleus

When considering the nucleus, a simple analogy is to think of it as the brain of the cell.

Prokaryotic cells do not have a nucleus, but eukaryotic cells do. Eukaryotic cells are found in animals and plants, whilst prokaryotic cells are very typical of bacteria. In many ways, prokaryotic cells are less complex and often smaller than eukaryotes.

However, not all human cells possess a nucleus. An example of a cell without a nucleus is the red blood cell. Chapter 7 describes the concave shape of the mature red blood cells. This is because the lack of a nucleus means the red blood cell 'collapses in' on itself. Also, just to make it more confusing, some cells can have more than one nucleus, e.g. some muscle fibre cells (see Figure 1.12).

Some facts about the nucleus are:

- The nucleus is the largest structure in the cell.
- It is surrounded by a nuclear membrane. This nuclear membrane has two layers and, like the cell membrane, is selectively permeable.
- The protoplasm within the nucleus is not called cytoplasm – it is called nucleoplasm.
- The nucleus assumes a great responsibility for both mitosis and meiosis (see later).
- Inside the nucleus is found the genetic material, consisting principally of deoxyribonucleic acid (DNA). When a cell is not reproducing, the genetic material is a threadlike mass called chromatin.

- Before cell division, the chromatin shortens, and coils into rod-shaped bodies called chromosomes.
- The basic structural unit of a chromosome is a nucleosome – composed of DNA and protein.
- DNA has two main functions:
  - It provides the genetic blueprint which ensures that the next generation of cells is identical to existing ones.
  - It provides the plans for the synthesis of protein by the cell.
- All this information is stored in genes.
- Inside the nucleus are little spherical bodies called nucleoli and these are responsible for the production of ribosomes from ribosomal ribonucleic acid (rRNA).
- In humans, there are 23 pairs of chromosomes in each cell with a nucleus, with the exception of the spermatozoa and ova (sperm and eggs).
- Sperm and ova only have 23 single chromosomes (i.e. one of each).
- The chromosomes are the same for males and females except for one pair – the X and Y chromosomes. It is these chromosomes that determine whether a baby is going to be male or female.

Mitosis and meiosis

These are the processes by which the cell reproduces itself. Most human cells reproduce asexually by mitosis, but the spermatozoa and ova reproduce by meiosis. Whereas the cells reproducing by mitosis finish up as exact copies of the parent cells with a pair of each of the 23 chromosomes, the cells reproducing by meiosis just finish up with one each of the 23 chromosomes.

Mitosis

In order for the body to grow, and also for the replacement of body cells that die, cells must be able to reproduce themselves, and in order for genetic information not to be lost, they must be able to reproduce themselves accurately. They do this by cloning themselves. In some organisms, this can occur by simple fission, where the nucleus in a single cell becomes elongated and then divides to form two nuclei in the same cell, each new nucleus carrying identical genetic information. The cytoplasm then divides in the middle between the two nuclei, and so two identical daughter cells result, each with its own nucleus and other essential organelles.

In humans, cell reproduction is a complex process called mitosis, in which the number of chromosomes in the daughter cells has to be the same as in the original parent cell.

Mitosis can be divided into four stages:

1. prophase
2. metaphase
3. anaphase
4. telophase.

- Before and after it has divided, the cell enters a stage known as interphase – this was thought to be a resting period for the cell, but the cell is actually very busy during this period because it has to get ready for replication.
- Extra organelles are manufactured by the replication of existing organelles.
- Also, the cell builds up a store of energy which is required for the process of division.

Prophase

The first stage after interphase is prophase:

- During prophase (Figure 1.6), the chromosomes become shorter, fatter and more easily visible, and each chromosome now consists of two chromatids, each containing the same genetic information (i.e. the DNA has replicated itself during interphase).
- The nucleolus and nuclear membrane disappear, leaving the chromosomes in the cytoplasm.

Metaphase

- During metaphase (Figure 1.7), the 46 chromosomes (two of each of the 23 chromosomes), each consisting of two chromatids, become attached to the spindle fibres.

Anaphase

- During anaphase (Figure 1.8), the chromatids in each chromosome are separated.
- One chromatid from each chromosome then moves towards each pole of the spindle.

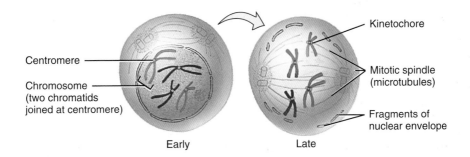

Kinetochore

Centromere

Chromosome
(two chromatids
joined at centromere)

Mitotic spindle
(microtubules)

Fragments of
nuclear envelope

Early   Late

Figure 1.6   Prophase.

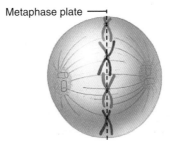

Metaphase plate

Figure 1.7   Metaphase.

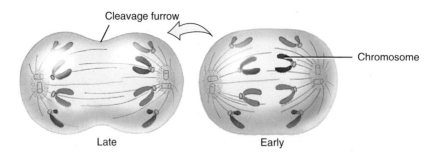

Cleavage furrow

Chromosome

Late   Early

Figure 1.8   Anaphase.

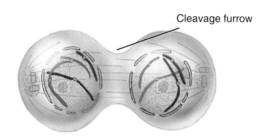

Cleavage furrow

Figure 1.9   Telophase.

Telophase

- There are now 46 chromatids at each pole, and these will form the chromosomes of the daughter cells.
- The cell membrane constricts in the centre of the cell, dividing it into two cells.
- The nuclear spindle disappears, and a nuclear membrane forms around the chromosomes in each of the daughter cells (Figure 1.9).
- The chromosomes become long and threadlike again, and are very difficult to see.

Cell division is now complete, and the daughter cells themselves enter the interphase stage in order to prepare for their replication and division.

Cell cycle

Looking now at the cell cycle (Figure 1.10) and supposing that one full cycle represents 24 hours, then the actual process of replication (mitosis) would only last for about 1 hour out of those 24 hours. The rest of the time, the cell is undertaking the replication of its DNA. It also has to produce two of everything that is in the cell. In addition, it has to go through the process of obtaining and digesting nutrients so that it has the raw materials for this duplication, as well as the energy required in order to carry out various functions of the cell.

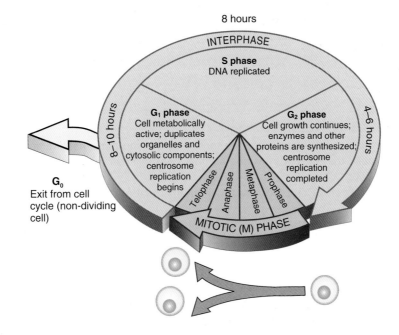

Figure 1.10 Cell cycle.

Table 1.1 Stages of meiosis.

First meiotic stage	Second meiotic stage
Prophase I	Prophase II
Metaphase I	Metaphase II
Anaphase I	Anaphase II
Telophase I	Telophase II

Meiosis

During the reproduction of humans, the egg is penetrated by a sperm, which then releases its DNA to combine with the DNA of the egg, so that the resulting embryo has two copies of each of the 23 chromosomes in nucleated cells. If the sperm and eggs had two copies of each chromosome (like other cells), the resulting fusion and developing embryo would have four copies of each chromosome. This means that the next generation would have four copies of each chromosome. The generation after that would have eight copies, and so on. This is obviously not practical, so the sperm and eggs undergo a process known as meiosis to ensure that the resulting embryo will only carry two copies of each chromosome in each cell with a nucleus.

For descriptive purposes, meiosis can be divided into eight stages (not the four of mitosis). However, they have the same names, but are known as either I or II (Table 1.1). As with mitosis, these phases are continuous with one another. However, there are differences as well as similarities between mitosis and meiosis.

First meiotic stage

Prophase I

- This is similar to prophase in mitosis.
- However, instead of being scattered randomly, the chromosomes are arranged in 23 pairs. For example, the two chromosome number ones will pair up, as will the two chromosome number twos.
- Within each pair of chromosomes, genetic material may be exchanged between the two chromosomes.
- It is these exchanges that are partly responsible for the differences between children of the same parents.
- This process is called 'gene cross-over'.

Metaphase I

As in mitosis, the chromosomes become arranged on the spindles at the equator. However, they remain in pairs.

Anaphase I

One chromosome from each pair moves to each pole, so that there are now 23 chromosomes at each end of the spindle.

Telophase I

The cell membrane now divides the cell into two halves, as in mitosis. Each daughter cell now has half the number of chromosomes that each parent cell had.

Second meiotic stage

- The cells produced by the first meiotic division now divide again.
- Prophase II, metaphase II, anaphase II and telophase II are all similar to their equivalent stage in mitosis, with the exception that the DNA has not been replicated before prophase II, so there are only 23 single chromosomes in each of the granddaughter cells.

Fusion of the gametes

- When the gametes, each with 23 chromosomes, fuse together, a cell known as a zygote with 23 paired chromosomes (i.e. 46 in all) is formed.
- One chromosome in each pair comes from the mother and one from the father.
- The zygotic cell then divides (by mitosis) many times to form the embryo.

The organelles

All cells contain many organelles (little organs).

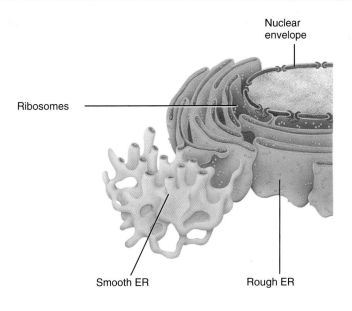

Nuclear
envelope

Ribosomes

Smooth ER   Rough ER

Figure 1.11   Endoplasmic reticulum (ER).

Endoplasmic reticulum

It is believed that the endoplasmic reticulum (ER; Figure 1.11) is formed from the nuclear membrane.

The ER consists of membranes that form a series of channels (called cisternae) dividing the cytoplasm into compartments. The cisternae are concerned with the transport of materials, primarily proteins. The alteration or addition of proteins for export from the cell can occur within the cisternae. They also contain a number of enzymes of importance in cell metabolism, such as digestive enzymes, enzymes involved in the synthesis of steroids, and enzymes responsible for a variety of reactions leading to the removal of toxic substances from the cell (McCance *et al.*, 2010). The ER present in liver cells has a role in drug detoxification.

There are two types of cisternae:

- granular (rough) ER – associated with ribosomes
- agranular (smooth) ER – free of ribosomes.

Granular ER is particularly well developed in cells that actively synthesise (produce) and export proteins. Agranular ER is found in steroid hormone secreting cells, such as the cells of the adrenal cortex or the testes. Ribosomes include tiny particles of RNA on which the synthesis of proteins needed by the cell takes place, and they are formed in the nucleoli.

Golgi apparatus

The Golgi apparatus is a collection of membranous tubes and elongated sacs – actually flattened cisternae stacked together. It plays a part in concentrating and packaging some of the substances that are made in the cell, e.g. lysosomal enzymes. The complex also plays a part in the assembly of substances for secretion outside of the cell. Secretory cells (such as those found in the mucous membrane) have many Golgi stacks, whereas non-secretory cells have few Golgi stacks per cell.

Proteins for export from the cell are synthesised on the ribosomes, and then travel through the ER to the Golgi vesicles (a vesicle is a fluid-filled sac). Vesicles leaving the Golgi fuse with the cell membrane by the process of exocytosis. The contents of the vesicles are then exported out of the cell. In addition, the Golgi is itself involved in the formation of glycoproteins.

Lysosomes

Lysosomes are organelles bound to the membrane and contain a variety of enzymes. Lysosomes have a number of functions:

- Digestion of material taken up by endocytosis, e.g. pathogenic organisms.
- Break down of cell components, e.g. during embryological development, the fingers and toes are webbed – the cells between the toes and fingers are removed by the lysosomal enzymes. After a baby's birth, the uterus, which weighs around 2 kg at full term, is invaded by phagocytic cells that are rich in lysosomes – these reduce the uterus to its non-pregnant weight of about 50 g within about 9 days.
- In normal cells, some of the synthesised proteins may be faulty – lysosymes are responsible for their removal.
- Contribute to hormone production, e.g. thyroxine – a hormone affecting a wide range of physiological activities, including metabolic rate.

It is important that lysosomes do not rupture and release their contents inside living cells; otherwise the lysosomal enzymes would start to digest the cell. In certain degenerative diseases, such as rheumatoid arthritis, enzymes released by the breakdown of lysosomes from macrophages may be a significant factor by attacking living cells and tissues.

Peroxisomes

These are organelles similar in structure to lysosomes, but are much smaller. They are particularly abundant in liver cells. They contain several enzymes that are toxic to body cells. The role of peroxisomes in cells appears to be one of detoxification of harmful substances, such as alcohol and formaldehyde. More importantly, they neutralise dangerous free radicals. Free radicals are highly reactive chemicals that contain electrons that have not been paired off, and so are 'free' to disrupt the structure of molecules (Marieb and Hoehn, 2010).

Mitochondria (single = mitochondrion)

Mitochondria (often known as the power houses of the cell) consist of three membranes. The inner membrane has many folds that increase the surface area available for chemical reactions to occur. This process is collectively known as internal respiration. The mitochondrial matrix (the space surrounded by the inner membrane) contains enzymes of the tricarboxylic acid (TCA) cycle, as well as enzymes involved in fatty acid oxidation. The inner membrane is of the same thickness as the outer membrane and is responsible for oxidative phosphorylation. The mitochondria themselves are often found concentrated in regions of the cell associated with intense metabolic activity.

By using ATP, the mitochondria are able to generate the energy needed by the cell for it to function by converting the chemical energy contained in molecules of food. The production of ATP requires the breakdown of food molecules, and it occurs in several stages, each requiring the appropriate enzyme. An enzyme is a protein that can initiate and speed up a chemical reaction (it acts as a catalyst). The enzymes in the mitochondria are stored in the membranes in the required order so that the reactions occur in the correct sequence. This is very important, as it would be disastrous if the chemical reactions occurred out of sequence.

Mitochondria are self-replicating – just like the cells. DNA that is incorporated into the mitochondrial structure controls the replication process.

Cytoskeleton

The cytoskeleton is a lattice-like collection of fibres and fine tubes in the cytoplasm, and it is involved in the cell's maintenance and alteration of its shape as required.

There are three components of the cytoskeleton:

- microfilaments
- microtubules
- intermediate filaments.

Microfilaments

These are rod-like structures, 6 nm in diameter, consisting of a protein called actin. In muscle, both actin (thick) and myosin – another protein (thin) are involved in the contraction of muscle fibres. In non-muscle cells, microfilaments help to provide support and shape to the cell, and also assist in the movement of cells as well as movement within the cells.

Microtubules

These are relatively straight, slender, cylindrical structures that range in diameter from 18 to 30 nm. They consist of a protein called tubulin. Microtubules, like microfilaments, help to provide shape and support for cells. They also provide conducting channels through which various substances can move through the cytoplasm, and assist in the movement of pseudopodia.

Intermediate filaments

These range in diameter from 8 to 12 nm and also help to determine the shape of the cell. Examples of intermediate filaments are neurofilaments found in the nerve.

Centrioles, cilia and flagella

Centrioles

These are found in most animal cells and are cylindrical structures. They are composed of nine sets of microtubules arranged in a circular pattern. They are involved in cell reproduction.

Cilia and flagella

These structures extend from the surface of some cells and can bend, thus causing movement. In humans, cilia generally have the function of moving fluid or particulates over the surface of cells. Ciliated cells of the respiratory tract move mucus that has trapped foreign particles over the surface of respiratory tissues. A flagellum is usually a much larger structure than a cilium and is often used like a tail to propel the cell forward. The only example of a cell in the human body with a flagellum is the sperm, where the flagellum acts as a tail and propels the sperm towards the ova.

Types of cells

Figure 1.12 illustrates some of the cells that make up certain tissues.

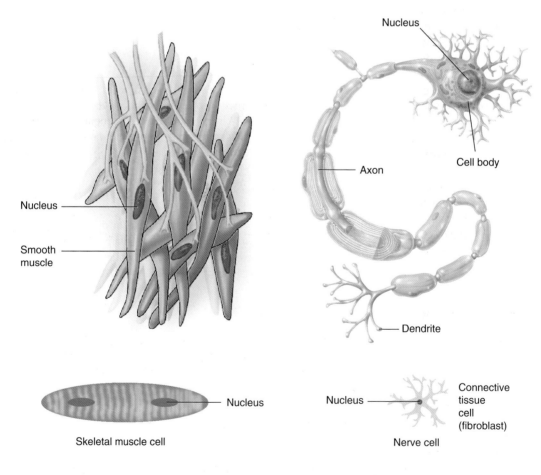

Figure 1.12 Types of cells.

Tissues

A human begins as a single cell – the fertilised egg. As soon as fertilisation takes place, the egg divides continuously. However, these cells do not divide endlessly and haphazardly. They divide and grow together in such a way that they become specialised, e.g. muscle cells, skin cells, cells of the lens of the eye and blood cells (Marieb, 2010). Cells group together to become tissues. Tissues are basically groups of cells that are similar in structure and generally perform the same functions (McCance *et al.*, 2010). There are four primary types of tissues:

- epithelial
- connective
- muscle
- nervous.

Most organs of the body contain all four types of tissue. All four have distinct functions that help to maintain homeostasis. For instance:

- Epithelial tissue is concerned with 'covering'.
- Connective tissue is concerned with 'support'.
- Muscle tissue is concerned with 'movement'.
- Nervous tissue is concerned with 'control' (Wheeldon, 2011).

Specialised cells form themselves into tissue in one of the two ways. The first way is by mitosis. Cells formed as a result of mitosis are clones of the original cell. Therefore, if one cell with a specialised function undergoes mitosis, and subsequent generations of daughter cells continue to undergo mitosis, then the resulting hundreds of cells will all be of the same type and have the same function – they will become tissue. For example, epithelial cell sheets (such as skin) are formed as a result of mitosis (McCance *et al.*, 2010).

The second way involves the migration of specialised cells to the site of tissue formation and then assembling there. This is particularly seen during the development of the embryo when, for example, cells migrate to sites in the embryo where they differentiate and assemble into a variety of tissues (McCance *et al.*, 2010). This movement of cells is known as chemotaxis. Chemotaxis is discussed in detail in Chapter 3, but put simply, it is the 'movement along a chemical gradient caused by chemical attraction' (McCance *et al.*, 2010).

Epithelial tissue

Epithelial tissue lines and covers areas of the body, as well as forming the glandular tissue of the body. So, the exterior of the body is covered by one type of epithelial tissue (the skin), whilst another type of epithelial tissue lines some digestive system organs, such as the stomach and the small intestines, and the kidneys. In effect, epithelial tissue covers most of the internal and external surfaces of the body.

Epithelial tissue is classified into two ways:

- the number of cell layers:
  - simple – where the epithelium is formed from a single layer of cells (Figure 1.13).
  - stratified – where the epithelium has two or more layers of cells (Figure 1.14).

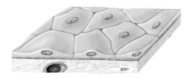

Figure 1.13   Simple epithelium.

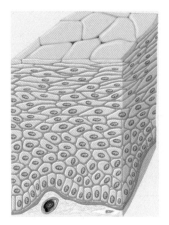

Figure 1.14   Stratified epithelium.

- shape:
  - squamous
  - cuboidal
  - columnar.

Simple epithelial tissues are most concerned with absorption, secretion and filtration, but because they are usually very thin, they are not involved in protection.

Simple squamous epithelium rests on a basement membrane (basal layer). The basement membranes provide a layer of cells that supports and separates epithelial tissue from underlying connective tissue. Squamous epithelial cells fit very closely together to form a thin sheet of tissue. It is this type of epithelial tissue that is found in the alveoli of the lungs and the walls of capillaries. Rapid diffusion of filtration can take place through this very thin tissue. Oxygen and carbon dioxide exchange takes place through the epithelial tissue lining the alveoli of the lungs, whilst nutrients and gases can pass through the epithelial tissue from the cells into and out of the capillaries. In addition, simple squamous epithelial cells form serous membranes that line certain body cavities and organs (Wheeldon, 2011).

Simple cuboidal epithelial tissue consists of one layer of cells resting on a basement membrane. However, because cuboidal epithelial cells are thicker than squamous epithelial cells, they are found in different places of the body and perform different functions. This epithelial tissue is found

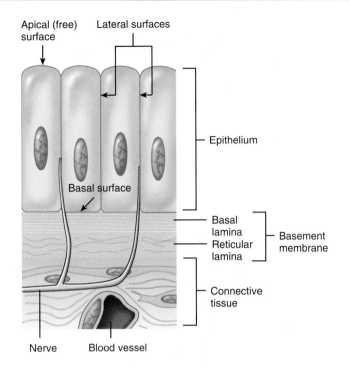

Apical (free)   Lateral surfaces
surface

Epithelium

Basal surface

Basal
lamina   Basement
Reticular   membrane
lamina

Connective
tissue

Nerve   Blood vessel

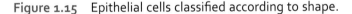

Figure 1.15   Epithelial cells classified according to shape.

in glands, such as the salivary glands and the pancreas, as well as forming the walls of kidney tubules and covering the surface of the ovaries (Marieb, 2010).

Simple columnar epithelium (Figure 1.15), whilst being composed of single layer of cells, is made up of a single layer of quite tall cells that, like the other two types, fit closely together. This epithelial tissue lines the entire length of the digestive tract from the stomach to the anus and contains goblet cells. Goblet cells produce mucus, and those simple columnar epithelial tissues that line all the body cavities that are open to the body exterior are known as mucous membranes (Marieb, 2010).

Stratified epithelial tissue, unlike the simple epithelial tissue, consists of two or more cell layers. Because these stratified epithelial tissues have more than one layer of cells, they are stronger and more robust than the simple epithelia. This means that a primary function of stratified epithelia is protection.

Stratified squamous epithelial tissue (Figure 1.14) is the most common stratified epithelium in the human body, and it consists of several layers of cells (Marieb, 2010). Although this epithelial tissue is called squamous epithelium, in actual fact, it is not made up entirely of squamous cells. It is the cells at the free edge of the epithelial tissue that are composed of squamous cells, whilst those cells that are close to the basement membrane are composed of either cuboidal or colum-nar cells. Squamous epithelium is found in places that are most at risk of everyday damage, including the oesophagus, the mouth and the outer layer of the skin (Marieb, 2010).

Stratified cuboidal epithelial tissue only has two cell layers and is fairly rare in the human body, only being found in the ducts of large glands. The same can be said of the stratified columnar epithelial tissue.

There is a fourth type of epithelial tissue, known as transitional epithelium. This is a highly modified stratified squamous epithelium and it forms the lining of just a few organs/structures – all of which form part of the urinary system – the urinary bladder, the ureters and part of the urethra. This type of tissue has been modified to cope with the considerable stretching that these organs undergo. So, when one of these organs or structures is not stretched, the tissue has many layers with the superficial (those in the top layer) cells being rounded and looking like domes. However, when distended with urine, the epithelium becomes thinner, the surface cells flatten and they become just like squamous cells. These transitional cells are able to slide past one another and change their shape, allowing the wall of the ureter to stretch as a greater volume of urine flows through. Similarly, it allows for more urine to be stored in the bladder (Marieb, 2010).

Glandular epithelium

Glandular epithelial tissue is found within glands. According to Marieb (2010), a gland consists of several cells that make and secrete a particular product.

Two major types of glands develop from epithelial sheets:

- exocrine glands
- endocrine glands.

Exocrine glands have ducts leading from them, and their secretions empty through these ducts to the surface of the epithelium. Examples of exocrine glands include the sweat glands, the liver and the pancreas.

Endocrine glands, on the other hand, do not possess ducts. Instead, their secretions diffuse directly into the blood vessels that are found within the glands. All endocrine glands secrete hormones. These glands include the thyroid, the adrenal glands and the pituitary gland.

Connective tissue

Connective tissue is found everywhere in the body and it connects body parts to one another. It is the most abundant and widely distributed of all four primary tissue types. It varies considerably in structure and has four main functions:

- protection
- support
- binding together other tissues (Marieb, 2010)
- acting as storage sites for excess nutrients (McCance *et al.*, 2010).

However, the most common structure and function of connective tissue is to act as the framework on which the epithelial cells gather in order to form the organs of the body (McCance *et al.*, 2010).

There are several common characteristics of connective tissue. One is that there are few cells in the tissue, but surrounding these few cells there is a great deal of what is known as extracellular matrix. This extracellular matrix is composed of ground substance and fibres and it varies in consistency from fluid to a semisolid gel. The fibres are made up of fibroblasts – one of the connective tissue cells, and are of three types:

- collagen (white) fibres
- elastic (yellow) fibres
- reticular fibres.

Collagen fibres have great strength, whilst elastic fibres are can stretch and then recoil. The reticular fibres form the internal 'skeleton' of soft organs such as the spleen.

The ground substance is composed largely of water plus some adhesion proteins and large polysaccharide molecules, and it is these adhesion proteins that serve as a glue that attaches the connective tissue cells to the fibres. The change of consistency within the ground substance from fluid to a semisolid gel depends upon the number of polysaccharide molecules that are present. An increase in polysaccharide molecules causes the matrix to move from being a fluid to being a semisolid gel. The ground substance can store large amounts of water, so it serves as a water reservoir for the body (Marieb and Hoehn, 2010).

Connective tissue forms a 'packing' tissue around organs of the body (very much like the packing that can surround a delicate object in a parcel in transit) and so protects them. It is able to bear weight and to withstand stretching and various traumas, such as abrasions. There is a wide variation in types of connective tissue, e.g. fat tissue is composed mainly of cells and a soft matrix. Bone and cartilage have very few cells but do contain large amounts of hard matrix and that is what makes them so strong (Marieb, 2010).

There are also variations in the blood supply to the tissue. Although most connective tissues have a good blood supply, there are some types, e.g. tendons and ligaments, that have a poor blood supply, whilst cartilage has no blood supply. That is the reason why these structures heal very slowly when they are injured – often a broken bone will heal much quicker than a damaged tendon or ligament (Marieb, 2010).

Bone

Bone is the most rigid of the connective tissues and it is composed of bone cells surrounded by a very hard matrix containing calcium and large numbers of collagen fibres. Because of their hardness, bones provide protection, support and muscle attachment (Marieb, 2010).

Cartilage

Cartilage, which is not as hard, but is more flexible than bone, is found in only a few places in the body, e.g. hyaline cartilage that supports the structures of the larynx. It attaches the ribs to the sternum and covers the ends of the bones where they form joints (Marieb and Hoehn, 2010). Other types of cartilage include fibrocartilage which, because it can be compressed, forms the discs between the vertebrae of the spinal column, and elastic cartilage where some degree of elasticity is required, e.g. in the external ear.

Dense connective tissue

Dense connective tissue forms strong, stringy structures such as tendons (which attach skeletal muscles to bones) and the more elastic ligaments (that connect bones to other bones at joints). Dense connective tissue also makes up the lower layers of the skin (known as the dermis). These tissues have collagen fibres as the main matrix element, with many fibroblasts found between the collagen fibres (Marieb, 2010). These fibroblasts are the cells that are involved in the manufacture of the fibres.

Loose connective tissue

Loose connective tissue is softer and contains more cells, but fewer fibres, than other types of connective tissue (with the exception of blood). There are four types of loose connective tissue:

- areolar tissue
- adipose tissue
- reticular tissue
- blood.

Areolar tissue

Areolar tissue is the most widely distributed connective tissue type in the body. It is a soft tissue that cushions and protects the body organs that it surrounds. It helps to hold the internal organs together. It has a fluid matrix that contains all types of fibres which form a loose network, so giving it its softness and pliability. It provides a reservoir of water and salts for the surrounding tissues. All body cells obtain their nutrients from this tissue fluid and also release their waste into it. It is also in this area that, following injury, swelling can occur (known as oedema) because the areolar tissue soaks up the excess fluid just like a sponge does, causing it to become puffy (Marieb and Hoehn, 2010).

Adipose tissue

This tissue is commonly known as 'fat' and is actually areolar tissue in which there is a preponderance of fat cells. It forms the subcutaneous tissue which lies beneath the skin where it insulates the body and can protect it from the extremes of both heat and cold (Marieb and Hoehn, 2010). In addition, adipose tissue protects some organs, such as the kidneys and eyeballs.

Reticular connective tissue

Reticular connective tissue consists of a delicate network of reticular fibres that are associated with reticular cells (similar to fibroblasts). It forms an internal framework to support many free blood cells – mainly the lymphocytes – in the lymphoid organs, such as the lymph nodes, spleen and bone marrow (Marieb and Hoehn, 2010).

Blood

'Blood, or vascular tissue, is considered a connective tissue because it consists of blood cells, surrounded by a non-living, fluid matrix call blood plasma' (Marieb and Hoehn, 2010). Blood is concerned with the transport of nutrients, waste material, respiratory gases (such as oxygen and carbon dioxide), as well as many other substances throughout the body.

Muscle tissue

There are three types of muscle tissue and these are responsible for helping the body to move, or to move substances within the body

- skeletal muscle
- cardiac muscle
- smooth muscle.

Skeletal muscle

This muscle is attached to bones and is involved in the movement of the skeleton. These muscles can be controlled voluntarily and form the 'bulk' of the body (the flesh). The cells of skeletal muscle are long, cylindrical and have several nuclei. In addition, they appear striated (have stripes). They work by contracting and relaxing, with pairs working antagonistically, i.e. one muscle contracts and the opposite muscle relaxes. So, for example, if the muscles in the front of the arm contract and the ones at the back of the arm relax, then the arm bends.

Cardiac muscle

Cardiac muscle is only found in the heart and it pumps blood around the body. It does this by contracting and relaxing, just like skeletal muscle, and it appears striated. However, unlike skeletal muscles, it works in an involuntary way – the activity cannot be consciously controlled. The cells of cardiac muscle do not have a nucleus.

Smooth muscle

Also known as visceral muscle, smooth muscle (see Figure 1.12) is found in the walls of hollow organs, e.g. the stomach, bladder, uterus and blood vessels (hence 'visceral' because these organs are also known as 'viscera'). Smooth muscle has no striations, and like cardiac muscle it works in an involuntary way. Smooth muscle causes movement in the hollow organs, i.e. as it contracts, the cavity of an organ becomes smaller (constricted) and when it relaxes the organ becomes larger (dilated). This allows substances to be propelled through the organ in the right direction, e.g. faeces in the intestines. Because smooth muscle contracts and relaxes slowly, it forms a wavelike motion (known as peristalsis) that pushes, in the case of the intestines, the faeces through the intestines (Figure 1.16).

Nervous tissue

Nervous tissue is concerned with control and communication within the body by means of electrical signals. The main type of cell that is found in nervous tissue is the neuron (see Figure 1.12). All neurons receive and conduct electrochemical impulses around the body. The structure of neurons is very different from that of other cells. The cytoplasm is found within long processes or extensions – some in the leg being more than a metre long. These neurons receive and transmit electrical impulses very rapidly from one to the other across synapses (junctions). It is at the synapses that the electrical impulse can pass from neuron to neuron, or from a neuron to a muscle cell. The total number of neurons is fixed at birth, and cannot be replaced if they are damaged (McCance et al., 2010).

In addition to the neurons, nervous tissue includes cells known as neuroglia-supporting cells. These supporting cells insulate, support and protect the delicate neurons. The neurons and supporting cells make up the structures of the nervous system:

- the brain
- the spinal cord
- the nerves.

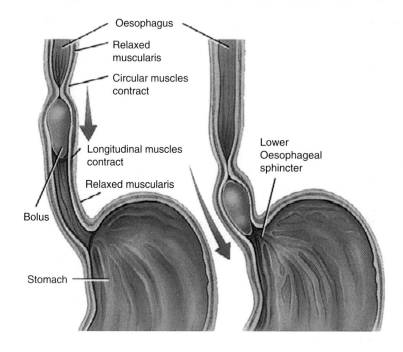

Figure 1.16   Peristalsis.

Tissue repair

The many tissues of the body are always at risk of injury or disease. Inflammation is the body's immediate reaction to tissue injury or damage, because when tissue injury or damage does occur, this stimulates the body's inflammatory and immune responses to spring into action so that the healing process can begin almost immediately.

There are four major signs and symptoms of an inflammatory response (Nairn and Helbert, 2002):

- pain
- swelling
- heat
- redness.

There may also be nausea, sweating, a raised pulse, a lowered blood pressure and even a loss of consciousness. These symptoms are the body's response to the pain and to shock.

Inflammation is usually initiated by damage to a cell. Following this damage, three simultaneous processes occur:

- Mast cell degranulation – mast cells are tissue cells which contain granules in their cytoplasm. These granules are similar to, but smaller than, the granules found in basophils in the blood.

These granules contain, amongst other substances, histamine which, during the process of degranulation, is released into the tissues. It causes some inflammatory symptoms and works with the two other processes listed here to provide full inflammatory symptoms.

- The activation of four plasma protein systems – these systems are the complement, clotting and kinin systems, and immunoglobulins (antibodies). The complement system activates and assists inflammatory and immune processes. It also plays a major role in the destruction of bacteria. The clotting system traps bacteria that have entered the wound and also interacts with platelets to stop any bleeding. The kinin system helps to control vascular permeability, whilst immunoglobulins help in the destruction of bacteria.
- The phagocytic cells move to the area of damage in order to phagocytose bacteria or any other non-self debris in the wound.

A typical inflammatory response to injured tissue is:

- Arterioles near the injury site constrict briefly, followed by vasodilation which increases blood flow to the site of the injury (redness and heat).
- Dilation of the arterioles at the site increases the pressure in the circulation, which increases the movement of plasma proteins and blood cells into the tissues in the area, so causing oedema (swelling).
- The nerve endings in the area are stimulated, partly by pressure (pain).
- The clotting and kinin systems, along with platelets, move into the area and block any tissue tears by commencing the clotting process.
- Phagocytes and lymphocytes move into the area and start to destroy any infectious organisms found there and remove pus.
- These blood cells remain in the area until tissue regeneration (repair) takes place – known as resolution.

Thus, inflammation can be summed up as the presence of:

- vasodilation – redness/heat
- vascular permeability – oedema
- cellular infiltration – pus
- thrombosis – clots
- stimulation of nerve endings – pain.

Conclusion

This chapter has looked at the building blocks of the human body, namely the cells. Cells are extremely complicated parts of the body, but an understanding of them and their functions is important in order to understand how the human body itself functions. Cells form tissues, which then form all the structures, systems and organs of the body. Therefore, it is necessary to also have an understanding of tissues. The remainder of this book will look at the various systems, structures and organs of the body – how they function as well as what can go wrong with them.

Test your knowledge

- How does the cell membrane control metabolism?

- Explain briefly the differences between phagocytosis, receptor-mediated endocytosis and pinocytosis.

- How does the process of cellular reproduction ensure that there are only 46 (23 pairs) chromosomes in a fetus?

- Describe the function of connective tissue.

- Briefly explain the roles of the four plasma protein systems in the process of tissue repair.

Activities

 Here are some activities and exercises to help test your learning. For the answers to these exercises, as well as further self-testing activities, visit our website at www.wiley.com/go/fundamentalsofappliedpathophysiology

Fill in the blanks

Connective tissue _____ body parts to one another. In addition to binding and storage its other main functions are _____ and _____. Connective tissue cells are surrounded by a collection of substances referred to as the _____ , which is composed of _____ and fibres. There are three types of fibre found in connective tissue. The _____ fibres provide strength, whereas elastic fibres are able to _____ and _____. _____ fibres form the internal _____ of _____ such as the spleen. There are several types of connective tissue. _____ is the most rigid, whereas _____ is more flexible. Dense connective tissue consists of stringy structures called _____, which attach _____ to bone. Loose connective tissue is much softer and comes in four main forms, _____, _____, _____ and _____.

Choose from:
Blood; Reticular; Stretch; Support; Areolar; Cartilage; Connects; Collagenous; Skeleton; Tendons; Adipose; Extracellular matrix; Protection; Ground substance; Recoil; Skeletal muscle; Reticular; Bone; Soft organs

Label the diagram

Using the list of words supplied, label the diagram:

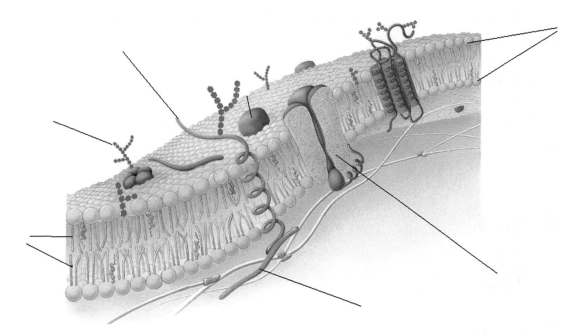

Glycolipid (carbohydrate lipid); Glycoprotein (Carbohydrate protein); phospholipid heads; Integral transmembrane protein; Peripheral protein; Fatty acid tails

Word search

C	M	U	S	C	L	E	K	V	F	C	W	D	O	P	O
S	I	Y	E	P	I	T	H	E	L	I	A	L	B	R	K
I	T	T	C	L	A	G	F	R	A	Y	M	W	G	O	L
S	O	I	X	A	W	S	D	R	G	O	M	A	R	P	L
O	C	S	E	S	O	U	L	E	E	D	N	U	I	H	Y
T	H	S	F	M	U	L	E	C	L	E	U	V	B	A	O
Y	O	U	D	A	R	E	Y	M	L	O	C	L	O	S	M
C	N	E	C	M	S	O	M	L	A	I	L	W	S	E	E
O	D	V	E	E	S	E	E	S	O	E	E	E	O	C	L
X	R	G	N	M	C	S	M	D	A	J	U	C	M	E	C
E	I	J	O	B	O	F	U	O	B	L	S	N	E	G	Y
J	A	S	B	R	H	S	R	Q	S	Y	P	B	N	U	C
M	I	H	E	A	O	D	O	W	I	O	K	O	M	O	L
S	V	C	A	N	T	S	D	Z	S	W	S	P	T	E	L
C	O	N	N	E	C	T	I	V	E	X	L	Y	F	Y	E
N	O	T	E	L	E	K	S	O	T	Y	C	N	L	C	C

Epithelial	Muscle	Osmosis
Plasma membrane	Lysosome	Exocytosis
Organelles	Bone	Cytoplasm
Connective	Mitochondria	Ribosome
Nucleus	Flagella	Cytoskeleton
Cell cycle	Prophase	Tissue

Glossary of terms

Active transport: the process in which substances move against a concentration gradient from an area of low concentration to one of higher concentration. It requires the release and use of energy.

Active transport pump: also known as a sodium pump, this is situated in the plasma membrane and uses the energy produced by the ATP reaction to pump sodium ions (Na^+) out of the cell and potassium ions (K^+) into it.

Adenosine diphosphate (ADP): found inside cells, it helps to produce ATP during reactions which produce cellular energy and is itself formed from ATP at a later stage. It is this continual synthesis and breaking down of ADP and ATP that produces the energy.

Adenosine triphosphate (ATP): a compound of an adenosine molecule with three attached phosphoric acid molecules. Essential for the production of cellular energy.

Amino acid: the building block of proteins. The type of protein that is produced depends upon the number and types of amino acids that are used to construct it.

Carbohydrate: an organic compound that is composed of carbon, hydrogen and oxygen. Sugars (including glucose) and starch are carbohydrates. They are very important as an energy store.

Carrier/transport protein: a small molecule that helps in the movement of ions across a cell membrane.

Catalyst: a substance that speeds up a reversible chemical reaction. Enzymes are catalysts.

Chemical reaction: a reactions in which molecules are formed, changed or broken down.

Chromatid: one of the two strands of chromatin. Two identical chromatids form a chromosome after nuclear reproduction.

Chromatin: the material which forms chromosomes. It consists of DNA and proteins.

Chromosomes: tightly coiled chromatin. This is the form in which the genetic material of all cells is organised.

Concentration gradient: the gradient that demonstrates the difference between an area of high concentration and one of low concentration of a substance.

Cytoplasm:	collective name for all the contents of the cell, including the plasma membrane, but not including the nucleus.
Deoxyribonucleic acid (DNA):	found in the nucleus, it contains all the genetic information of an organism.
Diffusion:	the passive movement of molecules or ions from a region of high concentration to one of low concentration until a state of equilibrium is achieved.
Endocytosis:	the general name for the various processes by which cells ingest foodstuffs and infectious micro-organisms.
Enzyme:	a protein that speeds up chemical reactions.
Eukaryotic cell:	a cell that normally includes, or has included, chromosomal material within one or more nuclei.
Exocytosis:	the system of transporting material out of cells.
Extracellular fluid:	the fluid outside of the cell and bathes the body's cells.
Extracellular matrix:	found in connective tissue, this is non-living material that is made up of ground substance and fibres. It separates the living cells found in this tissue.
Facilitated diffusion:	similar to diffusion, this requires the help of another substance – a carrier protein – for the process to take place (i.e. a facilitator).
Fibre:	are any long, thin structures. The body contains many of them, including nerve fibres and muscle fibres.
Fibroblast:	the most common connective tissue cell and only found in the tendons. It is responsible for the production and secretion of extracellular matrix materials.
Gene:	the smallest physical and biological unit of heredity that encodes for a molecular cell product.
Genetic material:	mainly DNA (deoxyribonucleic acid) that contains genetic information.
Glucose:	also known as dextrose, it is the principal sugar found in the blood. It is essential for life. An absence can lead to diabetes, coma and even death.
Glycoprotein:	a protein linked to carbohydrates.
Goblet cell:	a mucus-secreting cell found in epithelial tissue.
Ground substance:	the part of the extracellular matrix (found in connective tissue) that is composed mainly of water, with some adhesion proteins and large polysaccharide molecules.

Hormone:	a chemical messenger that is linked to the endocrine system, and that has a physiological control over the function of cells or organs other than those that created it.
Inorganic substance:	a compound that does not contain carbon (e.g. water).
Internal respiration:	the use of oxygen by cells in the enzymatic release of energy from organic compounds. This is known as aerobic respiration. Anaerobic respiration does not require oxygen, but does require a substance such as nitrate or iron to do the same job as oxygen (accept electrons during the chemical reaction). Only human cells with mitochondria can undertake aerobic respiration.
Ion:	an atom or group of atoms that carries either a positive or a negative electrical charge.
Lipid:	an energy-rich organic compound that is soluble in organic substances such as alcohol and benzene.
Lysosome:	an organelle within the cell that is an important part of the cell's digestive system because it secretes lysosyme and other similar enzymes, which are very important in the phagocytosis of micro-organisms.
Lysosyme:	a bacteria-destroying enzyme found in lysosomes, sweat, tears, saliva and other bodily secretions.
Meiosis:	the process by which the gametes (spermatozoa and ova) are reproduced.
Membrane:	the outer covering of a cell and of a nucleus within a cell.
Metabolism:	the collective name for all the physical and chemical processes occurring within a cell/living organism, but often referring only to reactions involving enzymes.
Metabolite:	a substance involved in the process of metabolism – either to cause it, assist it or occurring as a result of the process.
Mitosis:	the process by which cells (other than the gametes) are reproduced by simple division of the nucleus and the cell itself.
Neuroglia-supporting cell:	a cell found in nervous tissue; its role is to support the delicate neurons by insulating, supporting and protecting them.
Nuclear membrane:	the outer shell of the nucleus within the cell.

Nucleolus:	a small spherical body found in the cell nucleus that is involved in the production of ribosomes.
Nucleoplasm:	the protoplasm found within the nucleus.
Nucleosome:	the basic structural unit of a chromosome.
Organelle:	a structural and functional part of a cell that acts like human organs to fulfil all the needs of the cell so that it can grow, reproduce and carry out its functions.
Osmosis:	the passive movement of water through a selectively permeable membrane from an area of high concentration of a chemical to an area of low concentration.
Osmotic pressure:	the pressure that must be exerted on a solution to prevent the passage of water into it across a semipermeable membrane from a region of higher concentration of solute to a region of lower concentration of solute.
Oxidative phosphorylation:	the process by which energy released during aerobic respiration and is linked to the production of adenotriphosphate (ATP).
Passive transport:	the process by which substances move on their own down a concentration gradient from an area of high concentration to one of lower concentration. No cellular energy is required for this process.
Phagocytosis:	the method by which cells ingest large particles, including whole micro-organisms.
Pinocytosis:	the method by which cells ingest small particles and fluids.
Prokaryotic cell:	the opposite of eukaryote cell; their DNA/RNA is not contained within a discrete nucleus. They are generally very small bacteria for example.
Protoplasm:	the collective name for everything within the cell, including the cytoplasm, nucleus and the organelles, as well as the plasma membrane.
Ribosomal ribonucleic acid (rRNA):	a highly selective method by which the cell is able to ingest large particles (particularly proteins).
Receptor site:	also known as membrane receptor molecule. This is a protein on the membrane of cells that is able to receive certain other proteins that match them (e.g. hormones and antibodies).
Receptor-mediated endocytosis:	involved in the translation of the genetic material encoded in DNA into proteins. It works in conjunction with ribosomes and messenger RNA (mRNA) and transfer RNA (tRNA).

Ribosome:	an organelle found in cytoplasm that plays a major role in the synthesis of proteins from RNA.
Selective permeability:	the ability of the cell membrane to allow only certain substances to pass into or out of the cell.
Simple fission:	the asexual reproduction of cells by means of division of the nucleus and the cell body.
Solute:	a substance that is dissolved in a solution.
Transmembrane ion gradient:	the gradient in the concentration of ions on either side of a plasma membrane. It is involved in the production of cellular energy.
Tricarboxylic acid cycle:	also known as the Krebs cycle. This is an aerobic pathway that occurs in the mitochondria and is necessary for the production of energy there.
Vesicle:	a spherical space within the cell cytoplasm that is involved in the storage and transfer of substances for the cell.

References

Colbert, B.J., Ankney, J. and Lee, K.T. (2011). *Anatomy and Physiology for Health Professionals: An Interactive Journey*, 2nd edn. New Jersey: Pearson Prentice Hall.

Marieb, E.N. (2010). *Essentials of Human Anatomy and Physiology*, 10th edn. San Francisco: Pearson Benjamin Cummings.

Marieb, E.N. and Hoehn K.N. (2010). *Human Anatomy and Physiology*, 8th edn. San Francisco: Pearson Benjamin Cummings.

McCance, K.L., Huether, S.E., Brashers, V.L. and Rote, N.S. (2010). *Pathophysiology: The Biologic Basis for Disease in Adults and Children*, 6th edn. St. Louis: Mosby.

Nairn, R. and Helbert, M. (2002). *Immunology for Medical Students*. St. Louis: Mosby.

Watson, R. (2005). Cell structure and function, growth and development. In: Montague, S.E., Watson, R. and Herbert, R.A. (eds). *Physiology for Nursing Practice*, 3rd edn. Edinburgh: Elsevier, pp. 49–69.

Wheeldon, A. (2011). Tissue. In: Peate, I. and Nair, M. (eds). *Fundamentals of Anatomy and Physiology for Student Nurses*. Chichester: Wiley-Blackwell.

2

Cancer

Carl Clare

Senior Lecturer, Department of Adult Nursing and Primary Care, School of Health and Social Work, University of Hertfordshire, Hatfield, Hertfordshire, UK

Contents

Fundamentals of Applied Pathophysiology: An Essential Guide for Nursing and Healthcare Students, Second Edition. Edited by Muralitharan Nair and Ian Peate.
© 2013 John Wiley & Sons, Ltd. Published 2013 by John Wiley & Sons, Ltd.

Key words

- Cancer
- Tumour
- Oncogene
- Chemotherapy
- Carcinogen
- Malignant
- Radiotherapy
- Immunotherapy
- Carcinoma
- Neoplasm
- Cytotoxic

Test your prior knowledge

- What is the difference between a malignant tumour and a benign tumour?
- Name three methods of treating cancer.
- What can cause lung cancer?
- What is the aim of palliative treatment?

Learning outcomes

On completion of this chapter the reader will be able to:

- Discuss the process of carcinogenesis and explain the difference between benign and malignant tumours.
- List and explain the ways in which the body tries to prevent cancers from growing.
- Describe the role of genes and environmental factors in the development of cancers.
- Understand the staging of cancers and describe some of the more common cancers.
- Describe the signs and symptoms of cancer and explain what causes them.
- List and discuss the many ways in which cancers can be treated.

Don't forget to visit to the companion website for this book (www.wiley.com/go/ fundamentalsofappliedpathophysiology) where you can find self-assessment tests to check your progress, as well as lots of activities to practise your learning.

Introduction

According to Ferlay *et al.* (2010), approximately 157,275 people died of cancer in the UK in 2008, most of whom were over 65 years of age.

Cancer is a disease of abnormal cell growth, cell division and cell differentiation. The disease 'cancer' actually consists of a group of diseases, all of which are underpinned by (and caused by) uncontrolled abnormal cell growth. Cancers are always life-threatening but not always fatal. There are many causes of cancers, just as there are many types of cancers.

According to McCance (2010a), cells of multicellular organisms are not concerned just with the individual cell, but rather with the survival of the entire multicellular organism. These cells can be thought of as specialised members of a society – a cellular society. This means that all cells work for the good of the organism. Because of this, the processes of cell division, proliferation and differentiation are normally regulated so that they are in balance – particularly a balance between the rate of cell birth and the rate of cell death (see Chapter 1).

However, as in any society, there are always some abnormal cells that disobey all social control mechanisms; in this case, the social control mechanisms of cell division, proliferation and differentiation. These are the cells that will proliferate to form tumours in the body, and indeed, as McCance (2010a) points out, virtually every cell in the body has the potential to become a tumour if it mutates.

Carcinogenesis is a multistep mechanism and is caused by an accumulation of cellular and chemical errors, particularly concerning the deoxyribonucleic acid (DNA) of a cell. Altered DNA bases – known as mutations – are the cause of any changes that lead to cells becoming cancers, and several mutations within the DNA are required for carcinogenesis to happen. Carcinogenesis always begins with a single cell whose DNA has been damaged for some reason. This cell starts to grow in an abnormal and uncontrolled way. Following the process of division and reproduction, as discussed in Chapter 1, each new daughter cell, because it has inherited its parent's DNA, also grows in an uncontrolled way. Normally, a cell is programmed to stop growing when it reaches its correct size, but because of the DNA abnormality (mutation), it continues past this point and grows ever larger.

The body does have mechanisms to deal with cells that are abnormal, which means that these cells that carry a genetic mutation causing uncontrolled growth should either commit suicide (apoptosis) or should be killed by the body's own defences (see Chapter 3). In order to become a cancer, these abnormal cells have to multiply literally billions of times. It takes a long time for a single cell to develop billions of daughter cells, and this is why cancers are generally considered to be diseases of old age. Unfortunately, there are exceptions to this, and some cancers develop in children (some even in babies). Examples are some cancers of the eye – retinoblastoma, and of the blood – certain leukaemias. However, the idea that cancer is generally a disease linked with old age still holds true, and there is a high incidence of cancer occurring after the age of 40 years.

Cancer can occur in almost any cell, but the most common cancers are to be found in the:

- skin
- lung
- colon

- breast
- prostate gland.

Over the past few years, there have been some changes in the incidence rates of the various cancers. For example, the incidence of stomach and colon cancer has reduced, whilst the incidence of skin and lymphoid cancers has increased (Marieb and Hoehn, 2010). Marieb and Hoehn (2010) also point out that despite all the advances in diagnosis, care and treatment of cancer, the overall rate of cancer deaths has increased. This may be accounted for by the fact that life expectancy has also increased and, as already mentioned, cancers are more prevalent in older people.

Biology of cancer

For whatever reason, the DNA of a cell becomes altered, causing the cell to grow uncontrollably. This is known as the initiation period. What happens after the cell starts to grow uncontrollably determines whether or not cancer will occur.

Apoptosis (or cell suicide) is a process that is continually occurring within the body. This is because altered and damaged cells are constantly being produced in the body. To understand why this should be so, one only needs to look at the process by which DNA and cells are replicated. This process is an extremely rapid one (as it needs to keep pace with the needs of the body in terms of replacing altered and damaged cells). For example, skin cells are constantly being replaced because of damage caused by being worn away and dislodged every time the skin comes into contact with any surface. Because of the speed at which this very complicated process of DNA replication occurs, it can be no surprise when mistakes occur. There are several mechanisms by which cellular apoptosis can be induced (Figure 2.1), e.g. internal cell stresses can lead to apoptosis via the cell's own mitochondria.

Another mechanism that the body possesses in order to try and prevent the development of damaged cells is the destruction of these cells by the body's own immune system. One of the many functions of the immune system is called immune surveillance, and this does just what it says. Certain white blood cells of the immune system (including cytotoxic T lymphocytes) move through the body looking for any abnormal or 'alien' cells (e.g. bacteria and viruses). Each cell carries receptors on its outer membrane, and some of these receptors are specific identification (ID) receptors that identify them as belonging to that particular body. If these cytotoxic T lymphocytes come across a cell that does not carry these particular ID receptors for that body, then they will kill it. Either there is activation of death receptors on the cell wall or there is activation of apoptosis using an enzyme known as granzyme. Although cancerous cells will belong to the same body as the cytotoxic T lymphocytes, because of their alteration, due to the altered DNA, the ID receptors on these cancerous cells may have slight alterations to their formation. Luckily, even though there is only a slight alteration to the ID receptors carried by cancerous cells, they are still different enough for the T cells to recognise them as not being 'correct' cells, and to destroy them. However, unfortunately, some of the cells (known as precancerous cells) are able to develop strategies to hide their differences from the immune system, and so escape being destroyed by the T cells. Once the precancerous cells have achieved this evasion of the body's immune system, they can then proceed to divide and replicate in order to cause cancers, because all their daughter cells will also have this ability to evade the T lymphocytes (Gorczynski and Stanley, 2006; Vickers, 2005).

Once the precancerous cell has developed a strategy for avoiding both apoptosis and the T lymphocytes, it can then proceed to clone itself, and the cancer starts to develop. To transform

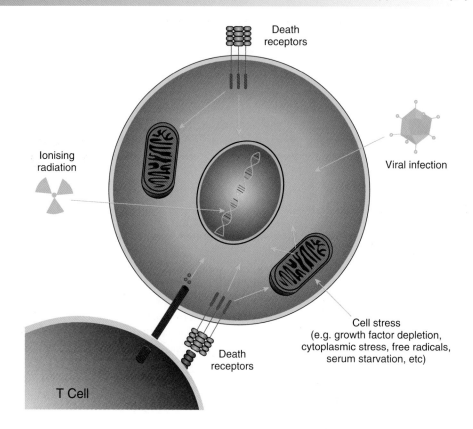

Figure 2.1   Apoptosis (Cell Migration Lab, University of Reading, http://www.reading.ac.uk/cellmigration/apoptosis.htm).

a single precancerous cell into a cancer requires more than just a straightforward cloning of this cell, because, in addition to the cell cloning itself, new blood vessels need to form (known as angiogenesis). These new blood vessels need to develop because all cells require a good blood supply so that oxygen and nutrients can reach them and keep them alive (as well as allowing for the removal of carbon dioxide and other toxins). In order for these new blood vessels to develop, the cancerous cell needs to produce angiogenic growth factors. The other thing to consider is that the cancerous cells need extra blood flow (more than a normal cell) because they are growing so rapidly and to such a great size that they require extra oxygen and nutrients for the growth to continue and for the extra metabolism that is required by the cancerous cell.

There are several models that demonstrate the development of cancers, and the two that are of most relevance are:.

● Molecular biology model – Figure 2.2 illustrates the process of the development of cancer from the cellular perspective. A normal cell can become precancerous as a result of DNA changes (1) during reproduction/cloning. The precancerous cell can then become a cancer as a result of further alteration in its DNA (2) during cloning, and the final DNA change (3) can cause the cancerous cell to become metastatic and to spread throughout the body. Thus, it

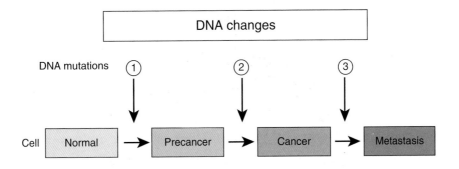

Figure 2.2   Molecular biology model (after King, 2000).

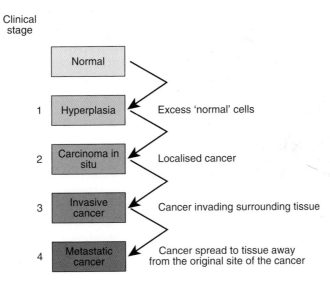

Figure 2.3   Clinical model (after King, 2000).

can be seen that the DNA needs to continue to mutate for a normal cell to reach the metastatic stage – it is not just a single mutation.
- Clinical model – in this model (Figure 2.3), which looks at the actual clinical disease as opposed
to the biochemical underpinning, the cancer commences with a normal cell, which starts to
overproliferate (i.e. reproduce/clone excessively), so that although these cells are 'normal',
they are dividing rapidly. The next stage occurs when there are sufficient cancerous cells to
be able to say that a cancer is present, although it is still only situated in one place within
the body. The third stage is when the cancerous cells start to invade the surrounding tissue
(aggressive behaviour), and finally the cancer spreads to other, often remote, parts of the
body – metastasis.

Often, once a cancer can be detected, it is already at an advanced stage and thus the prognosis
is poorer than if it had been diagnosed at an earlier stage.

Causes of cancer

The main causes of cancer appear to be linked to interactions between genes and the environment.

Genes

The role of genes in the development of cancer is very important, and there are three types of genes that are involved:

- proto-oncogenes
- oncogenes
- tumour suppressor genes.

Proto-oncogenes possess the genetic codes for the proteins that are needed for normal cell division and growth, whilst oncogenes are proto-oncogenes that have mutated and so have become cancer-causing genes that increase the rate at which cells divide and proliferate. One of the problems with proto-oncogenes is that many of them have fragile sites that can easily break once they are exposed to carcinogens. Once this occurs, then the proto-oncogenes are converted into oncogenes. Unfortunately, since oncogenes have been discovered in only 15–20% of cancers found in humans, there has to be something else which causes cancerous cells to develop, and tumour suppressor genes, e.g. *p53*, provide the answer. Tumour suppressor genes work to suppress or even prevent cancer by repairing any damaged cell DNA, as well as slowing down or even stopping cell division. These tumour suppressor genes also help to inactivate carcinogens as well as improving the ability of the immune system to destroy cancer cells (Marieb, 2010). When these mutated cancer-causing cells occur in germline cells (i.e. sperm and ova), then the cancer-causing genes can be inherited from one generation to the next, and so produce families in which there is a predisposition for certain cancers, such as breast cancer (Jorde *et al.*, 2009). Therefore, it is now known that certain forms of cancer oncogenes can be inherited within some families. However, if the oncogene is only to be found in somatic cells, then it would not be inherited by future generations. Examples of inherited cancers, for which a specific oncogene has been isolated, include:

- retinoblastoma – cancer of the eye (found in children)
- Wilms' tumour – cancer of the kidney (also found in children)
- familial breast cancer.

Environmental factors

Turning now to the link between cancer genes and environmental factors, the frequency of the cancer-causing mutations, and the seriousness of their effects, can be altered by a large number of environmental factors (Jorde *et al.*, 2009). Chemicals that cause mutations in cells can cause cancers, and so it is appropriate to describe these particular chemicals as carcinogens. In addition, there are other environmental agents that may enhance the development of genetically altered cells but do not cause new mutations. So, it would seem that it is often the interplay of genes with environmental factors that leads to carcinogenesis and they cannot be viewed in isolation (Jorde *et al.*, 2009).

Environmental factors, such as chemicals, radiation and viruses, can cause cancer by increasing the frequency with which cells mutate. Environmental agents that cause cancer are known as carcinogens, and most carcinogens are mutagens (they increase the frequency of mutations). What is apparent is that most of the agents that are known to cause cancer (carcinogenesis) also cause genetic changes (mutagenesis), whilst factors that cause genetic change also cause cancer. Many environmental agents are known to be carcinogenic, and include things such as:

- radiation
- alcohol
- chemicals
- some foods
- air pollution
- smoking
- viruses.

At the same time, however, most human cancers appear to arise spontaneously, and develop without any known prior exposure to a carcinogenic agent, but this may be because the carcinogenic agents have not yet been identified.

Radiation

- Ultraviolet radiation – ultraviolet (UV) sunlight (or solar radiation) causes basal cell carcinoma and squamous cell carcinoma (see Chapter 18). These are two common cancers that are found in people who have pale skin with a light complexion. This type of radiation causes mutations in two tumour suppressor genes. In addition, the very malignant pigmented moles known as melanomas are linked to the amount of exposure to UV light.
- Ionising radiation –the list of carcinomas caused by ionising radiation is extremely long, and includes:
  - acute leukaemias in adults and children
  - thyroid cancer
  - breast cancer
  - lung cancer
  - stomach cancer
  - cancer of the colon
  - oesophageal cancer
  - urinary tract cancer
  - multiple myeloma.

Ionising radiation is thought to inhibit cell division. This is of particular importance where the cells only live for a short time, which leads to rapid cell division, e.g.:

- lymphocytes
- cells of lymphoid tissue
- bone marrow cells
- intestinal epithelial cells.

The developing fetus is especially at risk, even at such low doses that may not cause any problems to adults. This is because during pregnancy, fetal organ development occurs very early and at an extremely rapid rate; therefore, even small doses of radiation can completely alter the integrity of the cells and hence normal development. This is why pregnant women – especially in the early stage of pregnancy – should not have X-rays taken (unless there is no alternative and their condition is life-threatening).

Smoking

It has been known for a long time that cigarette smoking is carcinogenic, and that it remains one of the most important causes of cancer. A hundred years ago, lung cancer was a rare disease, but as the incidence of cigarette smoking increased, so the incidence of lung cancer rose to epidemic proportions. Smoking not only leads to lung cancer, it also increases the incidence of cancer of the bladder, pancreas, kidney, larynx, oral cavity and oesophagus. The reason for this is that there are 20 carcinogens in tobacco smoke that can cause tumours.

Diet

Many toxic, mutagenic and carcinogenic chemicals can be found in the human diet. Sources of toxic carcinogenic substances within our diet include various compounds that are produced during the cooking of fat or protein. In addition, there are naturally occurring carcinogens that are associated with plant food substances, e.g. alkaloids and by-products of moulds/fungi.

Alcohol

Alcohol is linked with increased rates of incidence of oral cancer and cancer of the pharynx, larynx, oesophagus and liver – particularly if taken with large quantities of tobacco in the form of cigarettes, cigars and in pipes. Alcohol interacts with smoke, and this increases the risk of malignant tumours. Although the rationale for this is not proven, it is thought that it acts possibly as a solvent for the carcinogenic smoke products. Alcohol consumption has also been linked to breast cancer and colorectal cancer.

Sexual and reproductive behaviour

The possible mechanism for the carcinogenesis of cervical and other cancers of the sexual organs is a viral infection transmitted between sexual partners. According to Lowy et al. (2008), the age of first sexual intercourse allied to the number of sexual partners (or the number of sexual partners of a partner) are the major factors leading to the risk of the development of cervical cancer.

Certain types of the human papillomavirus (HPV) are known to be a cause of cervical cancer. HPV has also been identified with many other cancers of the anogenital region, such as cancers of the penis, vulva and anus (Lowy et al., 2008).

Environmental pollution

Because of the huge quantities of air that humans inhale every day (about 20 000 L), even small amounts of carcinogens and other pollutants in the atmosphere can cause problems. There is particular concern with the industrial emissions of pollutants, such as arsenic, benzene, chloroform and vinyl chloride, but there are many others (Chameides, 2010). Consequently, it is recognised that living close to certain industries is a risk factor for developing certain cancers, although, again, other factors have to be taken into account – particularly lifestyle factors (such as drinking and smoking as discussed earlier). According to McCance (2010b), indoor pollution is generally considered to be a greater risk than outdoor pollution, partly because of second-hand or environmental tobacco smoke.

Along with smoke, another indoor air pollutant of significance is radon gas – this is a natural radioactive gas that is present in certain soils (e.g. granite). It can become trapped in houses and produce carcinogenic radioactive decay products (Lubin, 2010).

Occupation

Exposures to carcinogenic substances as a result of one's occupation have been recognised for a long time as being a cause of cancer. In Victorian times, for example, there was a high incidence of testicular cancer amongst boy chimney sweeps.

Asbestos accounts for the largest number of occupational cancers in recent years, although that is improving as the risks of asbestos have become common knowledge. What is particularly of concern is that a combination of asbestos exposure and cigarette smoking can lead to a significant increase in the risk of lung cancer (Frost et al., 2011). In actual fact, a large percentage of cancers of the upper respiratory tract, lung, bladder and peritoneum can be linked causally to various occupational factors.

Hormones

The relationship between hormones and human cancer has been widely studied. Hormones, such as steroids, can be immunosuppressive. However, much of the current research on hormones and cancer focuses on the sex steroids, which include:

- oestrogen
- progesterone
- testosterone.

According to McCance (2010b), most evidence to date supports the role of hormones as promoters of carcinogenesis in target tissues rather than as primary carcinogens. However, oestrogen is now being seen as a cause of cancer, but its exact mechanism is unknown.

Oral contraceptives

Some studies have found that oral contraceptives have little effect on the risk of breast cancer in most women (Rosenberg et al., 2009), whilst other studies (Kabat et al., 2010) have identified subgroups of women using oral contraceptives who have an increased risk of breast cancer. These subgroups include:

- women who have used oral contraceptives for many years prior to the age of 25 years
- those who used them before 1971
- extended use before the first full-term pregnancy
- use at the age of 45 years or older
- history of biopsy-confirmed benign breast disorders
- nulliparous, premenopausal women, with an early menarche
- women with only one child
- family history of breast cancer.

In contrast, complete/incomplete pregnancies and the use of oral contraceptives reduce the risk of ovarian cancer. This is because ovarian cancer appears to develop from the epithelial cells on the ovarian surface, and the main stimulus for division of these cells is ovulation itself. What happens is that after each ovulation, epithelial cells then replicate in order to ensure that the exposed surface of the ovary (following ovulation and release of the egg) is covered. So, those factors that help to prevent ovulation also help to protect against ovarian cancers. The risk of endometrial cancer is reduced by 55% in women who have taken oral contraceptives for 5 years, as opposed to those who have not used oral contraceptives. In addition, it is also thought that oral contraceptive usage may reduce colorectal cancers (Long *et al.*, 2010).

Male hormones

The male sex hormone (i.e. testosterone) actually stimulates the growth of target tissues for cancers, such as the prostate – hence the risk of benign or malignant prostate tumours.

Viruses

There are a group of viruses, known as oncogenic viruses, that can cause cancers, e.g.:

- papovaviruses
- adenoviruses
- herpesviruses
- hepadenoviruses.

Burkitt lymphoma and nasopharyngeal carcinoma are caused by the Epstein-Barr virus (EBV), whilst HPV is found in cervical cancer (Moore and Chang, 2010).

Staging of cancers

Following the diagnosis of a cancer, the patient will be told the stage that the cancer has reached. The stage of a cancer at the time of diagnosis can give an indication of the likely prognosis for the patient. The staging system is linked to the spread of the cancer (metastasis). The common sites for the metastatic spread of cancer include the brain, the lungs, the bones and the liver (Figure 2.4).

There are four general cancer stages – although most types of cancer also have specific staging criteria (Colbert *et al.*, 2011):

- Stage 1 – no spread of the cancer from the original site of the cancer.
- Stage 2 – the cancer has spread to neighbouring tissues.
- Stage 3 – the cancer has spread to nearby lymph nodes.
- Stage 4 – the cancer has spread to tissues and organs in other parts of the body.

Cancers that have started to spread have a much poorer prognosis than cancers that are still confined to their original site. Stage 1 cancers have a much better chance of responding to treatment, whilst Stage 4 cancers are very often terminal. Consequently, the earlier a patient is diagnosed, the better the chances of overcoming cancer.

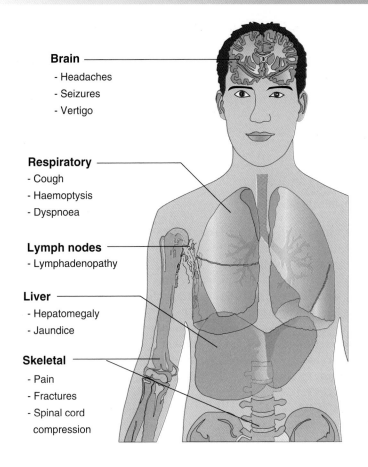

Brain
- Headaches
- Seizures
- Vertigo

Respiratory
- Cough
- Haemoptysis
- Dyspnoea

Lymph nodes
- Lymphadenopathy

Liver
- Hepatomegaly
- Jaundice

Skeletal
- Pain
- Fractures
- Spinal cord
  compression

Figure 2.4   Common sites and symptoms of cancer metastasis.

Signs and symptoms of cancer

Cancers can present in many ways depending upon the type of cancer and where it is situated, e.g. the brain, kidney, blood or breast, but there are some common factors to most of them:

- general run-down condition (general malaise, anorexia/loss of appetite, loss of weight)
- marked change in bowel or bladder habits
- nausea or vomiting for no apparent reason
- bloody discharge of any kind; failure to stop bleeding in the usual time
- presence of swelling, lump or mass anywhere in the body
- any change in the size or appearance of moles or birthmarks
- unexplained stumbling
- unexplained pain (or persistent crying of an infant or child).

The problem that the healthcare provider has in diagnosing cancer is that these signs and symptoms can be related to many other medical conditions. This is why there is sometimes a delay in diagnosing cancer until the cancer has developed and may have started to metastasise.

Treatment of cancer

Whilst there are different treatments for different cancers, there are certain principles and types of treatment that are generally accepted as standard. There are six types of treatment that are mainly used at the moment – depending upon the individual cancer and patient:

- drug therapy
- radiation therapy
- immunotherapy
- surgical removal
- hormone therapy
- photodynamic therapy.

The first, very important, point to make is that the earlier the cancer is diagnosed and treatment begins, the better will be the prognosis. If the cancer is still localised (i.e. it has not spread to other parts of the body) at the time of diagnosis, then the plan would be the removal of the primary cancer by surgery, accompanied by drug therapy and/or radiation therapy (King and Robins, 2006). Unfortunately, not all cancers are amenable to surgery, e.g. the blood cancers such as leukaemias and lymphomas.

If the cancer is detected late, or if surgery does not remove all of the primary cancer and metastasis occurs, then other forms of treatment are necessary – mainly drug therapy and radio-therapy. In this scenario, it is often not possible to cure the cancer and the treatment is based on preventing the growth of the cancer, or at least slowing it down.

Drug therapy

The other name for drug therapy is chemotherapy, and there are two different types of chemo-therapy that are used in the treatment of cancer:

- cytotoxic chemotherapy
- cytostatic chemotherapy.

The difference between the two types of chemotherapy is that cytotoxic chemotherapy has the potential to cure a patient, whereas cytostatic drugs are not able to get rid of the cancer but can prevent it growing too large.

Side effects

Unfortunately, because all these drugs affect normal cells as well as cancerous cells, treatment using these drugs can cause many severe side effects (Perry, 2008). These side effects can include:

- Secondary cancers, including leukaemia – these can occur because the normal blood cells, including the white blood cells which form a major part of the immune system (see Chapter 3), are particularly sensitive to many of these drugs, and a reduction in white blood cells can lead to further tumours arising because of a lack of immune surveillance.
- Infections – a reduction in white blood cells can leave the body open to serious infections, including septicaemia, because the immune system has been compromised.
- Sterility – the germ cells in the ovaries and testes are also very sensitive to these chemothera-peutic drugs and young people in particular can become sterile as a result of the treatment.

- Hair loss – this occurs because the cells of the hair follicles are rapidly dividing (as can be seen from the speed at which hair grows), and as some chemotherapeutic drugs target rapidly dividing cells because cancerous cells are themselves rapidly dividing cells, normal rapidly dividing cells are also destroyed.
- Nausea and vomiting – these are frequent side effects of chemotherapy because the drugs can activate the centres in the brainstem that can cause vomiting.
- Skin damage – these occur in the same way that hair loss occurs because skin cells have to rapidly replicate to replace the skin cells that are damaged with normal wear and tear.

Radiation therapy

Ionising radiation damages cell DNA. Once the DNA of a cell is damaged, one of three results can occur,:

- the death of the cancerous cell
- the cell becomes so severely damaged that any changes in its environment will cause it to die
- the cell becomes damaged but can eventually repair itself.

Radiation therapy attempts to kill the cancer cell, but as with chemotherapy, normal cells can also be killed by the radiation.

Immunotherapy

Current attempts at using immunotherapy to cure tumours are based on the idea that the immune system can eradicate existing tumours by means of immune surveillance and thus the modification of immune system cells may be a pathway to cancer therapy (Ljunggren and Malmberg, 2007). Immunotherapy is still not standard therapy in clinical practice, but recent advances show promising results in areas such as prostate therapy (Drake, 2010).

Surgical removal

Surgical therapy is used when the cancer has not yet spread. In addition, it is generally agreed that if there is any chance that local lymph nodes may be involved but there is no evidence that the disease has spread, then the lymph nodes should also be removed.

As with chemotherapy, there are two types of surgery – surgery to cure the disease and palliative surgery. Palliative surgery, which means alleviating the symptoms without curing the cancer, has two purposes:

- to prevent symptoms that would have occurred without the surgery
- to relieve symptoms that are already present.

Hormonal therapy

Hormonal therapy has been used for some years now. Although the way in which this works is not really known, but it is thought to work by blocking receptors on the cancerous cells, it prevents a cell from receiving normal growth stimulation signals.

Examples of hormones being used in cancer therapy include:

- corticosteroids – used in leukaemias, malignant lymphomas, Hodgkin's disease and breast cancer

- androgens – used in breast cancer
- oestrogens – used in breast cancer and prostate cancer.

Photodynamic therapy

Light on its own does not damage cells, whether they are malignant cells or normal cells. However, when light combines with oxygen, it can have a serious effect on photosensitive chemicals such as porphyrins (an example of a porphyrin is haemoglobin which binds and transports oxygen in the body). It is now possible to produce a drug consisting of a modified porphyrin and to give it systemically; then the target cancer can be eliminated by using a special light that is focused on the cancer and not the surrounding tissues. This can cause the death of the malignant cells of the cancer. Photodynamic therapy has now been successfully used to treat:

- cancers of the bladder
- head and neck cancers
- cancer of the oesophagus
- skin cancers
- non-small cell lung cancer.

Gene therapy

This is still experimental, but there is work ongoing that is looking at using the fact that genetics plays an important part in the causes of cancer. The eventual hope is that it will be possible to replace the affected genes with normal ones.

Prevention of cancer

Although the treatment of cancers has improved dramatically over the last 20 years or so, it is still better to try and prevent cancers occurring in the first place. As was discussed earlier, there are many environmental and lifestyle factors that play a part in causing the development of cancers. These include smoking, diet, alcohol, occupation, sexual behaviour and UV radiation. By reducing or even removing these factors it is possible, to a large extent, to prevent many cancers occurring, although, because of the genetic factors previously mentioned, cancers will never go away.

Increasing fruit and vegetable intake has the potential to reduce the risk of getting several cancers, including bowel cancer, breast cancer, cancer of the mouth, larynx and nasopharynx, and even lung cancer. In addition, bowel cancer and breast cancer, amongst others, can be prevented by reducing smoking as well as the intake of alcohol. A reduction in meat and alcohol intake, along with an increase in eating more fruits and vegetables, can reduce bowel cancer by as much as 70%. A diet that includes increased amounts of fruit and vegetables and reduced amounts of fat and alcohol can reduce breast cancer by as much as 40% if started before puberty (15% if started after puberty), whilst a diet high in fruit and vegetables can prevent an estimated 25% of lung cancers – in both smokers and non-smokers. So, it can be seen that diet is one environmental factor that can be used to reduce the incidence of many cancers.

For many years now, the link between smoking and lung cancer has been well known and well documented, although there are still many arguments about the role of passive smoking as a cause of lung cancer.

Taking sensible precautions in strong sunshine can prevent a lot of skin cancers, particularly the very malignant melanomas.

In addition to considering environmental factors as a means of preventing cancer, there are also certain drugs that can help to reduce cancers. For example, tamoxifen has been found to prevent breast cancers, particularly in women from families who carry a genetic defect that causes breast cancer. The major risk factor for breast cancer is excessive oestrogen production and tamoxifen is an anti-oestrogen drug, which is why it helps to prevent breast cancer. However, in a major trial in the United States, it was found that women who took tamoxifen had twice as many endometrial cancers than the control group, in addition to a higher-than-expected incidence of problems such as pulmonary embolus and deep vein thrombosis. However, because the risk probability of developing breast cancer for some women in families who carry the breast cancer gene defects is as high as 80%, many of them believe that the risk of developing these other problems is outweighed by the risk of developing breast cancer if tamoxifen is not taken (King and Robins, 2006).

The fifth most common cause of cancer deaths in women is ovarian cancer and oral contraceptive pills have been found to be effective against endometrial and ovarian cancer. In fact, it is so effective against ovarian cancer that oral contraceptive pills have now halved the risk of developing it.

Another drug that appears to prevent a particular type of cancer, colon cancer, is aspirin. Colon cancer is the third most important cause of cancer-related deaths in both men and women. It is not only aspirin that is effective, but also non-steroidal anti-inflammatory drugs that are taken for arthritis and similar diseases.

Finally, it is necessary to look at the potential role of vaccines in preventing various cancers. There have been many approaches that have been used to develop vaccines for use in the treatment of cancer. At present, prophylactic approaches to cancer focus on the use of vaccines that will induce immunity to viruses that are known to be associated with the development of a tumour, in the same way that any vaccination induces immunity to the causative organism, e.g. measles, mumps or rubella. An example of a vaccine in use to give immunity to a cancer is the HPV vaccine. HPV vaccines prevent the development of cervical carcinoma because HPV is a known cause of cervical cancer (Leggatt and Frazer, 2007).

Another possible vaccine against a virus that causes cancer would be a vaccine against hepatitis B, and such a vaccine would reduce the incidence of liver cancer. As we are able to identify other cancers that are caused by viruses, this prophylactic measure of vaccination against those particular viruses could help to prevent these cancers and save many lives.

In contrast to the use of vaccines against viruses that cause cancer, most other tumour vaccine approaches are designed to enhance or to initiate effective tumour immunity in patients who already have cancer.

Examples of cancers

Acute lymphoblastic leukaemia

Case study

Sarah Vaughan is a 34-year-old accountant who is married with no children. She has recently been diagnosed with acute lymphoblastic leukaemia (ALL) following a history of recurrent fevers, easily bruised skin and a general feeling of lethargy and weakness. Diagnosis was confirmed by blood tests and a bone marrow biopsy, which Mrs Vaughan found rather unpleasant. Mrs Vaughan has been advised that she will undergo treatment in three stages, including total body irradiation after which she will have to avoid going out in the sun for several months.

Take some time to reflect on this case and then consider the following.

1. Mrs Vaughan is slightly unusual in presenting with ALL. Which adult patient groups are most likely to develop ALL?
2. What are the three stages of treatment for ALL?
3. What is total body irradiation, why is it carried out and why will Mrs Vaughan need to avoid direct sunlight afterwards?
4. Mrs Vaughan is of child-bearing age. What should she be told about her fertility now and in the future?

ALL is a primary disorder of the bone marrow in which the normal marrow cells are replaced by immature or undifferentiated blast cells. When the quantity of normal marrow is depleted to below the level necessary to maintain peripheral blood cells within normal ranges, then the following occur:

- anaemia
- neutropaenia
- thrombocytopaenia.

The exact cause of ALL is unknown, but the following are suspected of being involved in the development of this disease:

- environmental causes
- infectious agents (especially viruses)
- genetic factors
- chromosomal abnormalities.

ALL is the most common malignancy in children, with over 400 new cases diagnosed in children under the age of 15 years each year in UK, with the incidence being higher amongst Caucasian children. ALL is classified according to the cell type involved.

ALL results from the growth of an abnormal type of leucocyte in the bone marrow, the spleen and the lymph nodes. These abnormal cells have little cytoplasm and a round nucleus – they resemble lymphoblasts. With ALL, the normal bone marrow cells may be displaced or replaced. The changes that occur in blood and bone marrow result from an accumulation of leukaemic cells and a deficiency of normal cells:

- Red cell precursors and megakaryocytes from which platelets are formed are decreased, leading to anaemia, bleeding and bruising.
- Normal white cells are decreased, which makes the patient liable to pick up infections.
- The leukaemic cells may infiltrate into the lymph nodes, spleen and liver, so causing a diffuse adenopathy and hepatosplenomegaly.
- The increase in the size and amount of marrow and/or this infiltration of leukaemic cells causes bone and joint pain.
- Invasion of the central nervous system (CNS) by leukaemic cells can lead to headaches, vomiting, cranial nerve palsies, convulsions and coma.

- Weight loss, muscle wasting and fatigue occur when the body cells are deprived of nutrients because of the immense metabolic needs of the proliferating leukaemic cells.

Therefore, the signs and symptoms of ALL are:

- an increase in lethargy and general malaise
- persistent fever of unknown cause
- recurrent infection
- prolonged bleeding (e.g. after dentistry)
- bruising easily
- pallor
- enlarged lymph nodes
- pain, particularly abdominal, bone and joint
- CNS involvement leading to headache and vomiting.

Treatment and prognosis

The treatment for ALL includes:

- supportive therapy, including:
    - control of infections, anaemia, bleeding, etc.
- specific therapy, including:
    - cytotoxic chemotherapy – e.g. dexamethasone, vincristine, imatinib, asparaginase, methotrexate
    - radiation therapy
    - bone marrow transplantation (BMT) to replace the damaged marrow with non-cancerous marrow.

The prognosis of ALL is good these days – almost 80% of children (Vrooman and Silverman, 2009) and 40% of adults survive more than 5 years. However, later relapses can still occur after long remissions.

Lung cancer

Case study

Geoffrey Simpson is a 72-year-old pensioner with a history of a non-productive cough and occasional chest pain. Recently he has noticed blood in his handkerchief when he coughs and he states he has been losing weight but puts it down to his loss of appetite. Following a CT scan and bronchoscopy he has been diagnosed with Stage 4 non-small cell lung cancer and bony metastases. The treatment plan is for chemotherapy to treat the primary tumour and biphosphonate drugs and radiotherapy for the bony metastases. Mr Simpson retired from the ship building industry 12 years ago and states he has never been a smoker, eats healthily enough and only drinks moderate alcohol.

Take some time to reflect on this case and then consider the following.

1. What is the difference between small cell lung cancer and non-small cell lung cancer?
2. Why is Mr Simpson's previous employment a potential risk factor for lung cancer?
3. Why does Mr Simpson's treatment plan include biphosphonate drugs and radiotherapy for the bone metastases?
4. What are the statistics on 5-year survival for the different stages and types of lung cancer?

Lung cancer is the most common cause of death from cancer in men and the second most common cause of death from cancer in women, and in 2008, it was calculated that it is responsible for 1.8 million deaths each year throughout the world.

The causes of lung cancer are:

*   The greatest cause is long-term exposure to inhaled carcinogens, particularly tobacco smoke.
*   People who do not smoke tobacco may still get lung cancer, due to a combination of genetic factors and exposure to passive smoking.
*   Radon gas may also play a part in the development of lung cancer, as may air pollution.

Signs and symptoms of lung cancer are (Longo *et al.*, 2011):

*   dyspnoea (difficulty in breathing)
*   haemoptysis (coughing up blood)
*   chronic cough and wheezing
*   chest or abdominal pain
*   cachexia, fatigue and loss of appetite
*   dysphonia (hoarse voice)
*   difficulty in swallowing.

Unfortunately, for many patients, by the time that they seek medical attention because the symptoms have become so apparent, the cancer has already metastasised.

Treatment of lung cancer depends upon the particular type of lung cancer and how far it has metastasised, but common treatments include:

*   surgery
*   chemotherapy, e.g. cisplatin and vinorelbine
*   radiation therapy.

The 5-year survival rate for all types of lung cancer is very low, although again the earlier it is diagnosed and treated, the better the long-term prognosis. Consequently, this makes the prevention of this particular cancer a real priority.

Breast cancer

Throughout the world, breast cancer is the fifth most common cause of death from cancer (after lung cancer, stomach cancer, liver cancer and colon cancer), whilst among women throughout the world, breast cancer is the most common cancer (Ferlay *et al.*, 2010). The incidence of breast cancer has increased significantly since the 1970s, and this is partly explained by modern lifestyles

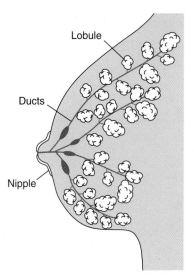

Figure 2.5   Diagram of breast showing lobules and ducts.

in the Western world. Breast cancer is not purely a cancer of women, because males can also have breast cancer, although this is less common than it is in females (Ottini *et al.*, 2010). The reason for this phenomenon is that the breast is composed of exactly the same tissues in both males and females. The lifetime risk for getting breast cancer is 1 in 11 for women and 1 in 1000 for men (King and Robins, 2006). The 5-year survival rates for breast cancer in Europe are 77% without metastasis, but only 40% once the cancer has metastasised (Sant *et al.*, 2009).

There are different sorts of breast cancer (although these can overlap), including (Figure 2.5):

- ductal carcinoma (where the milk ducts become cancerous)
- lobular carcinoma (cancer of the lobules attached to the ducts)
- inflammatory breast carcinoma (diffuse cancer of the breast).

The causes of breast cancer have been mentioned earlier, particularly with regard to hereditary breast cancer. In addition, the younger a woman is when her first child is born, the lower the risk of her developing breast cancer (Trichopoulos *et al.*, 2008).

Signs and symptoms of breast cancer can include (Figure 2.6):

- painless/painful lump in the breast
- a lump under the arm or above the collar bone (enlarged lymph nodes)
- nipple discharge/bleeding from the nipple
- oedema of the arms
- nipple retraction
- prominently visible veins in the breast
- pitting of the skin of the breast (known as 'peau d'orange' because it resembles the skin of an orange).

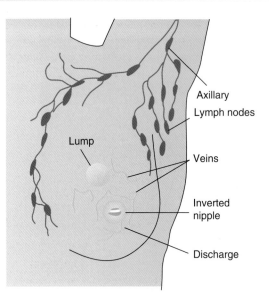

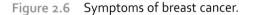

Figure 2.6   Symptoms of breast cancer.

The ideal treatment for breast cancer is surgery – the main treatment when the tumour is localised and has not metastasised, followed by:

- chemotherapy – before, after or instead of surgery where patients are unsuitable for surgery
- hormonal therapy (e.g. tamoxifen) – once chemotherapy has been completed
- immunotherapy – e.g. trastuzumab (Herceptin®; a monoclonal antibody that slows the growth of breast cancer cells)
- radiation therapy – to eliminate any microscopic cancer cells that may remain near the site of the primary tumour following surgery.

Surgery can range from a simple lumpectomy (just involving the cancerous lump itself) to a radical mastectomy – removal of the whole breast tissue and neighbouring lymph nodes (Marieb and Hoehn, 2010).

Conclusion

Cancer is always an emotional subject because of the historically very high mortality rate associated with it. Over the past few years, great strides have been made in the prevention and treatment of many cancers, but it still remains a tremendous challenge to researchers and clinical staff. Greater knowledge of the biochemical, economic, social and psychological aspects of these diseases has lead to a greater understanding of them and, in some parts of the world, an ability to defeat, or at least ameliorate, many of them. However, it is certainly true that the incidences of many of them are increasing (even though they can be better treated). This is related to the facts that many are diseases linked with old age, because they take so long to develop, and people in many countries are living much longer. In the past, they would have died from other causes before the cancers caused problems. So, there have been many triumphs in the treatment and prevention of cancers, but there is no room for complacency.

Test your knowledge

- How would the body normally prevent abnormal cells from growing and developing into cancer cells?

- What are the key steps in carcinogenesis (from a molecular biology standpoint as well as clinically)?

- Describe the contrasting roles of oncogenes and tumour suppressor genes in the development of cancers.

- What is the difference between cytotoxic and cytostatic chemotherapy?

- Briefly discuss how ionising radiation can cause cancers, particularly with regard to the fetus.

- Explain how cancer drug therapy is related to the cell cycle.

- Discuss the many ways of preventing cancer.

Activities

Here are some activities and exercises to help test your learning. For the answers to these exercises, as well as further self-testing activities, visit our website at www.wiley.com/go/fundamentalsofappliedpathophysiology

Fill in the blanks

Worldwide _____ is the most common cause of death from cancer in _____.
Cancer of the breast can be one of three types: _____ carcinoma which affects the
_____ ducts, _____ carcinoma (affecting the _____ attached to the ducts)
or _____ breast carcinoma, which is a _____ cancer of the breast _____.
The signs and symptoms of breast cancer include a _____ in the breast, _____
or _____ from the nipple, nipple _____ and _____ of the skin
(_____). Treatments for breast cancer include chemotherapy, _____
therapy (e.g. tamoxifen), immunotherapy and _____. A _____ in the chances
of developing breast cancer can be brought about by _____ changes such as reducing
_____ intake and increasing the amount of _____ and_____ in the diet.

Choose from: Pitting; Ductal; Lobular; Bleeding; Fruit; Dietary; Tissue; Milk; Breast cancer;
Reduction; Discharge; Alcohol; Inflammatory; Lobules; Lump; Surgery; Vegetables; Hormonal; Retraction; Diffuse; Women; Peau d'orange

Label the diagram

Using the list of words supplied,
label the diagram.

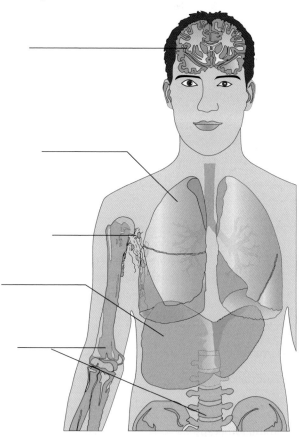

Lymphadenopathy; Haemoptysis; Vertigo; Hepatomegaly; Cough; Seizures; Pain; Headaches;
Fractures; Dyspnoea; Spinal cord compression; Jaundice

Word search

O	N	C	O	G	E	N	E	A	E	C	E	P	A	T	S	C
C	I	X	O	T	O	T	Y	C	I	T	I	R	C	C	N	S
S	M	U	O	I	N	T	I	E	Y	M	N	E	S	Y	V	I
I	M	V	A	M	U	T	M	C	N	C	E	C	E	N	S	A
S	U	R	I	V	A	M	O	L	L	I	P	A	P	D	M	M
E	N	U	U	M	N	H	C	D	Y	O	C	N	K	E	M	O
N	O	E	O	O	P	N	M	A	M	P	N	C	D	U	Y	N
E	T	S	G	M	M	M	E	E	P	P	C	E	A	Y	E	A
G	H	S	Y	A	P	U	R	G	H	C	O	R	C	V	N	L
O	E	L	M	P	T	P	T	A	O	A	S	O	N	I	I	E
I	R	G	C	O	A	U	L	E	B	N	N	U	U	I	L	M
G	A	A	C	P	O	P	M	D	L	I	I	S	T	E	M	E
N	P	H	O	T	O	D	Y	N	A	M	I	C	E	E	R	G
A	Y	S	U	O	M	A	U	Q	S	E	A	M	R	O	E	A
O	I	S	I	S	A	T	S	A	T	E	M	C	E	A	G	E
I	H	V	Y	I	N	C	Y	T	O	S	T	A	T	I	C	T
P	E	O	E	S	T	R	O	G	E	N	O	A	M	U	A	T

Angiogenesis	Leukaemia	Oncogene
Apoptosis	Lymphoblast	Papillomavirus
Carcinogen	Lymphocyte	Photodynamic
Clone	Melanoma	Precancerous
Cytostatic	Metastasis	Somatic
Cytotoxic	Mutagen	Squamous
Germline	Oederma	Tumour
Immunotherapy	Oestrogen	Vaccine

Further resources

BMC Cancer

http://www.biomedcentral.com/bmccancer
This is an open access (i.e. free) cancer journal. Here you will find peer-reviewed articles on topics ranging from cell biology to the psychological aspects of cancer.

British Cancer Journal

http://www.nature.com/bjc/index.html
This is a multidisciplinary cancer journal. Articles from each issue are available free of charge immediately upon publication and all content is free to access for 12 months after publication.

Cancer Research UK

http://www.cancerresearchuk.org/
This is the website of one of the leading cancer research charities in the UK. Here you will find a very useful and extensive information section and patient stories.

Cancer Symptoms

http://www.cancersymptoms.org/
This is a searchable website that includes the signs and symptoms of many forms of cancer and information on cancer prevention. It also has a useful section about the side effects of cancer treatments with tips on how to deal with them.

Inside Cancer

http://www.insidecancer.org/
This website provides multimedia presentations about cancer, including animated slide shows on the biology of cancer, causes and prevention, and interviews with researchers in the field. A good place to start.

Glossary of terms

Adenopathy:	the enlargement of lymph nodes.
Alkaloid:	a naturally occurring chemical that is basic (i.e. not acidic).
Allele:	a gene on one of a pair of chromosomes that codes for the same physical or other feature as its corresponding one on the other chromosome.
Anaemia:	blood lacking in iron. often used to mean a deficiency in red blood cells.

Angiogenesis: the growth of new blood vessels.

Angiogenic growth factor: substance within the body that is involved in the development
                                 of new blood vessels.

Anorexia: loss of appetite/weight.

Antibiotic: a drug used to kill bacteria.

Antibody: a protein in the blood that binds specifically to a particular
                                 foreign substance (its antigen). It is a major part of the immune
                                 system.

Antigen: a foreign substance (e.g. an infecting micro-organism) that can
                                 be recognised by the immune system and generates an
                                 antibody response.

Apoptosis: programmed cell death. It is a form of cell death in which the
                                 cell activates an internal death programme; it is a form of cell
                                 suicide.

Basal cell carcinoma: a cancer involving the surface epithelium of the skin.

Benign: causes no problem. In cancer, it means a growth that is not
                                 malignant.

Blast cell: an immature cell.

Cachexia: this is a syndrome that includes anorexia, weight loss,
                                 anaemia, marked weakness, and altered protein, lipid and
                                 carbohydrate metabolism. This most severe form of
                                 malnutrition is often associated with the later stages of cancer.

Cancer: unregulated growth of cells and tissue that are invasive and
                                 able to metastasise.

Carcinogen: something capable of causing cancer.

Cell differentiation: the process by which cells take on different roles.

Cell division: the reproduction of cells to produce two identical daughter
                                 cells. Also known as binary fission.

Colorectal cancer: a cancer that involves the colon and the rectum.

Cytoplasm: the collective name for all the contents of the cell, including
                                 the plasma membrane, with the exception of the nucleus.

Cytotoxicity: lethal to cells.

Cytotoxic T lymphocyte: a specialised white blood cell that is capable of destroying
                                 other cells of the body that are damaged or have become
                                 infected.

Daughter cell: the resultant cell following cell division.

Dysphonia:	hoarse voice.
Dyspnoea:	difficulty in breathing.
General malaise:	generally lethargic, with loss of appetite and loss of weight.
Germline cell:	a sperm or egg that possesses genes that can be passed on to offspring.
Gray:	the unit that defines the amount of energy released from radiation. It is usually abbreviated to Gy, and it replaces the older unit of radiation energy, the 'rad', which was equivalent to 0.01 Gy.
Haemoglobin:	a protein consisting of globin and four haem groups that is found within erythrocytes (red blood cells). Responsible for the transport of oxygen.
Haemoptysis:	coughing up of blood.
Hepatosplenomegaly:	enlarged liver and spleen.
Lymph node:	part of the lymphatic system, it contains many white cells to destroy bacteria that are trapped within the lymph node.
Lymphoblast:	an immature lymphocyte (a white blood cell).
Malignant:	invasive, has a tendency to grow and may spread to other parts of the body.
Megakaryocyte:	a large bone marrow cell that gives rise to platelets.
Melanoma:	a cancerous outgrowth of melanocytes (pigmented cells of the skin).
Menarche:	the time when the first menstruation occurs.
Metastasise:	the spread of cancerous cells to other parts of the body – often distant to the site of the original cancer.
Mutagen:	something that can affect genes and cause changes (mutations).
Mutation:	a change in one or several bases in DNA.
Neoplasm:	a new growth of tissue. It may or may not be malignant.
Nucleotide sequence:	the sequence of the bases of DNA that make up genes.
Nulliparous:	never having given birth to a viable infant.
Oncogene:	a gene that contains proteins that contribute to carcinogenesis.
Oncogenic virus:	a virus that causes cancers.
Ovulation:	the release of eggs from the ovary.
Palliative:	easing the situation – making it better, but not a cure.

Porphyrins:	an important group of several protein pigments involved in various processes – bound to the iron in haemoglobin.
Precancerous cell:	a cell that is at the stage before it becomes cancerous.
Precursor:	something that will eventually turn into something else (e.g. a red cell precursor will eventually become a red cell).
Premenopausal:	the period before the end of menstruation (i.e. the menopausal period).
Primary cancer:	the tumour that first appears; the site of this first cancer.
Prognosis:	a predication about how a person's disease will progress.
Prophylactic:	preventative.
Proto-oncogene:	a gene that, due to mutation, can become an oncogene.
Radiation therapy:	the use of ultraviolet or ionising radiation to treat cancer.
Solute:	a substance that is dissolved in liquid (solvent).
Solvent:	the liquid in which solutes are dissolved.
Somatic cell:	a cell that possesses genes that are not passed on to offspring (i.e. cells of the body other than the sperm and ova).
Spleen:	an organ in the abdomen that removes and destroys old, damaged or fragile red blood cells. Also, it has an important role to play in immunity.
Squamous cell carcinoma:	a cancer involving squamous cells, usually of epithelial tissue.
Terminal cancer:	cancer that cannot be cured and leads to death.
Thrombocytopaenia:	a deficiency in thrombocytes (platelets).
Toxic:	a substance that is poisonous or damaging to something else.
Tumour:	lump in or on the body caused by the abnormal growth of cells. It can be either malignant or benign.
Tumour suppressor gene:	a gene whose function is to suppress the growth and development of tumours.
Vaccine:	a substance that can be given to a host in order to provoke an immune response and therefore confer immunity on the host without making the host severely ill (e.g. polio vaccine).
Vector:	an organism that houses parasites and transmits them from one host to another. A prime example is the mosquito that transfers the malaria parasite to humans. Also, a means of carrying a substance so that it can be transferred to somewhere else. Viruses are often used as vectors to transfer genes to where they are required in gene therapy.

63

References

Chameides, V.L. (2010). Environmental factors in cancer: focus on air pollution. *Reviews in Environmental Health.* 25(1): 17–22.

Colbert, B.J., Ankney, J. and Lee, K.T. (2011). *Anatomy and Physiology for Health Professions: An Interactive Journey*, 2nd edn. Boston: Pearson/Prentice Hall.

Drake, C.G. (2010). Prostate cancer as a model for tumour immunotherapy. *Nature Reviews Immunology.* 10: 580–593.

Ferlay, J., Shin, H., Bray, F., Forman, D., Mathers, C. and Parkin, D.M. (2010). Estimates of worldwide burden of cancer in 2008, GLOBOCAN 2008. *International Journal of Cancer.* 127(12): 2893–2917.

Frost, G., Danton, A. and Harding, A. (2011). The effect of smoking on the risk of lung cancer mortality for asbestos workers in Great Britain (1971–2005). *The Annals of Occupational Hygiene.* 55(3): 239–247.

Gorczynski, R.M. and Stanley, J. (2006). *Problem-Based Immunology*. Philadelphia: Saunders Elsevier.

Jorde, L.B., Carey, J.C. and Bamshad, M.J. (2009). *Medical Genetics*, 4th edn. St. Louis: Mosby Elsevier.

Kabat, G.C., Jones, J.G., Olson, N. *et al.* (2010). Risk factors for breast cancer in women biopsied for benign breast disease: A nested case-control study. *Cancer Epidemiology.* 31(1): 34–39.

King, R.J.B. and Robins, M.W. (2006). *Cancer Biology*, 3rd edn. Harlow: Pearson/Prentice Hall.

Leggatt, G.R. and Frazer, I.H. (2007). HPV vaccines: The beginning of the end for cervical cancer. *Current Opinion in Immunology.* 19: 232–238.

Ljunggren, H. and Malmberg, K. (2007). Prospects for the use of NK cells in immunotherapy of human cancer. *Nature Reviews Immunology.* 7: 329–339.

Long, M.D., Martin, C.F., Galanko, J.A. and Sandler, R.S. (2010). Hormone replacement therapy, oral contraceptive use and distal large bowel cancer: A population-based case-control study. *American Journal of Gastroenterology.* 105(8): 1843–1850.

Longo, D.L., Fauci, A.S., Kasper, D.L., Hauser, S.L., Jameson, J.L. and Loscalzo, J. (2011). *Harrison's Principles of Internal Medicine*, 18th edn. New York: McGraw-Hill.

Lowy, D.R., Solomon, M.D., Hildesheim, A., Schiller, J.T. and Schiffman, M. (2008). Human papillomavirus infection and the primary and secondary prevention of cervical cancer. *Cancer.* 113(Suppl 7): 1980–1993.

Lubin, J.H. (2010) Environmental factors in cancer: Radon. *Reviews in Environmental Health.* 25(1): 33–38.

King, R.J.B. (2000). *Cancer Biology*, 2nd edn. Harlow: Pearson/Prentice Hall.

Marieb, E.N. (2010). *Essentials of Human Anatomy and Physiology*, 10th edn. San Francisco: Pearson/Benjamin Cummings.

Marieb, E.N. and Hoehn, K. (2010). *Human Anatomy and Physiology*, 8th edn. San Francisco: Pearson/Benjamin Cummings.

McCance, K.L. (2010a) Cellular biology. In: McCance, K.L., Huether, S.E., Brashers, V.L. and Rote, N.S. (eds). *Pathophysiology: The Biologic Basis for Disease in Adults and Children*, 6th edn. Missouri: Mosby Elsevier.

McCance, K.L. (2010b) Biology, cancer epidemiology. In: McCance, K.L., Huether, S.E., Brashers, V.L. and Rote, N.S. (eds), *Pathophysiology: The Biologic Basis for Disease in Adults and Children*, 6th edn. Missouri: Mosby Elsevier.

Moore, P.S. and Chang, Y. (2010). Why do viruses cause cancer? Highlights of the first century of human tumour virology. *Nature Reviews Cancer.* 10: 878–889.

Ottini, L., Palli, D., Rizzo, S., Federico, M., Bazan, V. and Russo, A. (2010). Male breast cancer. *Critical Reviews in Oncology/Haematology.* 73(2): 141–155.

Perry, M.C. (2008). *The Chemotherapy Source Book*, 4th edn. Philadelphia. Lippincott, Williams and Wilkins.

Rosenberg, L., Zhang, Y., Coogan, P.F., Strom, B.L. and Palmer, J.R. (2009). A case-control study of oral contraceptive use and incidental breast cancer. *American Journal of Epidemiology.* 169(4): 473–479.

Sant, M., Allemani, C., Santaquilani, M., Knijn, A., Marchesi, F., Capocaccia, R. and the EUROCARE Working Group. (2009). Eurocare-4. Survival of cancer patients diagnosed in 1995–1999. Results and commentary. *European Journal of Cancer.* 45(6): 931–991.

Trichopoulos, D., Adami, H., Ekbon, A., Hsieh, C. and Lagiou, P. (2008). Early life events and breast cancer risk: from epidemiology to etiology. *International Journal of Cancer*. 122(3): 481–485.

Vickers, P.S. (2005). Acquired defences. In: Montague, S.E., Watson, R. and Herbert, R.A. (eds). *Physiology for Nursing Practice*, 3rd edn. Edinburgh: Elsevier.

Vrooman, L.M. and Silverman, L.B. (2009). Childhood acute lymphoblastic leukaemia: update on prognostic factors. *Current Opinion in Paediatrics*. 21(1): 1–8.

3

Inflammation, immune response and healing

Janet G. Migliozzi

Senior Lecturer, Department of Adult Nursing and Primary Care, School of Health and Social Work, University of Hertfordshire, Hatfield, Hertfordshire, UK

Contents

Fundamentals of Applied Pathophysiology: An Essential Guide for Nursing and Healthcare Students, Second Edition. Edited by Muralitharan Nair and Ian Peate.

Key words

- Pathogen

- Virus

- Infectious response

- Phagocytes

- Micro-organism

- Reservoir of infection

- Immune system

- Inflammatory response

- Bacterium

- Vaccination

- Lymphocytes

Test your prior knowledge

- List the ways in which bacteria are transmitted.

- How does a virus cause disease?

- Describe the roles of tears within the immune system.

- What are the physical signs of inflammation?

Learning outcomes

On completion of this chapter the reader will be able to:

- List and describe the various types of infectious micro-organisms that affect humans.

- Discuss how infectious diseases are transmitted to humans.

- Outline the components of the immune system and their functions.

- Explain the process of inflammation and its role in tissue repair.

Don't forget to visit to the companion website for this book (www.wiley.com/go/ fundamentalsofappliedpathophysiology) where you can find self-assessment tests to check your progress, as well as lots of activities to practise your learning.

Introduction

From the moment that someone is born and for the rest of their life, they are constantly in danger. Some of the dangers come from inside the body and are known as genetic defects, whilst others come from external sources. Two of the dangers that beset everyone throughout life are infectious diseases and injuries. Fortunately, the human body has inbuilt mechanisms to protect it from these dangers, namely the immune system and wound healing.

Infectious diseases occur as a result of invasion of the body by micro-organisms, which cause damage to the tissues of the body. Every infectious disease is characterised by an interaction between the responses of both the infected human host and the infecting organism. Micro-organisms are everywhere – they colonise humans, animals, food, water and soil, and infectious diseases are acquired by humans following contact with an exogenous pathogen present within a reservoir of infection.

The immune system, which is actually an intricate system of cells, enzymes and proteins, is the system that has evolved within humans (and other animals) to protect against these infectious pathogenic micro-organisms. In particular, the white blood cells are essential to the functioning of the immune system. This chapter will describe these and the other elements of the body that constitute the immune system. It starts by looking at the micro-organisms that can cause disease and then at how the immune system fights these micro-organisms and how it helps to heal injuries.

Infectious micro-organisms

Micro-organisms are microscopic cells that either live in the environment, on the skin or inside bodies. They can cause infectious diseases if two conditions are met:

- they are in the right conditions to allow their growth and reproduction
- they are in the right location for their growth and reproduction.

These conditions are important because different micro-organisms have differing and sometimes exacting needs for their growth and reproduction. If environmental conditions are not right, they will not flourish. However, once the conditions are right for them, micro-organisms multiply at an astonishing rate within the host tissues, causing destruction or degeneration so that the host becomes unwell and cannot function properly.

It is not actually the presence of micro-organisms that is the problem, rather it is the fact that during their growth and reproduction (as well as part of the protection against the immune system) they produce waste products known as toxins, and it is these that cause the problems. However, not all of these micro-organisms pose problems for humans. In actual fact, humans need bacteria to help to break down food and digest it. These bacteria are known as commensal bacteria.

Unfortunately, even commensal micro-organisms can become pathogenic if they find themselves in the wrong place. For example, micro-organisms that live in the colon and are beneficial may invade the urinary bladder where they become pathogenic because they are in the wrong place. A good example of this is *Escherischia coli* (*E. coli*) which normally lives in the colon. If however it migrates to the bladder, then it causes cystitis. When infections are caused in this way, they are known as endogenous infections ('endogenous' means 'from within' – in this case the body). All other infections are known as exogenous infections – they come from outside of the body.

Spread of infection

The causative organisms of infectious disease in humans can be transmitted from the reservoir of infection in one of 10 ways:

- droplet spread
- air currents (airborne transmission)
- aerosol
- water
- direct contact
- soil
- inoculation
- faecal–oral route
- vector
- contaminated intermediates.

Droplet spread

Microbial organisms are spread in mucous droplet nuclei that travel only short distances – less than 1 m from the reservoir to the host. This spread can come from coughing and sneezing (as discussed later), but also by talking or laughing. In one sneeze, 20 000 droplets may be produced and expelled from the person who is the reservoir. Droplet transmission should not be confused with airborne transmission – although there are many similarities. Disease-causing organisms that do not spread more than 1 m from the host reservoir are not regarded as airborne, because they are not carried on currents of air, but instead rely upon the force of the expulsion to travel the short distance to a new host. Examples of disease spread by droplet transmission include:

- influenza
- pneumonia
- pertussis (whooping cough).

Air currents (airborne transmission)

Airborne transmission refers to the spread of agents of infection by droplet nuclei in dust. These droplets may spread by more than 1 m from the reservoir to the host.

A good example of droplet transmission is what happens during sneezing and coughing. When someone coughs or sneezes, they expel a fine spray into the air around them. That spray is made up of many, many droplets of mucus that could contain infectious micro-organisms. These droplets of mucus and bacteria/viruses are small and light enough to remain airborne for a long time. Consequently, anyone coming into contact is likely to breathe in the mucus/bacteria/virus droplets, and so become infected in turn. Infectious micro-organisms that can be spread in this way include:

- measles
- tuberculosis (TB)
- staphylococcal and streptococcal infections
- certain fungal diseases (spread by the spores), such as histoplasmosis.

Aerosol transmission

Both domestic and industrial water supplies are sources of aerosol transmission. It has a similar action to that which occurs with droplet transmission, except the reservoir is water, rather than another human. If someone with asthma is given salbutamol via an aerosol, this works quickly because the drug carried in the tiny droplets of water is able to get to the lining of the respiratory tract very quickly. The same thing happens with aerosol transmission of infectious organisms. Examples of diseases that are spread by this method include:

- Legionnaires' disease
- tuberculosis (TB).

Water transmission

In waterborne transmission, pathogens are usually spread by water that has been contaminated with untreated or poorly treated sewage. The pathogenic organisms enter the host by contact either with the mucosa or broken skin. Examples of infections spread through water include:

- leptospirosis – often picked up from rat urine whilst swimming in a river
- schistosomiasis (commonly known as bilharzia) – caused by a fluke (similar to a worm), which is a parasite found in fresh water snails that inhabit the edges of major waterways, such as the River Nile (Re, 2004).

Contact transmission

Contact transmission is the spread of an infectious organism by direct or indirect contact. Direct contact transmission is also known as 'person-to-person transmission'. This is the direct trans-mission of an infectious organism by physical contact between its present host and a susceptible recipient host. The most common forms of direct contact transmission are:

- touching
- kissing
- sexual intercourse.

There are many diseases that can be transmitted by direct contact:

- viral respiratory tract diseases (e.g. the common cold, influenza)
- staphylococcal infections (e.g. septicaemia)
- hepatitis A
- measles

- scarlet fever
- sexually transmitted infections (e.g. syphilis, gonorrhoea, genital herpes)
- infectious mononucleosis (glandular fever)
- human immunodeficiency virus (HIV).

Potential pathogens can also be transmitted by direct contact with animals (or animal products) to humans, e.g. rabies and anthrax.

Indirect contact transmission occurs when the infectious micro-organism is transmitted from its present reservoir to a potential susceptible host by means of a non-living object.

Soil

Soil has already been mentioned as a potential reservoir for infectious micro-organisms. The route of entry from the soil into the body is usually by a skin lesion. Infection can occur:

- when playing sport on a contaminated playing field
  whilst gardening or farming on soil that has been fertilised with animal manure
- any fall on contaminated ground in which the skin becomes broken.

Examples of infectious diseases that can occur from soil include:

- tetanus
- gas gangrene.

Inoculation

Inoculation can be accidental, e.g. by being bitten or scratched. Examples of infections caused in this way include:

- cat scratch disease
- rabies.

Inoculation happen following an injection as can occur with healthcare professionals not taking proper precautions, or by someone injecting themselves with drugs. Examples of infections contracted in this way include:

- HIV
- hepatitis B.

Faecal-oral route

This transmission of infectious micro-organisms can occur in several ways:

- Hand-to-mouth – this is seen particularly in young children who may be exploring their anal area, and then put their hands in their mouths.
- Sewage-contaminated food or water – this occurs particularly if fresh vegetables, salads and fruit are not properly washed before being eaten. It is a particular problem in certain places where human sewage is used to fertilise fields in which salads are grown.
- Certain sexual practices in which there is oroanal stimulation ('rimming').

Examples of infectious diseases transmitted via this route include:

- gastro-enteritis
- enteric fevers.

Vector transmission

This is commonly held to be inoculation by the bite of a sucking arthropod (such as a 'tick'), which is also a host, but there are other types of vector transmission. Vectors are animals that carry pathogens from one host to another. Arthropods are the most important group of disease vectors.

Contaminated intermediates

This is caused by indirect contact transmission, and it occurs when the infectious micro-organism is transmitted from its initial reservoir to a potential susceptible host by means of a non-living object. These non-living objects, or inanimate intermediates, are called fomites. Examples of fomites include:

- clothes, bedding and towels
- tissues and handkerchiefs
- drinking cups and eating utensils
- toys.

Fomites can transmit infections such as (Tortora *et al.*, 2011):

- chicken pox
- staphylococci and streptococci infections
- tetanus.

Case study

Mr Brian Hendrich, a 66-year-old retired town planner, was discharged from hospital 8 days ago following a large bowel resection for diverticular disease. He had been attending his GP practice for wound dressing changes as his wound was not healing well and had started to become painful, inflamed and to discharge purulent fluid. He has been admitted to a surgical ward for exploration and possible debridement of the infected wound. Swabs taken from the wound reveal that it is growing meticillin-resistant *Staphylococcus aureus* (MRSA).

Take some time to reflect on this case and then consider the following.

1. What is MRSA and what are its common causes?
2. What measures need to be taken whilst Mr Hendrich is in hospital to prevent cross-infection to other patients?
3. Outline the treatment protocol that Mr Hendrich will require to treat his MRSA infection.

Types of infectious micro-organisms

There are many different types of micro-organism that can infect humans, and each of them requires different environmental conditions in which to survive, grow and reproduce, as well as different modes of transfer to humans. Some of them are more well known to humans than others, and perhaps the three most well-known micro-organisms are:

- bacteria
- viruses
- fungi.

Bacteria

Bacteria come in a great many sizes and shapes (Figure 3.1), and their diameter ranges from 0.2 to 2.0 μm, whilst their length ranges from 2 to 8 μm.
There are three basic shapes of bacteria, namely:

- spherical (known as a coccus), e.g. streptococcus, staphylococcus
- rod-shaped (known as a bacillus), e.g. diplobacillus, streptobacillus
- spiral (known as a spiral), e.g. vibrio, spirochetes.

Cocci

Cocci are usually round, but they can also be oval, elongated or even flattened on one side. When cocci divide to reproduce, the cells can remain attached to one another. Cocci that remain in pairs after dividing are called diplococci. Cocci that divide and remain attached in chain-type patterns are called streptococci. Cocci that divide and form grape-like clusters are known as staphylococci (Figure 3.1).

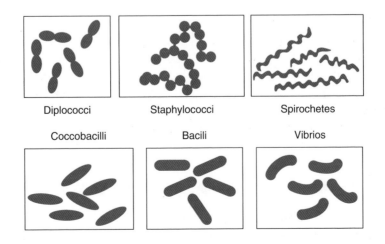

| Diplococci | Staphylococci | Spirochetes |
| Coccobacilli | Bacili | Vibrios |

Figure 3.1   Shapes of bacteria.

Bacilli

Most bacilli appear as single rods. However, those that appear in pairs after they have divided are called diplobacilli. Those that occur in chains are known as streptobacilli, whilst those that have a more oval shape are called coccobacilli (Figure 3.1).

Spiral

Spiral bacteria have one or more twists – they are never straight. Bacteria that look like curved rods are called vibrios. Spirella have a helical shape. Spirals that are helical and flexible are known as spirochetes (Figure 3.1).

Bacterial reproduction

Bacteria reproduce by means of simple fission, also known as binary fission (Figure 3.2). Initially in reproduction, the DNA divides into two and then a transverse wall or septum divides the cytoplasm of the cell. The cell then eventually divides into two, so that there are two daughter cells from each cell, which are clones of the parent cell (see Chapter 1).

Viruses

Viruses are obligate intracellular parasites, and they vary from 20 to 200 nm in size, e.g. the polio virus is 30 nm in size, whilst vaccinia virus (the cause of chicken pox) is 400 nm in size – as big as a small bacterium.

Viruses have varied shapes and chemical composition, but unlike bacteria (or human body cells), they do not contain RNA and DNA –containing onlyRNA or DNA.

Infection of host cells

Figure 3.3 illustrates the stages involved in viral replication.

First, the virus has to be transmitted, and the commonest ways are:

- via inhaled droplets (e.g. rhinovirus – causes the common cold)
- in food and/or water (e.g. hepatitis A – causes hepatitis)

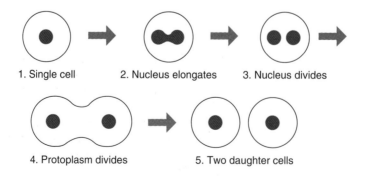

1. Single cell   2. Nucleus elongates   3. Nucleus divides

4. Protoplasm divides   5. Two daughter cells

Figure 3.2   Bacterial reproduction – simple fission.

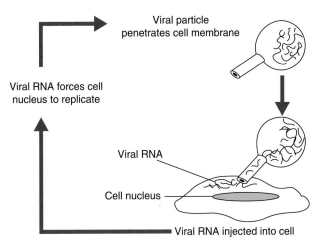

Figure 3.3   Viral replication.

- by direct transfer from other infected hosts (e.g. HIV)
- from the bites of arthropods (such as mosquitoes) that are acting as vectors (e.g. yellow fever).

Fungi

Fungi are characteristically multicellular organisms with a thick cell wall. They may grow as thread-like filaments known as hyphae, although there are many other forms of growth that occur with fungi. Of these other forms of fungi, the most familiar to us are the single-celled yeasts, and of course the mushrooms.

Fungi are free-living organisms and common causes of local infections on skin and hair. However, a number of fungi are also associated with significant disease, and many of these are acquired from the external environment. Pathogenic species invade tissues and digest material externally by releasing enzymes. They also take up nutrients directly from host tissues – as do all good parasites. The various forms of fungi are illustrated in Figure 3.4.

Protozoa

Protozoa are single-celled micro-organisms that range in size from 2 to 100 μm. Many species of protozoa are free-living (i.e. they can exist outside of a cell). Some protozoa are important parasites of humans. Infections are most prevalent in tropical and subtropical regions, but they can also occur in temperate regions.

Although protozoa can cause disease directly (e.g. by the rupture of red cells in malaria), usually the pathology of a protozoal infection is caused by the immunological response of the infected host. Most protozoal infections are actually not life-threatening, unless the infected host has a compromised immune system. The very obvious exception to the previous statement concerns malaria, which kills more than 1.5 million people every year (most of whom are young children, with an immature immune system).

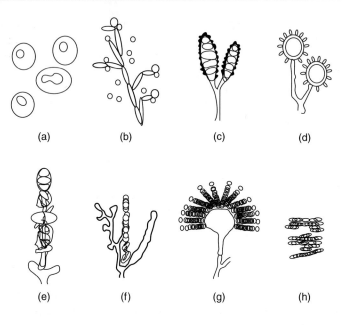

(a)   (b)   (c)   (d)

(e)   (f)   (g)   (h)

Figure 3.4   Typical fungi shapes. (a) *Cryptococcus neoformans*, (b) *Candida albicans*, (c) *Microsporum canis*, (d) *Histoplasma capsulatum*, (e) *Epidermophyton floccosum*, (f) *Trichophyton mentagrophytes*, (g) *Aspergillus fumigatus*, (h) ringworm infection of the hair.

Rickettsiae, chlamydiae and mycoplasmas

Rickettsiae

Rickettsiae belong to a group of pathogens that, whilst physically/anatomically belonging to bacteria, also have certain similarities with viruses. They are Gram-negative rod-shaped bacteria or coccobacilli. Perhaps the best-known disease that they cause is typhus. They are maintained in animal reservoirs and are transmitted by the bites of ticks, fleas, mites and lice.

Chlamydiae

Chlamydiae are very small bacteria that are also obligate intracellular parasites.

The majority of chlamydial infections are genital and acquired during sexual intercourse. Asymptomatic infection is common, especially in women; however, in men it is usually symptomatic. Chlamydiae enter the host through minute abrasions in the mucosal surface, where they bind to specific receptors on the host cells and enter the cells by 'parasite-induced' endocytosis.

Mycoplasmas

Mycoplasmas are also tiny bacteria (actually smaller than large viruses), which differ from normal bacteria by the fact that they lack cell walls, and consequently are not rigid structures. They can produce filaments that resemble fungi. Because of their small size and the fact that they lack rigid cell walls and therefore have a degree of plasticity, they were originally considered to be viruses. In fact, according to Tortora *et al.* (2011), viruses can be considered the smallest cell type and can replicate only in the living cells of an organism. There are several species of mycoplasma, and in humans, some species may cause atypical pneumonia, pelvic inflammatory disease, pyelonephritis and puerperal fever. *Mycoplasma pneumoniae* is transmitted from person to person by the airborne route, whilst *Mycoplasma hominis* and *Mycoplasma genitaleum* are transmitted by sexual contact (Goering *et al.*, 2012; Tortora *et al.*, 2011).

Helminths

'Helminth' is the correct term for all sorts of parasitic worms that infect the body. As far as the human body is concerned, there are three main groups of parasitic worms that cause disease:

- tapeworms
- flukes
- roundworms.

Tapeworms and flukes are also known as flatworms, because they have flattened bodies. They also have muscular suckers and/or hooks to enable them to attach themselves to the host. Roundworms, on the other hand, have long cylindrical bodies, and they generally lack any specialised attachment organs.

Helminth infestations are commonest in warmer countries, although intestinal species of helminth may also occur in temperate regions.

Transmission

Infestation by helminths can occur after:

- swallowing eggs or larvae via the faecal-oral route
- swallowing larvae in the tissues of another host (e.g. beef, pork, fish)
- active penetration of the skin by larval stages
- the bite of an infected blood-sucking insect vector.

Many helminths live in the intestines, whilst others live in the deep tissues, but almost any part of the body can be infested by these parasitic helminths. Flukes and nematodes actively feed on the host tissues or on the contents of the intestines. Tapeworms, on the other hand, have no digestive system and therefore have to absorb predigestive nutrients from the host.

Case study

Agnes Muretembi, a 24-year-old Nigerian woman, has been admitted to a medical ward complaining of joint and loin pain, generalised weakness and hair loss. On admission, her vital signs are: temperature 37.2 °C, pulse 90 beats/minute, respiratory rate 16 breaths per minute and blood pressure 100/65 mmHg. She is noted to have a butterfly-type rash on her face.

Following further investigation, a provisional diagnosis of systemic lupus erythematous (SLE) is made.

Take some time to reflect on this case and then consider the following.

1. What is SLE?
2. Plan the care that Miss Muretembi will require.

3. What ongoing health advice will Miss Muretembi require?

The immune system

Immunology is the study of the immune system and its effects on the body and on invading micro-organisms. However, the immune system does more than just protect the body from invasion by micro-organisms and it is linked to many different organs and cells of the body. The immune system is an intricate system of cells, enzymes and proteins, which together protect the body by making it resistant (i.e. immune) to infection by micro-organisms (bacteria, viruses, fungi) as well as larger organisms such as worms.

Organs, cells and proteins of the immune system

The lymphatic system consists of the:

- tonsils and adenoids
- thymus gland
- lymph nodes
- spleen
- appendix
- patches of lymphoid tissue in the intestinal tract.

The circulatory system consists of the:

- bone marrow
- lymphocytes (white blood cells)
- phagocytic cells (white blood cells)
- dendritic cells
- thrombocytes (platelets)
- complement proteins.

The lymphatic system

The lymphatic system is similar to the blood system and consists of a specialised system of lymph vessels (similar to blood vessels) and specialised lymph nodes and tissue. Unlike the circulatory system, the lymphatic system does not have a heart to pump the lymph around. Instead, the lymph (which fills the lymph vessels) is pushed around the body by a combination of contractions of the smooth muscular walls of the lymph vessels, as well as the flexing and relaxing of striated muscle in the body due to the movement of the individual.

The peripheral lymphatic system consists of lymphatic vessels, lymphatic capillaries and encapsulated organs. These organs include the:

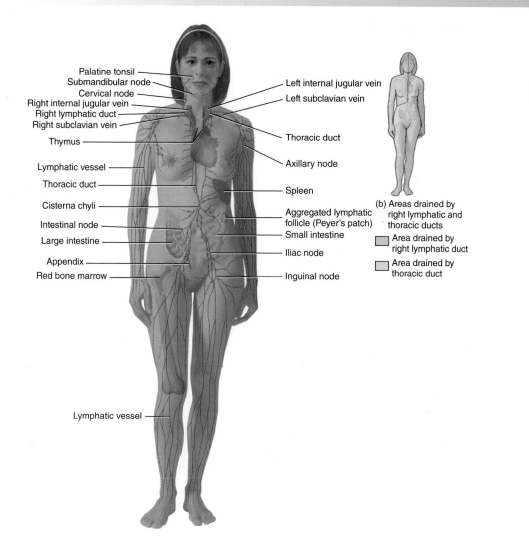

Figure 3.5   The lymphatic system.

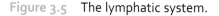

- spleen
- tonsils
- lymph nodes.

The lymph vessels and capillaries form an extensive network throughout the body (Figure 3.5) and connect the organs of the body to the lymphoid organs, such as the spleen, and the lymph nodes. Lymph originates from plasma that leaks from the blood capillaries, and it drains into the lymphoid organs from nearby organs of the body. The lymph nodes act like fishing nets that trap harmful toxins and infectious organisms from the blood, and allow the very high concentrations of immune cells (in this case lymphocytes) to destroy them.

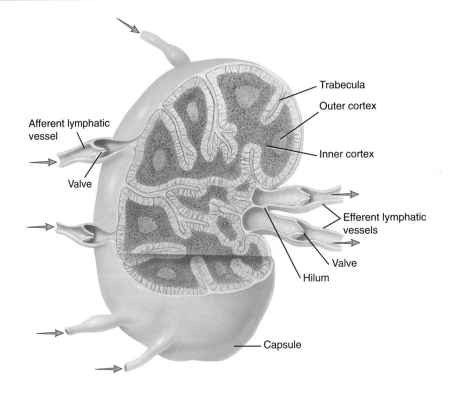

Afferent lymphatic
vessel

Valve

Trabecula

Outer cortex

Inner cortex

Efferent lymphatic
vessels

Valve

Hilum

Capsule

Figure 3.6   Lymph node.

The lymphatic capillaries join together to form larger lymphatic vessels, and lymph glands are
found throughout the lymphatic system – they are like railway stations on a railway network. All
the lymph eventually arrives at two large lymph glands – the thoracic duct and the right lymphatic
duct. These two lymph ducts then empty into the great veins of the neck, and this restores fluid
and proteins to the venous circulation.

Lymphoid tissue

Lymphoid tissue consists of lymph glands (lymph nodes; Figure 3.6), which are the size and shape
of a broad bean, and lymphoid tissue, which is found in specific organs such as the spleen, bone
marrow, lung and liver.

A lymph node is made up of a mesh of cells, and the lymph containing any antigens from
infected tissues and antigen-bearing cells passes through this mesh. Within the lymph gland,
lymphocytes and phagocytes are found in large numbers, so that they can destroy invading micro-
organisms that have been trapped in the lymph node.

Other lymphoid organs

The spleen collects antigens from the blood for presentation to phagocytes and lymphocytes. The
spleen also collects, and disposes of, dead red blood cells.

Types of immunity

There are two types of immune defence system:

- non-specific (or innate) immunity
- specific (or acquired) immunity.

Non-specific immunity

Non-specific immunity is the immunity with which we are born; hence its more common name 'innate immunity'.

The innate immune system can be divided into four different components, although there is some overlap of functions:

- physical barriers
- mechanical barriers
- chemical barriers
- blood cells.

Physical barriers

These include skin and mucosal membranes. The skin acts as a physical barrier to prevent infectious organisms and other material, such as dirt, from getting to the more delicate and undefended organs within our body. However, skin is not only a physical barrier, but also a chemical barrier in that sweat produced from the skin is bactericidal. Unfortunately, skin as a physical barrier does have weaknesses, namely the various orifices that connect the internal body to the outside, including the mouth, nose, urethral opening and anus.

There thus needs to be some other type of protection, and the body has that in the form of mucosal membranes, which coat all the passageways between the internal organs and the outside world. Mucosal membranes contain secretions that are also bactericidal as well as secreting large amounts of antibodies.

Mechanical barriers

Actions involving cilia, coughing, sneezing and tears are included in this section.

Cilia are the tiny hairs that are found in the nose. They are constantly moving like coral under the sea and they move mucus containing dirt and micro-organisms away from the inside of the body, where they can cause problems, to the outside of the body.

Sneezing and coughing work by pushing any micro-organisms or irritants out of the body and into the atmosphere. With each sneeze or cough, millions of viruses are expelled into the atmosphere, and this means that there are fewer viruses in the body to cause even worse problems. This is very effective for the person who is coughing and sneezing, but unfortunately it means that there are all these viruses in tiny droplets suspended in the air, just waiting for someone else to come along and breathe them in, and in turn becoming infected with these viruses.

Tears are also a mechanical barrier. They wash any dirt particles or micro-organisms away from the eyes. Tears are also a chemical barrier because they contain a bactericidal enzyme known as lysozyme.

Chemical barriers

Some of the components that are involved as chemical barriers have already been mentioned above. Chemical barriers include:

- tears
- breast milk
- sweat
- saliva
- acidic secretions, including stomach acid
- semen.

Most of these secretions contain either bactericidal enzymes, such as lysozyme, or antibodies. In addition, bacteria have great difficulty in surviving in acidic secretions and are often killed if the environment is too acidic.

Blood cells

As well as the defences mentioned above, the innate system includes certain blood cells, namely leucocytes (white cells) and thrombocytes (platelets).
The actual white cells involved in the innate immune system are:

- neutrophils
- monocytes and tissue macrophages
- eosinophils
- basophils
- mast cells.

There are several different types of cells that are involved with the innate immune system.

Phagocytic cells

Phagocytic cells include:

- mononuclear phagocytes (these are the monocytes and macrophages)
- polymorphonuclear phagocytes (neutrophils)
- eosinophils.

A phagocyte is a cell that ingests micro-organisms, such as bacteria, as well as other foreign matter, such as dirt in a wound and wood splinters, as well as any of the body's cells that are recognized by the immune system as being 'foreign' or 'non-self' cells through a process called phagocytosis (Figure 3.7). The neutrophils and eosinophils contain enzymes that are released when the phagocyte ingests a micro-organism. These enzymes help to break down the ingested micro-organism, so that the cell can utilise what it wants for its own needs, and expel the rest as waste matter.

Mediator cells

A second group of cells of the innate immune system (the basophils and mast cells) are more accurately described as the helper cells of the immune system. They do not actually destroy the

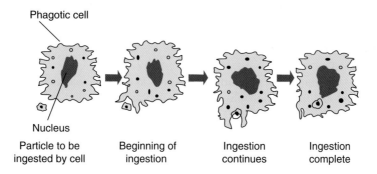

Figure 3.7   Phagocytosis.

invading micro-organisms by phagocytosis, but they help the phagocytes to do so. These mediator cells work by releasing various chemicals that have several actions. For example, some of these chemicals improve the inflammatory response to infection and injury, whilst others help the phagocytic cells to reach the micro-organisms. Although not usually thought of as being part of the immune system, platelets are included because they help to block off and close any cuts and breaks in the skin, and so prevent invading micro-organisms from getting inside the body.

Specific immunity

It is specific immunity that gives the body immunity to specific pathogenic micro-organisms, and it consists of lymphocytes (white blood cells) that target specific invading micro-organisms. This allows for a much more concentrated attack on pathogenic micro-organisms that have broken through the body's initial defences.

Immune problems

The immune system underpins just about all of health and so if anything goes wrong with it, then there can be serious problems for the body. The things that can go wrong include:

- Immunodeficiencies – the immune system is not working properly.
- Autoimmune diseases – the immune system in a person is working too well and attacking cells of the person's own body.

There are two types of immunodeficiency – primary and secondary. Primary immunodeficiency occurs as a result of genetic mutations, whilst secondary immunodeficiency has an external cause, such as infection (HIV) or chemicals. Both types of immunodeficiency can range from very mild to life-threatening, and the treatment consists of supportive care – antibiotics and other similar drugs, as well as improvement of nutrition and general well-being. In addition, some immunodeficiencies may be helped by the injection of immunoglobulins (antibodies) to replace the patient's own. With secondary immunodeficiencies, it may be possible to remove the cause of the immunodeficiency. For example, if the immunodeficiency is caused by a drug (such as is given in chemotherapy for cancer – see Chapter 2), once the drug has been discontinued, then the immunodeficiency resolves.

Autoimmunity is often caused by an overreaction of the immune system to an antigen, which can lead to the immune system attacking the body's own cells. Examples of autoimmune diseases include:

- Diabetes – the immune system attacks the cells in the pancreas that secrete insulin).
- Rheumatoid arthritis – the cells of joints, such as fingers and knees, are attacked by the immune system.

There is a third type of disease caused by a malfunctioning immune system – allergy. An allergy is a raised immune response to an allergen (something that causes an allergy, such as peanuts, dust, or pollen). As with immunodeficiencies, allergies can range from very mild to life-threatening.

Inflammatory response

Inflammation is the body's immediate reaction to tissue injury or damage. This damage can be caused by:

- physical trauma
- intense heat
- irritating chemicals
- infection by viruses, fungi or bacteria.

The inflammatory process (Figure 3.8) involves the movement of white cells, complement and other plasma proteins into a site of infection or injury (Rabson *et al.*, 2004).

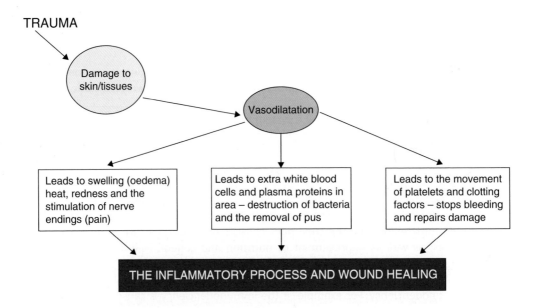

Figure 3.8   The inflammatory process.

There are fundamental signs and symptoms of any tissue or bony injury, and these include the following four classic signs of inflammation at the site of the injury:

- swelling
- pain
- heat
- redness.

There may also be:

- nausea
- sweating
- raised pulse
- lowered blood pressure.

These last few symptoms and signs are the body's response to the pain and to shock, but in terms of immunology, the first four signs and symptoms are important.

Although inflammation does cause pain and other problems, it actually has beneficial properties and effects (Marieb, 2011):

- Prevention of the spread to nearby tissues of infectious micro-organisms and other damaging agents.
- Disposal of killed pathogens and cell debris.
- Preparation for repair of the damage.

Inflammation can be defined clinically as the presence of swelling, redness and pain. It is usually initiated by injury to cells and tissues of the body. Following this injury/damage, three processes occur at the same time:

- Mast cell degranulation – the release from the mast cells into the tissues of granules containing serotonin and histamine. These work with the following two processes to provide the complete inflammatory signs and symptoms.
- The activation of four plasma protein systems:
  - complement (helps to orchestrate the inflammatory response)
  - clotting (stops bleeding and repairs damage)
  - kinin (involved in vascular permeability)
  - immunoglobulins (destroys bacteria)
  all of which work together to support the inflammatory process – activate and assist inflammatory and immune processes, and also play a major role in the destruction of bacteria.
- The movement of phagocytic cells to the area in order to phagocytose bacteria or any other non-self debris in the wound.

Summary of inflammation

The timetable of a typical inflammatory response to tissue in injury is:

- Arterioles near the injury site constrict briefly.
- This vasoconstriction is followed by vasodilatation which increases blood flow to the site of the injury (redness and heat).

- Dilation of the arterioles at the injury site increases the pressure in the circulation.
- This increases the exudation of both plasma proteins and blood cells into the tissues in the area.
- This exudation then causes oedema (swelling).
- The nerve endings in the area are stimulated, partly by pressure (pain).
- The clotting and kinin systems, along with platelets, move into the area and block any tissue damage by commencing the clotting process.
- White blood cells – phagocytes and lymphocytes – move into the area and start to destroy any infectious organisms in the vicinity of the trauma.
- These phagocytes and protein cells, along with the substances they produce, act at the site of the trauma in order to kill any bacteria or other micro-organisms in the vicinity, but just as importantly they will remove the debris that results from the coming together of the micro-organisms/other non-self matter and the forces of the immune system; this includes exudates and dead cells, also known more commonly as pus.
- These systems/blood cells/tissue cells will remain in the area until tissue regeneration (repair) takes place. This is known as resolution.

Thus inflammation can be summed up as the presence of (Traske *et al.*, 2009):

- vasodilation – redness/heat
- vascular permeability – oedema
- cellular infiltration – pus
- thrombosis – clots
- stimulation of nerve endings – pain.

Conclusion

This chapter commenced by looking at infectious diseases. An infection is the result of invasion of the body by micro-organisms, which cause damage to its tissues. Infectious disease are characterised by the interaction of the responses of both the infected human host and the infecting organism.

Micro-organisms are everywhere – they colonise humans, animals, food, water and soil. Infectious diseases are acquired by humans following contact with an exogenous pathogen present within a reservoir of infection. Such reservoirs include:

- active human carriers of the disease
- human carriers of the causative organism
- animal cases of disease or carriers of the organism
- the inanimate environment.

More than 70 bacteria, viruses, fungi and parasites have been identified as pathogenic infecting organisms that are capable of causing serious diseases in humans. Vaccines are available against some of these, and work continues to find vaccines for almost all the bacteria, and viruses and parasites .

Vaccines tend to mimic and enhance the body's own defences against invading micro-organisms – the immune system. The immune system is an extraordinary system, with the continued co-operation of all its components with each other being necessary for continued good health and protection against infecting micro-organisms.

Test your knowledge

- What are the differences between a pathogenic micro-organism and a commensal micro-organism?

- How are the following infectious diseases transmitted?

  - rabies

  - HIV

  - enteric fevers

  - tuberculosis

  - influenza

  - tetanus

- Discuss the effectiveness of physical, chemical and mechanical barriers to infection and what they consist of.

- What are the organs of the lymphatic system?

- Briefly discuss the signs and symptoms of an inflammatory response and explain what causes them.

Activities

Here are some activities and exercises to help test your learning. For the answers to these exercises, as well as further self-testing activities, visit our website at www.wiley.com/go/fundamentalsofappliedpathophysiology

Fill in the blanks

The body's immune system is a _____ and integrated collection of _____ and _____ that _____ the body against _____. It includes cells such as T cells, _____, B lymphocytes (the _____ that produce _____), macrophages and many more. Organs, _____ and _____ involved in the immune _____ include the _____, tonsils, _____, _____ and bone _____. Immune cells are _____ patrolling the body and _____ to any foreign _____, including _____, _____, _____, _____, or cancer cells.

Choose from:
Reacting; Bacteria; Complex; Protects; Tissues; Toxins; Thymus; Organs; Glands; Viruses; Spleen; Marrow; Cells; Disease; Phagocytes; White blood cells; Antibodies; Lymph nodes; Continually; Parasites; Substance; Response

Label the diagram

Using the list of words supplied, label the diagram.

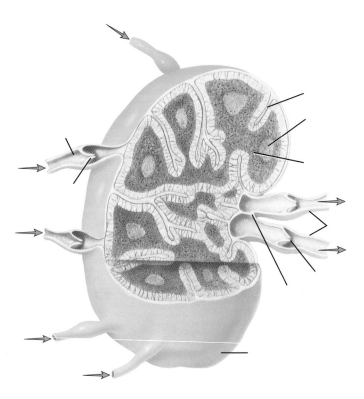

Trabecula; Capsule; Efferent lymphatic vessels; Outer cortex; Hilum; Valve; Afferent lymphatic vessel; Inner cortex

Word search

N	S	N	A	S	N	M	T	L	O	E	T	F	R	C	T	N
Y	S	U	M	I	H	M	I	E	I	I	O	Y	U	G	U	L
S	I	S	O	T	Y	C	O	D	N	E	P	T	S	N	M	O
I	M	M	U	N	O	G	L	O	B	U	L	I	N	S	G	T
S	I	M	M	M	E	T	S	Y	S	N	I	N	I	K	E	I
O	C	H	I	U	U	G	N	S	M	I	D	U	D	H	C	C
T	A	D	I	N	N	B	O	I	N	E	S	M	N	I	H	N
Y	N	V	C	S	T	I	S	D	T	L	E	M	A	C	E	M
C	M	E	O	S	T	C	S	R	N	U	S	I	L	T	M	R
O	E	C	M	S	C	A	N	A	M	E	R	D	G	E	O	T
G	P	T	M	E	L	R	M	I	T	I	O	R	O	N	T	N
A	H	O	E	I	L	A	D	I	C	I	R	E	T	C	A	B
H	M	R	N	R	P	P	A	N	N	N	O	H	S	D	X	I
P	E	S	S	O	N	O	M	R	M	E	N	N	O	A	I	L
E	E	I	A	N	T	I	B	O	D	I	E	S	R	O	S	T
A	S	E	L	M	M	U	S	N	C	S	S	E	P	H	U	S
P	A	R	A	S	I	T	E	E	O	M	I	O	E	O	N	D

Commensal	Prostoglandins	Chemotaxis
Herd immunity	Vectors	Fungi
Immunoglobuli	Pus	Antibodies
Complement	Bactericidal	Immunisation
Endogenous	Endocytosis	Phagocytosis
Kinin system	Histamine	Parasite

Further resources

AVERT

http://www.avert.org
This is the website of a charitable organisation that supports and builds partnerships with local organisations who are working directly to avert the spread of HIV and AIDS. Students will find it useful as it provides a wide range of information to educate people about HIV/AIDS across the world.

CELLS alive!

http://www.cellsalive.com/index.htmlCells alive!
Another useful website for students looking for visual images of human cells. CELLS alive! represents 30 years of capturing film and computer-enhanced images of living cells and organisms for education and medical research. The majority of the site is free to access. There is a stock video library on a range of subjects, both live recording and computer animation.

National Resource for Infection Control (NRIC)

http://www.nric.org.uk
This is a useful resource for students who wish to increase their knowledge in relation to healthcare-associated infection and its prevention. NRIC is an online project developed by healthcare professionals, and aims to be a single-access point to existing resources within infection control for both infection control practitioners and all other healthcare staff.

The Biology Project

http://www.biology.arizona.edu/immunology/tutorials/immunology/main.html
This online interactive resource for learning biology contains a good resource for immunology.

The Department of Health (DH)

http://www.dh.gov.uk
The DH exists to improve the health and well-being of people in England and the website provides policy, guidance and publications for NHS and social care professionals. There are a number of useful resources relating to HIV/AIDS for students wishing to understand more about this area.

HIV tutorial (University of Utah)

http://library.med.utah.edu/WebPath/TUTORIAL/AIDS/HIV.html
This is a short tutorial on HIV from the University of Utah's WebPath service. It covers prevention of infection, mechanism of infection, HIV structure and function, HIV-2, establishment and dynamics of HIV infection, immunodeficiency, genetic variability of HIV, transmission of HIV, primary HIV infection, onset of AIDS, persistent generalised lymphadenopathy (PGL), AIDS-related complex (ARC) and clinical AIDS.

Department of Health – *E. coli* outbreak

http://www.dh.gov.uk/en/Publichealth/index.htm
This website concerns public health – improving and safeguarding public health and well-being. The Department of Health is responsible for health protection, health improvement and health inequality issues in England. The most up-to-date issue discussed on this site is: Outbreak of Haemolytic Uraemic Syndrome in Germany - Verotoxin producing *Escherichia coli* (VTEC).

Glossary of terms

Antibody:	a protein in the blood that binds specifically to a particular foreign substance (its antigen). It is a major part of the immune system.
Antigen:	a foreign substance (e.g. an infecting micro-organism) that can be recognised by the immune system and generates an antibody response.
Asymptomatic:	an infection in which the infected person shows no symptoms of infection.
Autoimmunity:	an overreaction of the immune system to an antigen, which can lead to the immune system attacking the body's own cells.
Bacteria (single = bacterium):	a single-celled micro-organisms that can infect the body, but also may work with the body to the mutual benefit of both (symbiosis). *E. coli* is an example of a bacterium that can be both beneficial to the body and dangerous to it, depending upon the type of *E. coli* and where it is found within the body.
Bactericidal:	deadly to bacteria – kills them.
Commensal:	a micro-organism that does not cause any problems to a human and may even be beneficial. The opposite of a pathogen.
Complement:	a series of enzymatic proteins that work together to aid the immune system by means of being involved in the processes of opsonisation, chemotaxis and the death of bacterial cells.
Contaminated intermediate:	something that is itself contaminated and can contaminate something else. It acts as a 'go-between' for the infectious organism and the targeted potential host.

Cystitis:	inflammation of the urinary bladder – usually as a result of colonisation by an infectious micro-organism.
Degranulation:	the release of granules into the tissues from certain cells, particularly mast cells, eosinophils and basophils, which contain them. These granules contain, amongst other substances, serotonin and histamine, and these substances cause some of the signs and symptoms of inflammation
Dilate:	to widen.
Endocytosis:	the general name for the various processes by which cells ingest foodstuffs and infectious micro-organisms.
Endogenous:	from inside the body; in the case of infections, the infecting micro-organism is already present in the body before becoming infectious.
Enteric fever:	another name for typhoid or paratyphoid fever.
Enzyme:	a protein that speeds up chemical reactions.
Exogenous:	from outside the body (e.g. an infectious organism that comes from outside of the body).
Fluke:	a type of flattened worm (similar to helminths) that can cause schistosomiasis or liver fluke infestation.
Fungi:	micro-organisms that combine to form larger structures that can be seen by the naked eye. Include yeasts as well as fibrous forms.
Helminths:	also known as intestinal worms. These worms exist as parasites in the human intestines, although other types of helminth can live in the blood, lymph system or liver (some are even known to live in the eye).
Herd immunity:	a natural population of people (the herd) who are immune to a particular infection. This can be achieved by the population having natural immunity to the infectious organism, or it may be induced by means of vaccination. This means that anyone within that population who may not be immune to the infection will still have only a low chance of becoming infected because there is so little of the infecting organism in existence within that population.
Histamine:	a substance that causes constriction of smooth muscle, dilates arterioles and capillaries, and stimulates gastric juices. See serotonin.

Histoplasmosis:	a respiratory infection caused by inhaling the spores of the fungus *Histoplasma capsulatum* (found in soil contaminated with bird or bat droppings).
Hyphae:	tubular filament-like threads that make up certain fungi.
Immunodeficiency:	a deficiency in the structure or functioning of the immune system – it can be either secondary (with an external cause) or primary (usually with a genetic cause).
Immunoglobulin:	another name for antibody. Antibodies are opsonins that are manufactured by the B-cell lymphocytes and help the phagocytic cells to destroy invading micro-organisms.
Kinin:	a substance released during inflammation that causes vasodilation and increased capillary permeability; also attract phagocytes. The primary kinin is bradykinin.
Legionnaires' disease:	a form of pneumonia caused by the bacterium *Legionella pneumophila.* It breeds in warm, moist conditions, such as central heating water, and is transmitted via water droplets, such as occur when taking a shower.
Leptospirosis:	a disease that often affects the liver and kidneys and is caused by a bacterium found in the urine of rats. Also known as Weil's disease.
Micro-organism:	any living self-contained organism that can only be seen when under a microscope (e.g. bacteria and viruses).
Mucous membrane:	thin sheet of tissue lining a part of the body that secretes mucus. Cover all the passageways leading into or out of the body (e.g. the mouth, nose, bronchi, urethra).
Obligate intracellular parasite:	a micro-organism that is obligated to reproduce inside cells.
Oedema:	the abnormal collection of fluid in the tissues. It may be localised (following an injury = swelling) or generalised (as in heart failure).
Parasite:	an organism living on or in another organism, and obtaining nourishment at the expense of the organism that is not parasitic.
Passive immunisation:	rather than stimulating the person's own immune system to produce antibodies, the actual antibodies are given to the person.
Pathogen:	a micro-organism that causes problems – is 'infectious'.
Pelvic inflammatory disease:	an inflammation of the internal female reproductive organs.

93

Phagocytosis:	the method by which some cells ingest large particles, including whole micro-organisms.
Prostaglandin:	complex unsaturated fatty acid produced by the mast cells and acting as a messenger substance between cells. Intensify the actions of histamine and kinins. They cause increased vascular permeability, neutrophil chemotaxis and can induce pain.
Protozoa:	the simplest and most primitive type of micro-organism, although bigger than a bacterium. Examples of protozoa include those that cause malaria and sleeping sickness.
Puerperal fever:	also known as puerperal sepsis, this is an infection of the female genital tract. It occurs within 10 days of childbirth, a miscarriage or abortion.
Pus:	a thick green or cream fluid found at the site of a bacterial infection. It consists of millions of dead white blood cells of the immune system as well as dead bacteria.
Pyelonephritis:	inflammation of the kidney – usually as a result of bacterial infection.
Reservoir of infection:	the place where infectious micro-organisms reside before infecting people (e.g. human or animal carriers of the disease, or certain environments). For a disease to perpetuate itself there must be a continual source of the organisms that cause that disease.
Salbutamol:	a bronchodilator drug used in the treatment of asthma – it widens the bronchial tubes to allow asthmatics to breathe more easily.
Schistosomiasis:	a tropical disease caused by a fluke (schistosoma) and contracted by bathing in a river infested by such schistosomes.
Serotonin:	a neurotransmitter found in the central nervous system that is released from platelets in response to injury, trauma or infection. Along with other substances, such as histamine, it causes temporary, rapid constriction of the smooth muscles of large blood vessel walls and dilation of the small veins (venules). This results in increased blood flow and increased vascular permeability. Associated with pain sensation.
Submandibular area:	the area just below the jaw (or lower mandible).
Symptomatic:	the infected person shows the signs and symptoms of the infection, such as a raised temperature and respirations.

Trypanosomiasis: a tropical disease caused by protozoa (Trypanosoma) that is spread by the Tsetse fly that bites humans (and cattle); also known as sleeping sickness after its main symptom.

Vascular permeability: the widening/dilating of blood vessels to allow fluid and other matter to pass through easily.

Vector: an organism that houses parasites and transmits them from one host to another. A prime example of a vector is the mosquito that transfers the malaria parasite to humans.

Virus: a very tiny micro-organisms that is parasitic in that it can only multiply and survive within a cell that it has infected.

References

Marieb, E.N. (2011). *Human Anatomy and Physiology*, 9th edn.. San Francisco: Pearson Benjamin Cummings.

Goering, R., Dockrell, H., Zuckerman, M. *et al.* (2012), *Mims Medical Microbiology*, 5th edn. Edinburgh: Elsevier Saunders.

Re, V.L. (2004). *Hot Topics: Infectious Diseases*. Philadelphia: Hanley & Belfus.

Rabson, A., Rolitt, I. and Delves, P. (2004). *Really Essential Medical Immunology*, 2nd edn. Oxford: Wiley-Blackwell.

Tortora, G.J., Funke, B.R. and Case, C.L. (2011). *Microbiology: An Introduction*, 13th edn. San Francisco: Pearson Benjamin Cumming.

Traske, B.C., Rote, N.S. and Huether S.E. (2009). Innate immunity: Inflammation. In: McCance, K.L., Huether, S.E., Brashers, V.L. and Rote, N.S. (eds). *Pathophysiology: The Biologic Basis for Disease in Adults and Children*, 6th edn. St. Louis: Mosby.

4
Shock

Janet G. Migliozzi

Senior Lecturer, Department of Adult Nursing and Primary Care, School of Health and Social Work, University of Hertfordshire, Hatfield, Hertfordshire, UK

Contents

Fundamentals of Applied Pathophysiology: An Essential Guide for Nursing and Healthcare Students, Second Edition. Edited by Muralitharan Nair and Ian Peate.
© 2013 John Wiley & Sons, Ltd. Published 2013 by John Wiley & Sons, Ltd.

Key words

- Anaphylactic shock
- Anaerobic metabolism
- Cardiac output
- Distributive shock
- Homeostasis
- Hypovolaemic shock
- Hypoperfusion
- Neurogenic shock
- Obstructive shock
- Peripheral vasodilatation
- Septic shock
- Toxic shock syndrome

Test your prior knowledge

- What does the cardiovascular system consist of?
- What is homeostasis?
- How is blood pressure maintained at a constant level?
- List the different types of shock.

Learning outcomes

On completion of this chapter the reader will be able to:

- Describe the different types of shock and their causative factors.
- Describe the clinical presentation of the different types of shock.
- Describe the pathophysiology and three stages of shock.
- Understand the care of the patient in shock.

Don't forget to visit to the companion website for this book (www.wiley.com/go/ fundamentalsofappliedpathophysiology) where you can find self-assessment tests to check your progress, as well as lots of activities to practise your learning.

Introduction

The cardiovascular system consists of the heart, blood and a vascular network composed of arteries, veins, arterioles, venules and capillaries that work together to maintain tissue survival by ensuring that an adequate and constant supply of oxygen and nutrients reaches the cells and that metabolic waste products are removed.

Under normal circumstances, homeostasis is maintained by the four essential circulatory components:

- blood/interstitial fluid volume
- blood flow
- vascular resistance
- the ability of the heart to contract (myocardial contractility).

When one of these circulatory components fails, the others compensate. However, as compensatory mechanisms fail or if more than one of the circulatory components is affected, the cardiovascular system will fail to function, resulting in a state of circulatory shock (Sole *et al.*, 2008).

Case study

Mr Raj Kumar is an 84-year-old man with carcinoma of the stomach who returned to the ward an hour ago following surgery for a total gastrectomy. He has a Robinson's drain *in situ* that is draining small amounts of blood-stained fluid, a urinary catheter on hourly measurements of urine output and an intravenous infusion of normal saline in progress. He is currently on half-hourly observations of his vital signs and has been stable since his return from theatre.

Forty-five minutes later, Mrs Kumar asks you to check on her husband as she is worried about him. On examination his pulse is rapid, weak and thready, and he is breathless and hypotensive. His wound is oozing slightly, the Robinson's drain is now full of blood-stained fluid and there is approximately 5 mL of dark coloured urine in the urometer.

Take some time to reflect on this case and then consider the following.

1. What type of shock is Mr Kumar likely to be experiencing?
2. Discuss the signs and symptoms that Mr Kumar is experiencing.
3. Discuss the role of fluid therapy in managing Mr Kumar's condition.
4. Outline the immediate care that Mr Kumar will require to prevent deterioration.

Types of shock

Any condition that leads to a reduction in cardiac output can lead to circulatory shock; consequently, the effects of shock are not limited to one organ system and can be considered to be a general systemic reaction. However, shock is typically classified by its causative factors (Table 4.1).

Table 4.1   Types of shock and common causative factors (Docherty and Hall, 2002).

Type of shock	Common causative factors
Hypovolaemic shock	External and internal fluid volume loss
Anaphylactic shock	Repeated exposure to an antigen
Septic shock	Gram-negative bacteria Gram-positive bacteria
Neurogenic shock	Spinal cord injury Spinal anaesthetic Brain injury Vasomotor depression Drug overdose Severe pain
Cardiogenic shock	Myocardial infarction Cardiomyopathy Valvular disease Structural defects Cardiac arrhythmias
Obstructive shock	Cardiac tamponade Pulmonary embolism

Hypovolaemic shock

Hypovolaemic shock is the most common type of shock (Monahan and Phipps, 2007) and occurs as a result of fluid loss, including both blood loss, plasma loss and/or loss of interstitial fluid. Blood can be lost from a bleeding organ or wound; however, the circulating volume can also be reduced as a result of plasma loss, e.g. from extensive burns or damaged tissues, or excessive loss of fluids from either renal impairment or inadequate fluid intake, e.g. dehydration. This loss of fluid reduces the circulatory fluid in the blood vessels, leading to insufficient quantities of blood returning to the heart. This poor venous return results in a decrease in cardiac output and subsequent decrease in blood pressure, leading to a decrease in tissue perfusion and resulting in impaired cellular metabolism and shock. Figure 4.1 outlines the physiological events leading to hypovolaemic shock.

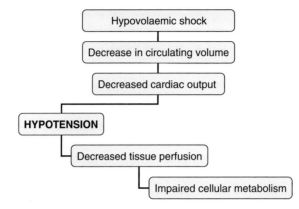

Figure 4.1   Hypovolaemic shock.

Cardiogenic and obstructive shock

Cardiogenic shock occurs when the heart 'fails' as a pump, resulting in abnormal cardiac functioning. Obstructive shock occurs when a mechanical or physical obstruction impedes the flow of blood, e.g. a pulmonary embolism or tension pneumothorax.

Distributive shock

Three types of shock – anaphylactic, septic and neurogenic – are collectively known as distributive shock (Figure 4.2). In these types, irrespective of the causative factors, widespread vasodilatation

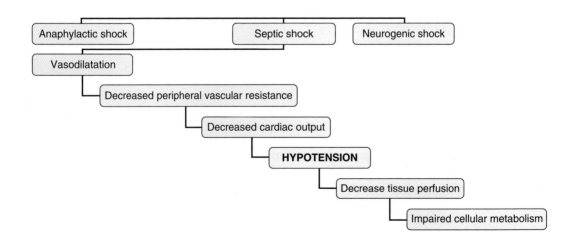

Figure 4.2   Distributive shock.

and decreased peripheral vascular resistance are common features (Kanaparthi and Pinsky, 2011). This type of shock differs from hypovolaemic shock in that the circulating blood volume remains normal (Martini, 2011). However, cardiac output and blood pressure are impaired due to the blood vessels losing their vasomotor tone, which leads to an increase in their diameter (vasodilatation). This leads to a decrease in peripheral vascular resistance, resulting in the blood collecting or 'pooling' in the large veins and causing circulating blood volume to be abnormally distributed. This results in blood pressure in the systemic circulation falling to such a low point that venous return is so decreased that cardiac output becomes insufficient to perfuse the tissues adequately and shock ensues (Figure 4.2).

Case study

Mr David Carter, a 29-year-old old builder, was working with others on a new construction at a local district general hospital. Mr Carter had been tearing down some old guttering when he encountered a wasp's nest, and was stung several times by a large number of swarming wasps. Immediately after this, he commented to his colleagues that, in addition to the pain of the stings, he had begun to feel generally unwell, weak, lightheaded and nauseous. His work colleagues have brought him into the hospital's accident and emergency department. On arrival, Mr Carter reports that he has begun to feel worse and is complaining of increased weakness and nausea, a tightness across his chest and some difficulty breathing. He also has several raised hives on his face and arms.

Take some time to reflect on this case and then consider the following.

1. What type of shock is Mr Carter likely to be experiencing?
2. Discuss the signs and symptoms that Mr Carter is experiencing.
3. Discuss the role of epinephrine in Mr Carter's care.
4. What health promotion advice would you give Mr Carter for the future?

Anaphylactic shock

This form of shock (also known as anaphylaxis) occurs following a widespread allergic or hypersensitivity reaction to the presence of an allergen or antigen that can lead to severe circulatory collapse within seconds (Resuscitation Council UK, 2012). Some common causes of anaphylaxis are (Docherty and Hall, 2002):

- antibiotics (penicillins and cephalosporins)
- anaesthetic agents and muscle relaxants
- aspirin and non-steroidal anti-inflammatory drugs, e.g. ibuprofen
- blood products and plasma expanders
- intravenous radiocontrast media
- latex
- food allergies, e.g. shellfish, eggs, nuts and dairy products
- insect stings.

Anaphylactic reactions can be either immunoglobulin E (IgE)-mediated or non-IgE mediated and occur as a result of repeated exposure to an antigen or allergen (to which the individual has previously produced an antibody response), which results in an allergic response (Johnson and Peebles, 2004). The subsequent release of histamine causes vasodilatation of blood vessels, increases vascular permeability (which results in loss of intravascular fluid volume) and constricts respiratory smooth muscle (Smith and Bullock, 2010).

Signs and symptoms of anaphylactic shock can include:

- sense of impending doom, anxiety and restlessness
- altered levels of consciousness
- severe air hunger
- bronchospasm and dyspnoea
- stridor caused by laryngeal oedema
- urticaria (hives)
- pruritus (itching)
- rhinitis and conjunctivitis
- abdominal pain, vomiting and diarrhoea
- oedema of the lips, eyes, hands, neck and throat.

Septic shock

Septic shock is the most common type of distributive shock (Smeltzer and Bare, 2010) and occurs as a result of widespread infection. This form of shock is most commonly associated with the release of Gram-negative and Gram-bacteria into the bloodstream – a condition known as bacteriaemia in which the pathogen's release of toxins into the bloodstream results in massive vasodilatation and hypotension.

Toxic shock syndrome is a form of septic shock that can occur in women who use tampons during menstruation or in individuals who have body piercings, and is caused by *Staphylococcus aureus*.

Neurogenic (vasogenic) shock

This is a rare form of shock which can occur following major brain or spinal trauma, emotional trauma, severe pain or a drug overdose. The loss of sympathetic impulses causes a significant decrease in peripheral vascular resistance. This results in massive vasodilatation, which affects venous return to the heart and leads to a decrease in cardiac output, low blood pressure and a reduction in blood flow (Table 4.1).

Pathophysiology of shock

Shock is a severe, life-threatening clinical syndrome that can result in death, and is characterized by inadequate tissue perfusion that results in impaired cellular metabolism. Shock manifests itself as a syndrome within many diseases or traumatic injuries that may be life threatening and is a state of insufficient oxygenation and perfusion to vital organs and tissues throughout the body. Therefore, whilst the causes of shock are varied and the individual's presentation may differ according to this (Table 4.2), the end results (at a cellular level, e.g. cellular hypoxia/damage) are the same (Jenkins and Tortora, 2013).

Table 4.2   A summary of the clinical presentation of different types of shock.

Manifestation	Hypovolaemic	Anaphylactic	Septic	Neurogenic
Heart rate	Tachycardia	Tachycardia	Tachycardia	Bradycardia
Respiratory rate	Tachypnoea	Tachypnoea and dyspnoea	Tachypnoea	Tachypnoea
Blood pressure	Hypotension	Hypotension	Hypotension	Hypotension
Urine output	Decreased	Decreased	Increased initially then oliguria	Decreased
Temperature	Within normal range	Within normal range	Initially raised and then within normal range	Regulation disrupted, therefore may be experiencing hypo/hyperthermia
Skin	Cool, pale	Cyanosis, swollen oedematous face, hands	Initially flushed and warm (warm shock), then cool and pale	Cool, pale
Mental state	Restless and anxious	Restless and anxious	Restless and anxious	May be unconscious due to fainting or head injury

Stages of shock

Although the patient's initial response to shock may vary as it is dependent on the individual's age and general state of health prior to the event leading to the shock state, three distinct stages of shock are recognized and occur regardless of the type of shock experienced (Sole *et al.*, 2008).

Stage 1: Compensatory (non-progressive) stage of shock

A sufficient blood pressure is essential to adequately perfuse cells with oxygen and nutrients. Shock begins when the blood pressure is unable to do this and the body then initiates a series of compensatory mechanisms. During this stage, although the individual will be experiencing symptoms of shock, they are not at imminent risk of death and shock may be reversed if appropriate interventions are initiated. In the early stages of compensatory shock, a set of neural, hormonal and chemical compensatory mechanisms are initiated in an attempt to restore homeostasis and maintain blood flow to vital organs, such as the heart, brain and kidneys.

Neural compensatory mechanisms

The sympathetic nervous system regulates blood flow and pressure through its ability to increase heart rate and total peripheral resistance. In the shock state, the baroreceptors and chemoreceptors located in the carotid sinus and aortic arch detect the reduction in blood pressure, and impulses are relayed to the vasomotor centre in the medulla oblongata.

Hormonal compensatory mechanisms

Stimulation of the sympathetic nervous system causes the adrenal medullae to release the catecholamines (epinephrine and norepinephrine), which increase the heart rate and force of contractions to improve cardiac output. The coronary arteries vasodilate to increase blood flow to the heart and meet its increasing demand for oxygen. The rate and depth of respirations will also increase to try and increase gaseous exchange and oxygen levels in the blood (Sole *et al.*, 2008).

A fall in cardiac output will also impact on the renal system, which detects a decrease in blood flow and pressure to the kidneys. This causes the kidneys to release renin, which converts angiotensinogen into angiotensin I, and the latter is metabolised into angiotensin II – a powerful vasoconstrictor. The presence of angiotensin II leads to the release of the hormone aldosterone from the adrenal gland, which causes the reabsorption of sodium from the renal tubule. This leads to the retention of water in the hope of increasing the falling blood volume (Figure 4.3). Stimulation of the posterior pituitary gland causes the release of antidiuretic hormone (ADH), also known as vasopressin hormone, which increases the amount of water reabsorbed by the kidney tubules; hence the patient may produce small volumes of concentrated urine or in more severe cases, no urine (anuria).

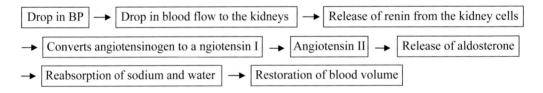

Figure 4.3   Renin–angiotensin mechanism.

Chemical compensatory mechanisms

A reduction in cardiac output leads to a decrease in the blood flow to the lungs, which is detected by the chemoreceptors located in the aorta and carotid arteries. This leads to an increase in the rate and depth of respirations; however, this hyperventilation causes a reduction in carbon dioxide, which impacts on blood flow and oxygen levels to the brain, and in turn this can lead to confusion and restlessness. The individual will move to the next stage of shock if the physiological adaptations that the body has initiated to overcome shock start to fail.

Stage 2: Progressive (decompensated) stage of shock

Progressive shock occurs when the body's initial compensatory responses fail to restore an adequate blood pressure and tissue perfusion (Smith and Bullock, 2000). In the early stages of progressive shock, the individual's life can usually be saved if treatment is timely and appropriate. However, if the originating problem, e.g. haemorrhage, has not been corrected, the body's compensatory mechanisms can no longer cope with the continuing decreased cardiac output and blood pressure; consequently vital organs are not sufficiently perfused (hypoperfusion) and tissue damage can occur. The systemic circulation continues to vasoconstrict in the hope of shunting blood to vital organs; however, this is at the expense of the microcirculation, resulting in ischaemia of the extremities. Impaired cellular metabolism occurs as a result of an inadequate supply of oxygen and nutrients, and the decreased level of oxygen causes the cells to switch from aerobic metabolism to anaerobic metabolism, which results in the production of lactic acid and leads to metabolic acidosis.

Prolonged anaerobic metabolism results in a reduction in the production of adenotriphosphatase (ATP), which leads to failure of the sodium–potassium pump, causing sodium ions to accumulate inside the cell, resulting in swelling and a deterioration in the cell's function.

As shock progresses, histamine and bradykinin (both of which have vasodilating properties) are released, and decrease the peripheral vascular resistance further, resulting in a continued reduction in blood returning to the heart. This leads to a further decrease in cardiac output and blood pressure, resulting in cellular hypoxia.

Hypoxia can lead to depression of the vasomotor centre in the medulla and the sympathetic nervous system. Levels of consciousness decrease and the patient may become restless, disorientated and confused. Abdominal distension and paralytic ileus are common, and the pancreas may become ischaemic (Smith and Bullock, 2010).

Stage 3: Irreversible (refractory) stage of shock

At this stage, the continued decrease in blood pressure and heart rate means that the inadequate tissue perfusion leads to the subsequent failure of the body to respond to any form of therapy. Multiple organ failure and death result within a matter of hours (Collins, 2000).

Table 4.3 summarizes the stages of shock, the physiological changes that occur and how the individual may present clinically.

Care of the patient in shock

Due to the life-threatening nature of shock, it is essential that the condition is recognized and treated in a prompt manner if inadequate tissue perfusion and subsequent organ failure are to be avoided. Therefore, the shocked patient requires close and careful monitoring within an intensive care or high-dependency unit. Common interventions include oxygen, fluid and/or drug therapy (Bench, 2004), and care of the patient should be the focus whilst they are undergoing these restorative measures. Key clinical considerations include:

- Close monitoring of vital signs (blood pressure, pulse, temperature, respiratory rate, urine output and oxygen saturation [SpO_2]) to ensure the early detection of any deterioration in the patient's condition. The frequency of monitoring will be determined by the patient's progress; however, half-hourly observations should be considered in the first instance unless the patient is at risk of deteriorating rapidly, in which case continuous monitoring should be instigated. Where there is a risk of neurological deterioration, e.g. if the patient is in neurogenic shock or experiencing fluctuations in levels of consciousness, then assessment of the

Table 4.3 Physiological changes that occur at each stage of shock (adapted from Sole *et al.*, 2008).

Stage of shock	Physiological changes	Clinical presentation
1. Compensatory	Neural and hormonal compensation Mild to moderate vasoconstriction Some anaerobic metabolism	Normal blood pressure Increased pulse rate (tachycardia) and respiratory rate (tachypnoea) Increased thirst Decreased urinary output Altered level of consciousness/dilated pupils
2. Progressive	Overall aerobic metabolism Decreased oxygen levels (hypoxia) to vital organs Little or no oxygen (anoxia) to non-vital organs Impaired blood flow (ischaemia) to tissues Failure of sodium–potassium pump	Low blood pressure (hypotension) Raised pulse rate Pulmonary oedema Peripheral oedema Decreased urinary output Altered level of consciousness Abdominal distension Paralytic ileus Cold, ashen skin
3. Irreversible	Severe tissue hypoxia, ischaemia and necrosis (tissue death) Build-up of toxic metabolites	Severe hypotension Respiratory failure Acidosis Peripheral oedema Acute renal failure (oliguria) Alterations in the blood clotting cascade

patient's neurological status using the Glasgow Coma Scale (see Chapter 10) may also be required.

- Administration of oxygen therapy as an imbalance between oxygen supply and tissue demand is fundamental to the nature of shock (Edwards, 2001). For patients who are conscious and able to breathe spontaneously, oxygen should be administered via a face mask or nasal cannulae. However, if the patient is unable to maintain their airway/sufficient oxygen levels in the blood, then they may have to be intubated and ventilated. The rate/percentage of oxygen required should be guided by regular measurements of pulse oximetry and blood gas analysis. As oxygen therapy is very drying to the mucosa, it should be humidified with sterile water and the patient should be given regular mouth care.

- Administration of prescribed intravenous fluid to improve the patient's blood pressure and cardiac output, as an adequate cardiac output and a systemic blood pressure that is sufficient to maintain perfusion of vital organs is essential to meet the body's metabolic requirements. Therefore, the patient will require intravenous fluid replacement to correct the decreased circulating volume (hypovolaemia). If the patient has lost blood, e.g. through a haemorrhage, then a blood transfusion is indicated to raise the haemoglobin level to a point that ensures that there is adequate oxygen-carrying capacity in the blood. Whilst the choice and volume of fluid given, e.g. blood, colloid or crystalloid infusion, is dependent on the type of shock the patient is experiencing, strict monitoring of fluid balance is required to ensure effectiveness of the fluid therapy and the early detection of complications related to fluid therapy, e.g. fluid overload. This will require the insertion of a urinary catheter and hourly monitoring of urine output to check an output of at least 30 mL of urine per hour is being produced, and regular monitoring of vital signs (see earlier) for early detection of any adverse reactions.

- Psychological care for the patient and their family. The patient in shock is a medical emergency and this situation is very frightening for both the patient and their family. Therefore, they should be kept fully informed about any changes/progress in the patient's condition, the purpose of any equipment used and any interventions given as this will help to reduce anxiety and alleviate fear.
- Maintaining adequate nutrition as the patient in shock will have increased demand for energy to support metabolic processes. As the patient may be nil by mouth due to their need for possible surgery or to impairment in digestive function, e.g. paralytic ileus, enteral or total parenteral feeding may be required, depending on the patient's condition.
- Ensuring the skin remains intact as the poor tissue perfusion and immobility will increase the risk of pressure sore formation. The patient will require regular pressure area care and should be nursed on a pressure-relieving mattress.

Pharmacological management of shock

In the shocked patient, drug therapy is primarily directed at enhancing the heart's ability to pump and to improve tissue perfusion (Monahan *et al.*, 2006). The common drugs used to manage the patient in shock are summarized in Table 4.4. Additional measures that may be taken according to the type of shock being experienced are provided in Table 4.5.

Table 4.4   Common drugs used to manage shock (adapted from Sole *et al.*, 2008).

Drug	Action
Dopamine Dobutamine Amrinone Norepinephrine	Increase the heart's ability to contract
Epinephrine Norepinephrine	Increase venous return to the heart by causing vasoconstriction
Atropine Isoproterenol	Increase heart rate and force of contraction

Conclusion

Shock is a common threat to patients and represents a medical emergency. The causes and treatment of the patient in shock are varied and complex. The overall aim of this chapter has been to

Table 4.5   Additional management of shock according to type.

Classification		Management
Hypovolaemic		Eliminate and treat cause of hypovolaemia
Distributive	Anaphylactic	Antihistamines Steroids Bronchodilators
	Septic	Establish and treat source of infection with appropriate antimicrobial agents
	Neurogenic	Treat cause Adequate pain relief

explore the different types of shock and the resulting pathophysiology these create. The prompt recognition of the signs and symptoms of shock are critical to the patient's prognosis and healthcare professionals play a central role in the early detection of any deterioration in the patient's condition.

Test your knowledge

- Outline the mechanisms the body uses to regulate and maintain blood pressure.

- Compare and contrast the signs and symptoms of hypovolaemic and distributive shock.

- Describe the mode of action of three pharmaceutical agents used in the treatment of circulatory shock.

- Outline a plan of care for the patient in circulatory shock.

- Which patients are at most risk of developing septic shock and why? Describe how these risks can be prevented.

Activities

Here are some activities and exercises to help test your learning. For the answers to these exercises, as well as further self-testing activities, visit our website at www.wiley.com/go/fundamentalsofappliedpathophysiology

Fill in the blanks

Under _____ circumstances, _____ is _____ by the four essential circulatory components – blood/interstitial fluid volume, _____, _____ resistance and _____. Any _____ that leads to a _____ in cardiac _____ can lead to _____ shock and the _____ of shock are not limited to one organ system – rather it is a general _____ reaction.

Choose from:
Myocardial contractility; Effects; Systemic; Circulatory; Normal; Homeostasis; Condition; Maintained; Blood flow; Vascular; Reduction; Output

Word search

N	U	T	I	E	N	B	C	V	V	C	O	T	U	E	C
T	I	S	O	S	I	H	R	H	O	L	E	I	R	U	E
P	I	A	S	V	E	N	O	U	S	R	E	T	U	R	N
L	A	I	I	Y	R	O	T	A	S	N	E	P	M	O	C
S	R	M	S	M	C	I	B	O	R	E	A	N	A	U	E
U	T	E	A	I	E	T	T	R	S	E	N	O	I	V	O
A	I	A	T	A	N	A	P	H	Y	L	A	X	I	S	R
E	M	R	S	L	E	T	L	S	M	D	D	T	T	T	B
E	E	E	O	L	U	A	T	O	R	I	U	Y	O	I	S
T	L	T	E	E	R	L	E	U	V	B	P	E	E	A	A
S	C	C	M	R	O	I	P	I	I	O	D	I	B	P	A
R	O	A	O	G	G	D	O	R	N	S	P	H	S	R	X
I	P	B	H	E	E	O	T	I	I	A	O	Y	T	O	Y
U	S	G	A	N	N	S	H	V	A	R	U	U	H	I	I
A	C	A	R	D	I	A	C	O	U	T	P	U	T	S	S
A	I	T	L	D	C	V	G	N	D	D	H	C	L	E	I

Anaphylaxis	Hupovolaemia	Distributive
Vasodilatation	Anaerobic	Bacteraemia
Cardiac output	Allergen	Compensatory
Neurogenic	Venous return	Homeostasis

Further resources

Resuscitation Council (UK)

http://www.resus.org.uk/pages/guide.htm
This is a useful resource for students wishing to understand more about the treatment of anaphylactic reactions and basic life support. The website is free to access and contains the latest guidance as well as links to other useful medical information, science worksheets and an application for the iPhone called iResus.

NHS Clinical Knowledge Summaries

Podcast on the treatment and management of anaphylaxis
http://www.cks.nhs.uk/knowledgeplus/podcasts/anaphylaxis#-350698
This is a useful website for students wishing to understand more about the treatment and management of anaphylaxis. The NHS Clinical Knowledge Summaries (formerly PRODIGY) are a reliable source of evidence-based information and practical 'know how' about the common conditions managed in primary care. This link provides two podcasts on anaphylactic shock.

Trauma and shock factsheet

http://www.nigms.nih.gov/Publications/Factsheet_Trauma.htm
This is a useful resource that provides factsheets on the different kinds of trauma and shock that health professionals may encounter, including symptoms and causes. It is one in a series of factsheets published by the National Institute of General Medical Sciences (NIGMS), which supports basic biomedical research to aid advances in the diagnosis, treatment and prevention of disease.

Toxic shock syndrome

http://www.mckinley.illinois.edu/Handouts/toxic_shock_syndrome.html
This is part of a series that students will find useful for information resources on common medical conditions and diseases. This resource focuses on toxic shock syndrome (TSS) and tampons. It provides details of the causes, symptoms, treatment and prevention of TSS.

Food Allergy & Anaphylaxis Network (FAAN)

http://www.foodallergy.org/
This is a useful resource for students wishing to understand more about food allergies and anaphylaxis. The FAAN website includes information about FAAN and their work; information about common food allergens and anaphylaxis; hot topics; allergy alerts; resources aimed at managing food allergies; and details of food allergy research.

British Society for Allergy and Clinical Immunology

http://www.bsaci.org/index.php?option=com_content&task=view&id=117&Itemid=1
This is a useful website containing guidance on a range of allergens. It is mostly free to access. There are also links to other useful resources relating to allergy.

Glossary of terms

Aerobic:	requiring the presence of oxygen.
Anaerobic:	without oxygen.
Allergen:	a compound that produces a hypersensitivity response.
Anaphylaxis:	a sudden, acute allergic reaction to a material (e.g. food, environment, drug or biological substance).
Antibody:	a protein in the blood that binds specifically to a particular foreign substance (its antigen). It is a major part of the immune system.
Antigen:	a foreign substance (e.g. an infecting micro-organism) that can be recognised by the immune system and generates an antibody response.
Anuria:	a condition in which no urine is produced.
Bacteriaemia:	the presence of bacteria in the bloodstream.
Bradykinin:	a substance derived from plasma proteins; its prime action is in producing dilatation of arteries and veins.
Dyspnoea:	shortness of breath; laboured breathing.
Histamine:	a substance that causes constriction of smooth muscle, dilates arterioles and capillaries, and stimulates gastric juices. See serotonin.
Homeostasis:	maintenance of relatively constant conditions within the body's internal environment despite external environment changes.
Hypersensitivity reaction:	an overreaction to an allergen that results in inflammation and tissue damage.
Hyperventilation:	abnormally deep and prolonged breathing.
Hypoperfusion:	abnormally low blood flow through a tissue.
Hypoxia:	reduced levels of oxygen in the tissues.
Immunoglobulin:	another name for antibody. Antibodies are opsonins that are manufactured by the B-cell lymphocytes and help the phagocytic cells to destroy invading micro-organisms in the immune response.
Interstitial fluid:	the fluid in the tissues that fills the spaces between cells.
Ischaemia:	a low oxygen state in a part of the body. Usually the result of obstruction to the blood supply to tissues.

| Peripheral vascular resistance: | the resistance blood encounters at it flows through the systemic circulation. |

Vasoconstriction: a decrease in the diameter of a blood vessel due to the relaxation of smooth muscle in the vessel wall; may occur as a result of hormones or after stimulation of the vasomotor centre leading to increased peripheral resistance.

Vasodilatation: an increase in the diameter of a blood vessel due to relaxation of smooth muscle in the vessel wall; may occur as a result of hormones or after decreased stimulation of the vasomotor centre leading to decreased peripheral resistance.

References

Bench, S. (2004). Clinical skills: assessing and treating shock: a nursing perspective. *British Journal of Nursing.* 13(12): 715–721.

Collins, T. (2000). Understanding shock. *Nursing Standard.* 14(49): 35–39.

Docherty, B. and Hall, S. (2002). Anaphylaxis in adults. *Professional Nurse.* 18: 73–74.

Edwards, S. (2001). Shock: types, classifications and explorations of their physiological effects. *Emergency Nurse.* 9(2): 29–38.

Jenkins, G.W. and Tortora, G.J. (2013). *Anatomy and Physiology*, 3rd edn. New Jersey: John Wiley and Sons.

Johnson, R.F. and Peebles, R.S. (2004). Anaphylactic shock: Pathophysiology, recognition, and treatment. *Seminars in Respiratory Critical Care Medicine.* 25(6): 695–703.

Kanaparthi, L.K. and Pinsky, M.R. (2011). Distributive shock. www.emedicine.com/med/article/168689

Martini, F. (2011). *Fundamentals of Anatomy and Physiology*, 9th edn. London: Prentice Hall.

Monahan, F.D., Neighbors, M., Sands, J.K. and Marek, J.F. (2006). *Phipps' Medical and Surgical Nursing – Health and Illness Perspectives*, 8th edn. St Louis: Mosby.

Resuscitation Council UK (2012). *Emergency Treatment of Anaphylactic Reactions – Guidelines for Healthcare Providers*. London: Resuscitation Council (UK).

Smeltzer, S. and Bare, B. (2010). *Brunner and Suddarth's Textbook of Medical – Surgical Nursing*, 12th edn. Philadelphia: Lippincott.

Smith, M.A. and Bullock, B.L. (2010). In: Bullock, B.L. and Henze, R.L. (eds). *Focus on Pathophysiology*. Philadelphia: Lippincott.

Sole, M.L., Klein, D.G. and Moseley, M.J. (eds) (2008). *Introduction to Critical Care Nursing*, 5th edn. St. Louis: Elsevier Saunders.

113

5

The heart and associated disorders

Muralitharan Nair

Senior Lecturer, Department of Adult Nursing and Primary Care, School of Health and Social Work, University of Hertfordshire, Hatfield, Hertfordshire, UK

Contents

Fundamentals of Applied Pathophysiology: An Essential Guide for Nursing and Healthcare Students, Second Edition. Edited by Muralitharan Nair and Ian Peate.

Key words

- Pericardium
- Chambers
- Systemic circulation
- Atria
- Myocardium
- Valves
- Pulmonary circulation
- Ventricles
- Endocardium
- Impulses
- Conducting systems
- Pacemaker

Test your prior knowledge

- What are the layers of the heart called?
- How many chambers does the heart have and what are they called?
- Can you trace the blood flow through the heart?
- Name the conducting systems of the heart.
- List the possible causes of myocardial infarction.

Learning outcomes

On completion of this section the reader will be able to:

- Describe the structure and functions of the heart.
- Outline the conducting system(s) of the heart.
- Describe the blood flow through the heart.
- Trace the systemic and pulmonary circulations.

Don't forget to visit to the companion website for this book (www.wiley.com/go/ fundamentalsofappliedpathophysiology) where you can find self-assessment tests to check your progress, as well as lots of activities to practise your learning.

Introduction

In order for water to flow through a pipe, it must be under pressure or a force pushing the water through the pipe. When the pressure is increased, water will flow with greater force and when the pressure drops the flow is decreased. The same principle can be applied to the heart and blood flow. In the human body, the heart is the muscular pump that provides the pressure necessary to propel the blood throughout the body. It must continue its cycle of contraction and relaxation; otherwise blood will stop flowing and the cells in the body will be unable to obtain nutrients from food sources and get rid of waste such as carbon dioxide and other products. Thus, a healthy and efficient heart is essential for cellular function. This chapter discusses the structure and functions of the heart, the conducting system and the blood flow through the heart. It also includes cardiac diseases such as myocardial infarction, heart failure (left and right heart failure) and cardiogenic shock and angina, and their related care and management.

Location of the heart

The heart is a muscular organ that rests on the diaphragm near the midline of the thoracic cavity in the mediastinum (Jenkins and Tortora, 2013), which is the space in the middle of the thorax between the right and the left lungs. It lies more to the left than the right side of the chest and the base of the heart is over its apex (Figure 5.1). It is about the size of the owner's closed fist

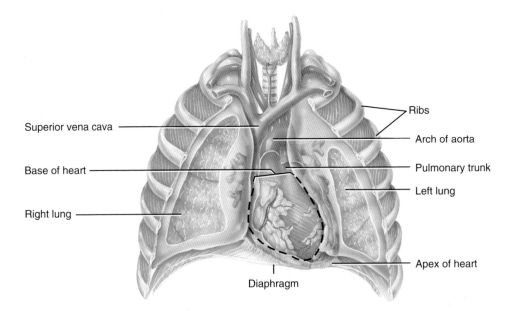

Figure 5.1   Location of the heart.

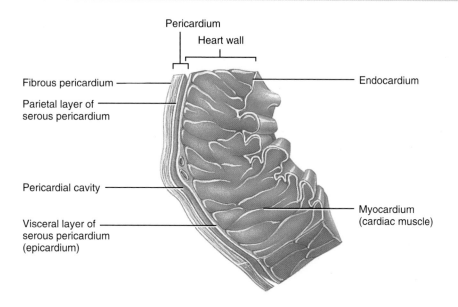

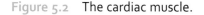

Figure 5.2   The cardiac muscle.

and is approximately 12 cm long and 9 cm wide. In men, it weighs approximately 250–390 g and in women, it is 200–275 g (Marieb and Hoehn, 2010).

Structures of the heart

The heart is composed of specialised cardiac muscle and is surrounded by a membrane called the pericardium. The pericardium is divided into parietal and visceral pericardium. The parietal pericardium, which is the outer layer, is a fibrous sac. The inner layer, called the visceral pericardium or the epicardium, is a serous membrane, which is close to the heart (Figure 5.2). The two layers are separated by a thin film of serous fluid which allows the heart to move freely. The cardiac muscle is called the myocardium and is only found in the heart. The fibres of the myocardium branch and join with each other (Figure 5.2). The endocardium lines the chambers and the valves of the heart. It is a thin, smooth and shiny membrane which allows the smooth flow of blood (Waugh and Grant, 2010). Thus, the heart can be described as having three layers:

- the pericardium – the outer layer
- the myocardium – the middle layer
- the endocardium – the inner layer.

Chambers of the heart

The heart is divided into two sides, right and left, which are separated by a muscle called the septum. The septum ensures that the oxygen-rich blood from the left side of the heart does not mix with the oxygen-depleted blood on the right side (Tortora and Derrickson, 2011). Each side

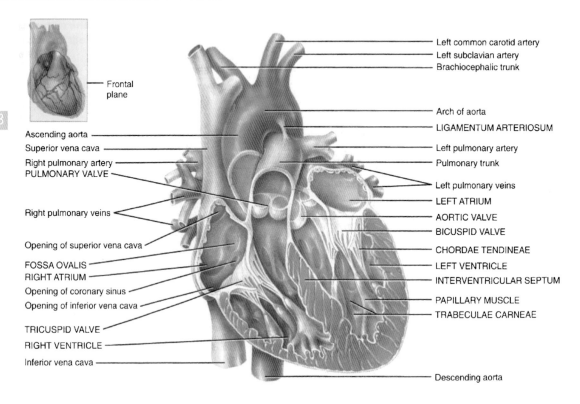

Figure 5.3   The chambers and the valves of the heart.

of the heart is divided into two chambers. The upper chambers are called the atria (the right and left atrium) and the lower chambers are called the ventricles (the right and left ventricle) (Figure 5.3). The walls of the atria are much thinner than the walls of the ventricles.

Valves of the heart

The valves between the atria and the ventricles are called the atrioventricular valves. The right atrioventricular valve is known as the tricuspid valve because it has three cusps, and the left has two cusps and is also known as the bicuspid (mitral) valve (McCance *et al.*, 2010). These valves only allow the flow of blood from the atria to the ventricles and prevent the blood from flowing in the opposite direction. Similarly, there are no valves in the aorta and pulmonary artery and these are known as semilunar valves (Figure 5.3).

Vessels of the heart

Blood flows in and out of the heart through several large vessels. The right atrium receives venous blood through the superior and inferior venae cavae. Oxygen-depleted blood from the right

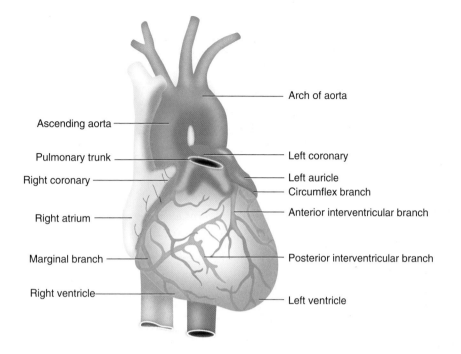

Arch of aorta

Ascending aorta

Pulmonary trunk

Right coronary

Right atrium

Marginal branch

Right ventricle

Left coronary

Left auricle

Circumflex branch

Anterior interventricular branch

Posterior interventricular branch

Left ventricle

Figure 5.4 The vessels of the heart.

ventricle is carried to the lungs by the pulmonary artery and the pulmonary veins return oxygen-rich blood from the lungs to the left atrium. The aorta transports oxygenated blood from the left ventricle to the whole body (McCance *et al.*, 2010). However, the heart has its own blood supply and this is delivered by the coronary arteries and the coronary veins return oxygen-depleted blood from the heart tissue to the right atrium (Figure 5.4). Table 5.1 summarises of the vessels and their functions.

Blood flow through the heart

The right atrium receives oxygen-depleted blood via the superior and inferior venae cavae and the coronary sinus. The right atrium then empties the blood into the right ventricle via the tricuspid valve. By opening the pulmonary artery, the right ventricle then pumps the blood to the lungs via the pulmonary arteries (right and left) and by opening the pulmonary semilunar valve. In the lungs, carbon dioxide is exchanged for oxygen molecules. The blood returning to the lungs has a higher content of carbon dioxide, which diffuses out of the lung capillaries into the alveolar sac and is disposed of during expiration. During inspiration, oxygen diffuses from the alveolar sac into the lung capillaries where it attaches itself to the haemoglobin molecules in the red blood cells. The oxygen-rich red blood cells are then transported in the blood to the left atrium by four sets of pulmonary veins. The short circulation from the right ventricle to the lungs and from the lungs to the left atrium is called the pulmonary circulation (Marieb and Hoehn, 2010).

From the left atrium, the blood is then pumped into the left ventricle via the bicuspid (mitral) valve. From the left ventricle, the blood is then pumped to the whole body via the aorta through

Table 5.1 Summary of the vessels and their functions.

Vessel	Function
Superior vena cava	Returns oxygen-depleted blood to the right atrium from the thoracic organs, head, neck and both arms
Inferior vena cava	Returns oxygen-depleted blood to the right atrium from the rest of the body
Pulmonary artery (divides into the right and left pulmonary artery)	Takes oxygen-depleted blood from the right ventricle to the lungs
Pulmonary veins (two from the right lung and two from the left lung)	Returns oxygen-rich blood from the lungs to the left atrium
Aorta	Takes oxygen-rich blood from the left ventricle to the whole body
Coronary arteries	Takes oxygen-rich blood to the heart tissues
Coronary veins	Returns oxygen-depleted blood from the heart tissues to the right atrium via the coronary sinus

the aortic semilunar valve (Figure 5.5). The aorta and its branches then transport the oxygen-rich blood to all parts of the body. The blood is then returned to the right atrium via the venae cavae. This loop is called the systemic circulation (Marieb and Hoehn, 2010). The role of the systemic circulation is to transport oxygen and nutrients, and to remove waste products, e.g. carbon dioxide, from the tissues.

Conducting systems of the heart

The heart has a built-in regulatory mechanism which produces a co-ordinated myocardial contraction of the four chambers. This is achieved by the cardiac conducting system (Figure 5.6), which is composed of the:

- sinoatrial (SA) node
- atrioventricular (AV) node
- bundle of His
- right and left bundle branches
- Purkinje fibres.

The SA node

The SA node is situated in the right atrium just below the opening of the superior vena cava. It is also known as the pacemaker, so called because it initiates impulses much faster than other groups

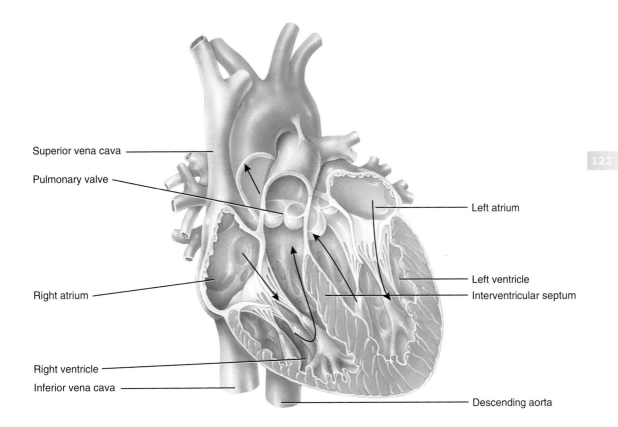

Superior vena cava

Pulmonary valve

Left atrium

Right atrium

Left ventricle
Interventricular septum

Right ventricle

Inferior vena cava

Descending aorta

Figure 5.5   Blood flow through the heart. The arrows indicate the direction of blood flow.

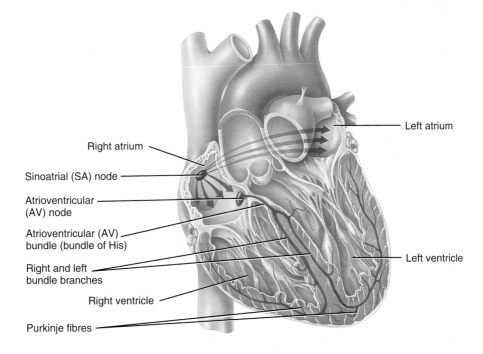

Right atrium

Sinoatrial (SA) node

Atrioventricular (AV) node

Atrioventricular (AV) bundle (bundle of His)

Right and left bundle branches

Right ventricle

Purkinje fibres

Left atrium

Left ventricle

Figure 5.6   The conducting system of the heart.

of neuromuscular cells (Waugh and Grant, 2010). Impulses from the SA node cause the atria to contract.

The AV node

The AV node is situated at the base of the right atrium. This is the last region of the atria to be stimulated, thus allowing time for the atria to empty the blood into the ventricles before the ventricles start to contract again. This ensures that the blood will flow in one direction only.

Bundle of His

This is a set of fibres that originate from the AV node.

Right and left bundle branches

From the bundle of His the nerve fibres split into the right and left bundle branches (Figure 5.6).

Purkinje fibres

These tiny nerve fibres innervate both the right and left ventricular myocardial cells.

Nerve supply of the heart

The pumping action of the heart is rhythmic. In other words, the cardiac muscle has the inherent ability of automatic rhythmic contraction, independent of its nerve supply. However, the rate of contraction is influenced by the nerve supply to the heart.

The nerve supply originates from the cardioregulatory centre in the medulla oblongata which is situated in the brainstem (Figure 5.7). These nerves are a branch of the autonomic nervous system and are called the sympathetic and parasympathetic nerves (Waugh and Grant, 2010).

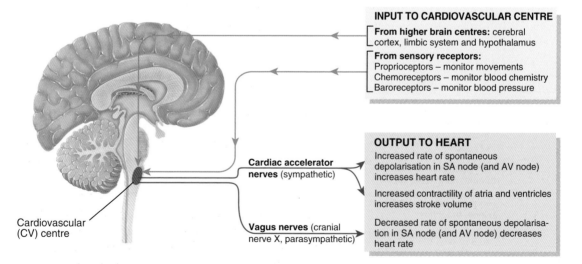

INPUT TO CARDIOVASCULAR CENTRE

From higher brain centres: cerebral cortex, limbic system and hypothalamus

From sensory receptors:
Proprioceptors – monitor movements
Chemoreceptors – monitor blood chemistry
Baroreceptors – monitor blood pressure

OUTPUT TO HEART

Increased rate of spontaneous depolarisation in SA node (and AV node) increases heart rate

Increased contractility of atria and ventricles increases stroke volume

Decreased rate of spontaneous depolarisation in SA node (and AV node) decreases heart rate

Cardiac accelerator nerves (sympathetic)

Cardiovascular (CV) centre

Vagus nerves (cranial nerve X, parasympathetic)

Figure 5.7   The cardioregulatory centre.

The sympathetic nerve increases heart rate; it innervates the SA node, AV node and the myo-cardium of the atria and ventricles. The parasympathetic (vagus) nerve slows down the heart rate and it supplies the SA and AV nodes, and the atria muscles. Factors affecting heart rate include (Waugh and Grant, 2010):

- hormones such as epinephrine, steroids
- stress
- age
- drugs such as propranolol, dopamine
- body temperature
- autonomic nervous system
- circulating volume of blood
- electrolyte imbalance
- levels of oxygen and carbon dioxide in the blood.

Diseases of the heart

Learning outcomes

On completion of this section the reader will be able to:

- List some of the common heart diseases.
- Describe the pathophysiology of the common heart diseases.
- List the possible investigations.
- Outline the care and management of some heart conditions.

Case study

Mr Suresh Patel is a 46-year-old married man who works as a bus driver. This morning, while he was having breakfast, Mr Patel felt unwell and collapsed but regained consciousness. His wife called for an ambulance. He is admitted to A&E complaining of chest pain spreading to the shoulders, neck and arms. His wife states that he complained of not feeling well when he got up that morning and that he vomited a couple of times in the toilet. His wife indicates that generally he is a fit man but does suffer from hypertension for which he takes medications to control his blood pressure. She informs you that Mr Patel has a family history of diabetes and hypertension and that he is under stress as he fears he will lose his job as a result of cuts and that they are behind in their mortgage payments.

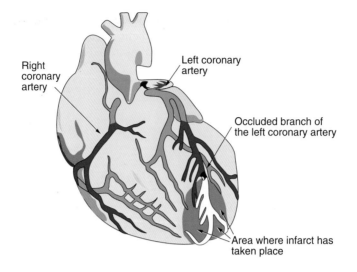

Figure 5.8   Myocardial infarction.

Take some time to reflect on this case and then consider the following.

1.   What is the possible diagnosis for Mr Patel?
2.   List the investigations that may be carried out and the rationale to confirm diagnosis.
3.   What medical treatment will Mr Patel have in A&E?
4.   What advice will you give Mr Patel and his wife when he is discharged from hospital?

Myocardial infarction

Myocardial infarction (MI) is commonly referred to as a 'heart attack', which results from oxygen starvation of the myocardium (Figure 5.8). When the coronary blood flow is occluded as a result of a blood clot or fatty deposits (atheromatous plaque) over a period of time, death of the myocardium will take place (McCance *et al.*, 2010), resulting in MI. Porth (2010) states that MI occurs more frequently in the early morning (between 0600 and 1200) than during the evening.

Aetiology

MI is a medical emergency that needs quick intervention; it is a major cause of death for both men and women (Bullock and Henze, 2010). Individuals at risk include:

- People who have a medical history of vascular disease such as atherosclerosis, a condition where fatty deposits build up in the arteries, causing them to narrow and restrict the blood flow to the tissues.
- Previous heart attack or stroke.
- Older age group (men over the age of 40 years and women over the age of 50 years).
- Smokers because the nicotine in cigarettes causes narrowing of the arteries.

- People who drink excessive amounts of alcohol because a high intake of alcohol increases the level of low-density lipoprotein (LDL).
- People with a family history.
- The misuse of drugs such as cocaine.
- Diabetics with or without insulin resistance.
- People with hyperlipidaemia and obesity.

Investigations

The following investigations may be carried out to confirm diagnosis:

- chest X-ray
- blood chemistry (urea and electrolytes, cardiac enzymes, e.g. creatine kinase, full blood count)
- electrocardiogram (ECG) to detect any abnormal changes in the rhythm
- angiogram.

Pathophysiology

An occluded coronary artery results in myocardial ischaemia due to a lack of oxygen to the myocardial cells. If the heart tissue is deprived of oxygen for a prolonged period of time, approximately 20–45 minutes, this can lead to cell death (necrosis) distal to the occlusion (Figure 5.8) (Hogan and Hill, 2004). The extent of the ischaemia depends on the location, extent of occlusion, amount of heart tissue supplied by the blood vessel and duration of the occlusion. It may affect one of the three layers of the heart (pericardium, myocardium and endocardium) or a combination of these layers (Porth, 2010).

Where the infarct has taken place, a collagen scar forms and the damaged muscle does not contract efficiently. Collagen is a bundle of inelastic fibres that do not stretch or contract effectively. Damaged heart tissue conducts electrical signals much more slowly than normal heart tissue, which can result in inefficient contraction of the myocardium. This can result in decreased:

- volume of blood ejected by the left ventricle with each heartbeat
- cardiac output (volume of blood pumped out by the left ventricle each minute)
- blood pressure
- tissue perfusion.

Signs and symptoms

- Central chest pain that radiates down the left arm and also to the lower jaw, neck, back and right arm. The pain may be described by the patient as crushing or tightness in the chest. Pain may last for more than 20 minutes.
- Rapid, irregular pulse, hypotension and dyspnoea (shortness of breath).
- Diaphoresis (excessive sweating), nausea, vomiting, palpitations, loss of consciousness and even sudden death.
- Signs of shock.
- Cyanosis.
- McSweeney et al. (2003) suggest that women often experience markedly different symptoms compared to men. Symptoms such as dyspnoea, fatigue, sleep disturbances and weakness are more common in women than men.

Care and management

When symptoms of MI occur, it is a medical emergency and prompt action is needed because time is an important factor in the prevention of extended damage to the heart muscle (Elton, 2003). Key care considerations are:

- The patient must be kept pain free as it presents as a result of myocardial ischaemia. Accurate pain assessment should be carried out using pain assessment tools such as the Numerical Rating Scale or the Verbal Rating Scale (Alexander *et al.*, 2007). Patients should be encouraged to report their pain as it occurs.
- Bed rest for the first 24 hours is important to reduce the effort and strain on the heart.
- Administer prescribed oxygen to treat tissue hypoxia, which helps to reduce ischaemia and pain (LeMone *et al.*, 2011).
- Monitoring of all the vital signs (heart rate, blood pressure, temperature and respirations) is important to detect early complications or changes in the patient's condition. This is normally carried out 1–2 hourly depending on the patient's condition.
- Observe for signs of shock, such as lethargy, bradycardia or tachycardia, cyanosis, hypotension and excessive sweating (diaphoresis).
- Document any care given to the patient in accordance with the Nursing and Midwifery Council (2009) Record Keeping: Guidelines for Nurses and Midwives.

Pharmacological and non-pharmacological treatment

Some of the pharmacological and non-pharmacological interventions are:

- Drugs to dissolve clots such as reteplase or streptokinase are administered within 2 hours of developing MI to limit tissue damage.
- Continuous ECG monitoring is carried out to detect abnormal cardiac rhythms and to allow prompt action to be taken.
- A urinary catheter may be inserted to monitor urine output.
- Drugs such as morphine or morphine derivatives are administered to control pain. Sublingual or intravenous nitrates such as glycerine trinitrate (GTN) are also considered (Adams *et al.*, 2008).
- An anticoagulant such as heparin is commenced to minimise the risk of a thrombus developing.
- In some patients, an emergency coronary angioplasty may be required to increase blood flow to the coronary arteries. This involves insertion of a catheter into the obstructed coronary artery under local anaesthesia. The balloon in the catheter is then inflated for 15 seconds to 2 or 3 minutes (Porth, 2010), which dilates the artery.

Heart failure/congestive heart failure

Heart failure (HF) is a general term used to describe several types of cardiac disease that lead to poor perfusion of tissues. Congestive heart failure is a progressive and debilitating disease that is accompanied by congestion of body tissues. Heart failure may affect either side of the heart; however, as all the chambers are part of the heart structure, if one side fails then it affects the other side (Waugh and Grant, 2010). Nevertheless, left heart failure (LHF) is more common than right heart failure (RHF).

Case study

Mr Martin Goldsmith, a 58-year-old married man with two children, collapsed while he was walking his dog. A passerby went to his aid and called for an ambulance to take him to the local hospital. At the local hospital, Mr Goldsmith was examined by the duty doctor. During the assessment the doctor noticed that Mr Goldsmith was breathless and his ankles were swollen. Mr Goldsmith refused to lie down and insisted that he would rather sit in the chair. The nurse in charge rang his wife to inform her that her husband had been admitted to the hospital after collapsing on the road. Mrs Goldsmith rang one of her children and they went immediately to the hospital.

Take some time to reflect on this case and then consider the following.

1. What are the possible reasons why Mr Goldsmith collapsed in the road?
2. What are the assessments that should be carried out to confirm diagnosis?
3. Why is Mr Goldsmith refusing to lie down?
4. What might the treatment options be for his condition?

Aetiology

Heart failure may be caused by a variety of conditions:

- acute MI where there is a loss of myocardial muscle, which can lead to poor contraction
- hypertension
- valvular heart disease
- inadequate emptying from the left ventricle due to poor contraction of the myocardium
- anaemia resulting from reduced red blood cells.

Pathophysiology

The onset of HF may be acute or chronic. It is often associated with systolic and diastolic congestion and with myocardial weakness. This weakness impairs the ability of the heart to pump efficiently. In acute HF, there is a sudden decrease in the amount of blood pumped out from both ventricles, which leads to a reduction in oxygen supply to the tissues. However, in chronic HF the progression of the disease is gradual and in the early stages there may be no symptoms of heart failure.

Investigations

The following investigations may be carried out to confirm diagnosis:

- electrocardiogram
- chest X-ray

- full blood chemistry and cardiac enzymes
- physical examination
- echocardiogram.

Pathophysiology of right heart failure

RHF is associated with the right ventricle being unable to pump the blood into the pulmonary artery leading into the lungs. This leads to an increase in volume of the right ventricle during the end-diastolic phase, which causes an increase in volume of the right atria (Bullock and Henze, 2010). This in turn increases the volume of blood and pressure in the systemic venous system. There is accumulation of blood in some of the major organs – the liver, the kidneys and the spleen (Nowak and Handford, 2010), resulting in enlargement of these organs and their eventual destruction.

Signs and symptoms of right heart failure

- Pitting oedema may be observed in the sacral area of a patient confined to bed, as well as on the feet and legs when the patient is sitting. This is due to the impaired pumping ability of the heart and as a result fluid accumulates in the tissues.
- Enlargement of the organs such as the liver (hepatomegaly) and the spleen (splenomegaly) can cause pressure on the surrounding organs such as the stomach.
- Pleural effusion may occur due to the increased capillary pressure.
- Distended jugular veins are a visible sign in patients who suffer from RHF.
- Patients have difficulty in breathing due to ascites.
- Fatigue.
- Jaundice and coagulation problems may be present due to liver damage.

Pathophysiology of left heart failure

LHF results from damage to the left ventricular myocardium. The contraction of the left ventricle is ineffective and it cannot pump out all the blood it receives from the left atrium (Hogan and Hill, 2004). This results in pooling of blood in the left atrium and raised pressure in the pulmonary veins, which leads to pulmonary oedema. Patients with pulmonary oedema may experience symptoms such as dyspnoea, orthopnea, productive cough, frothy sputum and pallor. Failure of the left ventricle also results in poor cardiac output. As the cardiac output decreases, perfusion to the tissues also diminishes, resulting in poor delivery of oxygen and nutrients to the tissues (McCance et al., 2010).

Left heart failure (backward effects)

- Emptying of the left ventricle is diminished.
- There is an increase in volume and end-diastolic pressure of the left ventricle.
- Pressure in the left atrium increases.
- Volume and pressure in the pulmonary veins increase.
- Volume of fluid in the pulmonary capillary bed increases.
- Movement of fluid from the lung capillaries to the interstitial space of the alveoli.
- Rapid filling of alveoli spaces with fluid leading to pulmonary oedema.

Left heart failure (forward effects)

- Cardiac output decreases.
- Perfusion to tissues of the body decreases.
- Blood flow to the kidneys and other organs decreases.
- This leads to reabsorption of sodium and water by the kidneys to increase the circulating fluid volume.

Signs and symptoms of left heart failure

- Patients with LHF may develop dyspnoea in the early stages due to fluid accumulation in the pulmonary capillary bed, resulting in poor exchange of gases (oxygen and carbon dioxide) in the lungs.
- Dizziness, fatigue and weakness due to the poor oxygenation of the body tissues resulting from the low cardiac output and oxygen saturation. The dizziness is the result of low oxygen to the brain, which may result in disorientation, confusion and unconsciousness.
- Orthopnoea – the patient's inability to breathe in a supine position.
- Productive cough and frothy sputum.
- Tachycardia.
- Cyanosis – the bluish discolouration of the mucous membranes around the lips and in the nail bed.
- Wheezing due to bronchospasm.
- Crackles at the lung bases due to pulmonary oedema.

Care and management

In order to provide high-quality care, healthcare professionals need to undertake a full and accurate assessment and to devise a care plan for all the problems identified. Vital signs are monitored hourly until they are stable. Early detection of changes in vital signs and prompt treatment may save the patient's life. Key care considerations are:

- Patients with heart failure may experience breathing problems such as breathlessness, especially on exertion. Prescribed oxygen should be administered to improve oxygenation of the blood.
- Patients with LHF may expectorate large amounts of frothy sputum due to pulmonary oedema and therefore they will need a sputum mug/carton to expectorate into, and be provided with tissues and a waste receptacle to put the used tissues in.
- The patient should be nursed in the upright position in bed supported by pillows to assist breathing unless contraindicated.
- Accurate monitoring of daily fluid intake and output is important in patients with HF. Output should be in excess of 30 mL/hour (Kozier et al., 2008) and this should be recorded hourly (if a urinary catheter is in situ) and any changes in output reported immediately.
- The patient should be encouraged to reduce salt intake in the diet as salt promotes fluid retention.
- Carers should provide assistance when bathing or showering.
- Carers must ensure that all treatment and care is explained to the patient in a way that the patient will understand.
- Patients may need laxatives to avoid straining when defaecating.

Pharmacological and non-pharmacological treatment

The treatment of HF focuses on treating the signs and symptoms, and improving the quality of life. Such measures include:

- Moderate physical activity when symptoms are mild or moderate.
- Weight reduction is important through physical activity and healthy eating, as obesity is a risk factor for heart disease.
- Reduction in salt intake is essential as excessive intake can cause fluid retention and lead to an exacerbation of cardiac problems.
- Patients with HF will need their fluid intake monitored carefully to prevent fluid overload.

The pharmacological interventions for HF include:

- Antihypertensive drugs, e.g. quinapril 2.5–5 mg daily or captopril 6.25 mg three times per day should be prescribed for patients with heart failure (National Institute for Health and Clinical Excellence, 2010).
- Diuretics such as furosemide (maximum recommended dose is 250–500 mg) or matolazone (maximum dose 10 mg) are used to decrease fluid load in patients with HF (National Institute for Health and Clinical Excellence, 2010).
- Beta-blockers are also used in the treatment of HF. Bisoprolol 10 mg daily is used to improve left ventricular function (National Institute for Health and Clinical Excellence, 2010).

Cardiogenic shock

Cardiogenic shock is a physiological state in which inadequate tissue perfusion occurs from cardiac failure mainly caused by acute MI. It can occur relatively quickly due to the effect of infarction on the myocardial tissue. It is a medical emergency and if not treated quickly the patient will die.

Aetiology

There are numerous causes of cardiogenic shock but the most common cause is acute MI. The severity of the shock is associated with myocardial damage. Low cardiac output due to cardiogenic shock also impairs perfusion of the coronary arteries and the myocardium, thus further increasing myocardial damage. Although MI is the most common cause of cardiogenic shock, several other factors may be implicated:

- acute pulmonary embolism
- myocarditis
- acute mitral valve regurgitation
- right ventricular infarction
- septic shock
- mitral stenosis
- complications of cardiac surgery
- valvular heart disease.

Investigations

The following investigations may be carried out to confirm diagnosis:

- chest X-ray
- ECG
- arterial blood gas analysis
- full blood chemistry
- cardiac enzymes, e.g. troponins.

Pathophysiology

Cardiogenic shock results from the diminished ability of the heart to function effectively. In MI, cardiogenic shock usually develops when approximately 40% of the myocardium is damaged. This leads to decreased blood pressure, poor cardiac output and inadequate perfusion to the tissues (Alexander *et al.*, 2007). The sympathetic nervous system's response is to increase the heart rate and induce vasoconstriction. This causes unwanted stress on the heart, which results in further damage to the cardiac muscle, leading to poor cardiac output and hypotension, and it becomes a vicious cycle of cardiogenic shock (Figure 5.9). Poor cardiac output reduces blood flow to essential body organs, thus affecting their functions. The sympathetic stimulation also causes decreased renal blood flow, which could lead to acute renal failure.

As the perfusion to the tissues is reduced, the peripheral cells utilise anaerobic metabolism to produce energy. Anaerobic metabolism is the process in which cells use carbohydrates to produce

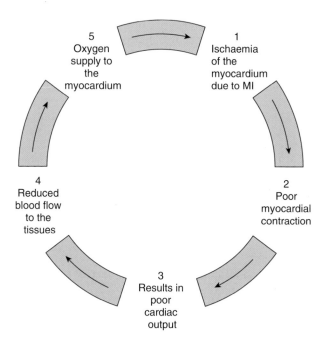

Figure 5.9 Vicious cycle of cardiogenic shock.

energy in the absence of oxygen. The effect of this energy production is to keep the cells functioning; however, the production of lactic acid leads to metabolic acidosis, which in turn depresses cardiac function.

Signs and symptoms

Signs and symptoms of cardiogenic shock include the following:

- pulmonary oedema
- severe hypotension
- oliguria/anuria
- pale and cold skin
- raised jugular venous pressure
- chest pain
- nausea and vomiting
- dyspnoea
- profuse sweating
- confusion/disorientation.

Care and management

Patients in cardiogenic shock will require precise and immediate care and management; if the condition is not treated immediately, it could lead to severe complications and the death of the patient. The priority in the management of cardiogenic shock is to prevent further damage to the myocardium.

- Maintaining a clear airway and monitoring respiration is important in patients with cardiogenic shock. Carers should observe the patient for signs of restlessness, breathlessness, dyspnoea and confusion. Oxygen must be administered as prescribed either by nasal cannulae or a Ventimask.
- Patients in cardiogenic shock and their relatives are very anxious and frightened. They will need support and reassurance from healthcare professionals.
- Vital signs must be monitored hourly and they include temperature, heart rate, blood pressure and respiratory rate. Any changes in the vital signs must be reported immediately to allow prompt action to be taken.
- Carers must observe and report any side effects of the drugs administered.

Pharmacological interventions

Some of the medications include:

- analgesia for pain relief
- antihypertensive drugs to treat hypertension and decrease effort on the heart
- diuretics to decrease fluid load.

Angina

Angina is chest pain that occurs when the heart muscle does not receive enough oxygenated blood. It is also described as a crushing pain in the chest. The term is derived from a Latin word meaning to choke. The pain can radiate through to the back and shoulder, or down one or both arms, or into the neck and jaw. However, not all patients present with such extensive pain.

Investigations

These include:

- physical examination
- medical history
- ECG
- full blood analysis
- stress test.

Pathophysiology

Angina pain closely resembles the signs and symptoms of MI; thus it is vital that carers are able to differentiate the two conditions, as the treatment differs in both cases. If a patient has angina pain, this is usually relieved by vasodilators, e.g. GTN, but the angina pain is rarely fatal.

Angina results from a blockage in the coronary arteries, which reduces blood supply to the affected part of the heart muscle (Figure 5.10). At rest the blood supply may be sufficient to provide nutrients and oxygen to the heart muscle; however, during activity, e.g. walking or running, the heart rate increases which puts more effort on the heart. During exertion, if the blood flow to the heart muscle is inadequate, the oxygen supply is also diminished, leading to severe

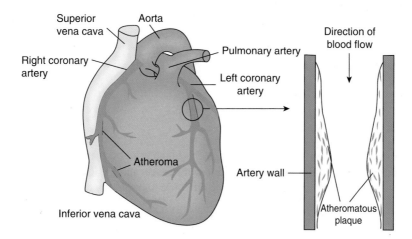

Figure 5.10   Blockage of the coronary arteries.

pain. The patient may present with pallor, dyspnoea, cyanosis, diaphoresis and tachycardia (Adams *et al.*, 2008).

Types of angina

There are three types of angina:

- stable angina
- unstable angina
- variant angina.

Stable angina is the most common type and it occurs when there is a greater demand on the heart than usual. It is estimated that over 1.2 million people in the UK suffer from angina. Stable angina is mainly caused by myocardial ischaemia. The pain usually lasts about 3–5 minutes. If the blood flow is restored by immediate treatment, no permanent damage results (McCance *et al.*, 2010).

Unstable angina (also known as crescendo angina) is characterised by a change in frequency, intensity and duration of pain. It is more serious than stable angina and is unpredictable. It can also occur when the person is at rest and is not relieved by rest or medication. Patients who develop unstable angina are at risk of having an MI (Hogan and Hill, 2004).

Variant angina is a rare form of angina. It is thought to occur as a result of coronary artery vasospasm resulting in diminished blood flow. Variant angina is very painful and occurs from midnight to early morning. It usually occurs at rest and the same time each day (Hogan and Hill, 2004).

Signs and symptoms

- crushing pain in the chest
- pain radiates to arms, jaw, neck and back
- shortness of breath on exercise
- sweating
- light headedness
- hypotension
- irregular pulse
- indigestion

Care and management

Healthcare professionals play a crucial role in the management of patients with angina. An accurate assessment of the patient must be carried out to ascertain the location, duration and intensity of the pain. Risk factors must be identified to provide high-quality care. The care will include:

- controlling pain
- reducing anxiety
- advising the patient on the possible risks and preventative measures
- providing health promotion where appropriate.

Non-pharmacological interventions

- Advise the patient to eat a healthy diet and avoid saturated fat. This will help lower cholesterol as high cholesterol could lead to vascular complications.
- Encourage the patient to take up leisure pursuits such as walking and swimming as physical activity aids circulation and improves cardiac function unless contraindicated.
- Patients who are overweight should be encouraged to lose weight through individual programmed activity unless contraindicated.
- Advice on the consumption of excessive alcohol and smoking should be offered as these are risk factors associated with cardiac problems.
- Patients should be advised to have their blood pressure monitored regularly by the practice nurse.

Pharmacological interventions

The following medications could be prescribed for angina; it is the nurse's responsibility in the safe administration of these medicines to recognise and advise patients on the side effects of these drugs (Nursing and Midwifery Council, 2008).

- GTN is administered as tablets (sublingual), IV, patches and spray. It is a quick-acting drug that dilates blood vessels and improves blood flow.
- A statin such as simvastatin may be prescribed to lower blood cholesterol (Scottish Intercollegiate Guidelines Network, 2007).
- Aspirin may be prescribed to reduce platelet aggregation (sticking together).
- Beta-blocker drugs may be prescribed to decrease heart rate and to reduce the workload of the heart (Scottish Intercollegiate Guidelines Network, 2007).

Other treatments such as bypass surgery and balloon angioplasty may be performed if the medications are ineffective in controlling the angina or if the condition gets progressively worse.

Conclusion

The overall aim of this chapter was to provide the reader with insight into some problems related to the heart. In order to help patients with cardiac problems, healthcare professionals need an in-depth knowledge of the normal anatomy and physiology of the heart to allow them to recognise the related dysfunctions and to provide the appropriate care. There are numerous dysfunctions associated with the heart and it is not the remit of this chapter to address all of these dysfunctions. Some of the common conditions were discussed with their associated care and management. Healthcare professionals are often in the forefront in delivering high-quality care for patients with cardiac problems, and it is their duty to ensure that they have a sound knowledge base and are confident in delivering safe and effective individualised care. Healthcare professionals care for patients with cardiac problems in both hospital and community settings. Healthcare professionals need to recognise various signs and symptoms quickly and take immediate action to prevent any further complications arising from the illness. Ongoing assessment and evaluation of interventions are important in order to respond to the changing needs of the patient, which may have implications for patient outcomes.

Test your knowledge

- How does the heart rate affect the cardiac output?

- Explain the differences between ischaemia and infarction.

- Explain how the backward effect causes pulmonary oedema.

- Define cardiogenic shock and list the possible causes.

- What advice would you give a patient with congestive heart failure?

Activities

Here are some activities and exercises to help test your learning. For the answers to these exercises, as well as further self-testing activities, visit our website at www.wiley.com/go/fundamentalsofappliedpathophysiology

Fill in the blanks

The heart has a mass of between 250 and 350 g and is about the size of a _____. It is located _____ to the vertebral column and _____ to the _____. It is enclosed in a double-walled sac called the _____. The superficial part of this sac is called the _____ pericardium. This sac _____ the heart, anchors its surrounding struc-tures, and prevents overfilling of the heart with blood.

   The outer wall of the heart is composed of three _____. The outer layer is called the _____ pericardium since it is also the inner wall of the pericardium. The middle layer is called the _____ and is composed of muscle which _____. The inner layer is called the _____ and is in contact with the _____ that the heart pumps. Also, it merges with the _____ of blood vessels and covers _____.

Choose from:
Layers; Sternum; Anterior; Endocardium; Heart valves; Pericardium; Protects; Fist; Poste-rior; Endothelium; Blood; Contracts; Myocardium; Fibrous; Visceral

Label the diagram

Using the list of words supplied, label the diagram.

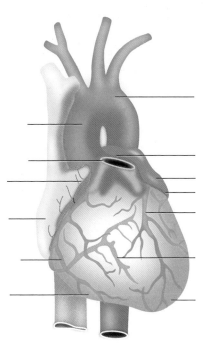

Left ventricle; Arch of aorta; Left coronary; Left atria; Circumflex branch; Anterior interventricular branch; Posterior interventricular branch; Ascending aorta; Pulmonary trunk; Right coronary; Right atrium; Marginal branch; Right ventricle

Word search

A	M	U	R	D	Y	S	P	N	O	E	A	Y	E	M	R	I
E	U	I	E	E	E	I	I	M	A	D	T	P	O	R	M	D
B	I	C	U	S	P	I	D	P	A	R	H	P	N	E	E	N
O	D	T	T	I	M	M	E	U	R	T	E	R	E	M	D	S
Y	R	A	N	O	M	L	U	P	P	S	R	E	R	R	I	T
R	A	L	U	C	I	R	T	N	E	V	O	I	R	T	A	T
D	C	R	R	T	M	M	M	L	R	N	S	P	A	I	S	S
A	O	A	T	O	R	T	C	E	A	A	C	E	P	I	T	M
S	Y	E	E	E	D	I	K	S	E	T	L	C	P	N	I	C
A	M	U	I	D	R	A	C	O	D	N	E	L	I	T	N	U
K	C	I	R	T	M	I	S	U	P	R	R	I	U	A	U	R
I	S	K	N	E	U	N	E	C	S	B	O	I	R	D	M	M
R	P	E	C	U	I	A	S	S	O	P	S	U	A	A	E	U
M	V	A	P	E	R	I	C	A	R	D	I	U	M	P	P	M
S	P	T	V	N	T	E	E	L	I	M	S	D	D	R	R	S
I	E	V	B	A	O	T	U	T	A	P	I	V	T	Y	R	M
U	S	I	O	D	D	M	I	Y	I	L	R	R	R	I	A	C

Arteries	Bicuspid	Medulla
Atherosclerosis	Dyspenoea	Pacemaker
Veins	Endocardium	Pulmonary
Ventricles	Myocardium	Septum
Atria	Pericardium	Tricuspid
Atrioventricular	Mediastinum	Parietal

Further resources

Online nutritional information and facts

http://www.second-opinions.co.uk/index.html
This website discusses dietary and medical misinformation on congestive heart failure. It includes nutritional information about the various government recommendations. It also lists a wide range of over 70 diseases from the serious such as cancer, to the less serious such as acne, all of which are caused or exacerbated by a so-called 'healthy' diet and it looks at other scams and misinformation.

NHS Choices

http://www.nhs.uk/conditions/heart-failure/Pages/Introduction.aspx
Students will find this NHS website useful. This site discusses heart failure, symptoms, causes, diagnosis, treatment and prevention.

BUPA

http://www.bupa.co.uk/individuals/health-information/directory/h/heartfailure
This is a useful website for students to browse for health-related topics. Like the NHS Choice site, it gives a quick overview of health-related topics.

National Institute for Health and Clinical Excellence (NICE)

http://www.nice.org.uk/CG005
Here students should find NICE guidelines related to healthcare issues, such as heart failure, stroke and care in the community.

Department of Health – Policy, guidance and publications for NHS and social care professionals

http://www.dh.gov.uk/en/index.htm
This is a useful website for students and healthcare professionals to browse. Policy, guidance and publications for NHS and social care professionals can be found on this website.

Glossary of terms

Aetiology:	the cause of a disease.
Alveolar sac:	a small sac structure in the lungs where gas exchange takes place.
Anaerobic metabolism:	metabolism by the body cells in the absence of oxygen.
Antidiuretic hormone:	a protein hormone produced in the hypothalamus and stored in the posterior pituitary gland; it aids reabsorption of water by the kidneys.
Artery:	a blood vessel that carries blood away from the heart.
Ascites:	accumulation of fluid in the peritoneal cavity.
Atherosclerosis:	a condition where cholesterol and lipid deposits accumulate on the inner layer of the medium and large blood vessels, leading to narrowing of these vessels.
Athromatous plaque:	a collection of lipids and cholesterol that accumulates in large- and medium-sized vessels.
Atria:	the upper chambers of the heart.
Atrioventricular valve:	a heart valve made up of membranous flaps that allow blood to flow in one direction only; also known as the bicuspid valve.
Bicuspid valve:	as its name suggests it contains two cusps; also known as the atrioventricular valve.
Bronchospasm:	constriction of the walls of the bronchi.
Collagen:	a protein that is the main organic component of connective tissues.

Dyspnoea:	shortness of breath; laboured breathing.
Endocardium:	the endothelial membrane that lines the inner surface of the heart.
Inferior vena cava:	the large vein that returns oxygen-depleted blood from all parts of the body below the diaphragm to the right atrium.
Interstitial space:	the space between the cells.
Intracellular space:	the space found within the cell.
Lactic acid:	the product of anaerobic metabolism, especially in the muscle.
Mediastinum:	a subdivision of the thoracic cavity.
Medulla oblongata:	the lowest portion of the brain; concerned with the control of internal organs.
Mitral valve:	the left atrioventricular valve.
Molecule:	a particle containing two or more atoms joined together by chemical bonds.
Myocardial infarction:	death of an area of heart muscle due to an interruption of the blood supply to the affected area.
Myocardium:	the middle layer of the heart.
Oliguria:	deficient secretion of urine; less than 30 mL per hour.
Orthopnoea:	difficulty in breathing unless in an upright position.
Pacemaker:	the sinoatrial node.
Parasympathetic nerve:	a division of the autonomic nervous system.
Parietal:	pertaining to the walls of a cavity.
Pericardium:	a double-layered sac that encloses the heart.
Pulmonary artery:	the vessel that takes oxygen-depleted blood from the right ventricle to the lungs.
Pulmonary circulation:	the flow of blood from the right ventricle to the lungs.
Pulmonary oedema:	the abnormal collection of fluid in the tissue space and the alveolar sac.
Pulmonary vein:	the vessel that returns oxygenated blood from the lungs to the left atrium.
Semilunar valve:	a valve that prevents the backflow of blood to the ventricles after contraction.
Septum:	a wall dividing the two cavities.
Sinoatrial node:	also known as the pacemaker of the heart.
Superior vena cava:	the large vein that returns oxygen-depleted blood superior to the diaphragm to the right atrium.
Sympathetic nerve:	a division of the autonomic nervous system.

Systemic circulation:	the flow of blood from the left ventricle to all parts of the body.
Tissue perfusion:	blood flow through the body tissues and organs.
Tricuspid valve:	the right atrioventricular valve.
Vasoconstriction:	a decrease in the diameter of a blood vessel due to the relaxation of smooth muscle in the vessel wall; may occur as a result of hormones or after stimulation of the vasomotor centre leading to increased peripheral resistance.
Ventricle:	the two larger lower cavities of the heart.

References

Adams, M.P., Holland, L.N. and Bostwick, P.M. (2008). *Pharmacology for Nurses: A Pathophysiologic Approach*, 2nd edn. New Jersey: Pearson Prentice Hall.

Alexander, M.F., Fawcett, J.N. and Runciman, P.J. (eds.) (2007). *Nursing Practice: Hospital and Home: The Adult*, 3rd edn. Edinburgh: Churchill Livingstone.

Bullock, B.A. and Henze, R.L. (2010). *Focus on Pathophysiology*. Philadelphia: Lippincott.

Elton, J. (2003). *Care Deliver: The Needs of the Mature Adult*. London: Arnold.

Hogan, M.A. and Hill, K. (2004). *Pathophysiology – Reviews and Rationales*. New Jersey: Prentice Hall.

Jenkins, G.W. and Tortora, G.J. (2013). *Anatomy and Physiology*. New Jersey: John Wiley & Sons.

Kozier, B., Erb, G., Berman, A., Snyder, S.J., Lake, R. and Harvey, S. (2008). *Fundamentals of Nursing: Concepts, Process and Practice*. Harlow: Pearson Education Ltd.

LeMone, P., Burke, K. and Bauldoff, G. (2011). *Medical – Surgical Nursing; Critical Thinking in Client Care*, 4rd edn. New Jersey: Pearson.

Marieb, E.N. and Hoehn, K. (2010). *Human Anatomy and Physiology*, 8th edn. San Francisco: Pearson Benjamin Cummings.

McCance, K.L., Huether, S.E., Brashers, V.L. and Rote, N.S. (2010). *Pathophysiology: The Biologic Basis for Disease in Adults and Children*, 6th edn. St. Louis: Mosby.

McSweeney, J.C., Marisue, C., O'Sullivan, P., Elberson, K., Moser, D.K. and Garvin, B.J. (2003). Women's early warning symptoms of acute myocardial infarction. *Circulation*. 108: 2619–2623.

National Institute for Health and Clinical Excellence (2010). *Management of Chronic Heart Failure in Adults in Primary and Secondary Care*. National Clinical Guidelines for diagnosis and management in primary and secondary care. London: NICE.

Nowak, J. and Handford, A.G. (2010). *Essentials of Pathophysiology: Concepts and Applications for Health Care Professionals*, 3rd edn. Boston: McGraw-Hill.

Nursing and Midwifery Council (2008). *Standards for Medicines Management*. London: NMC.

Nursing and Midwifery Council (2009). *Record Keeping: Guidance for Nurses and Midwives*. London: Nursing and Midwifery Council.

Porth, C.M. (2010). *Pathophysiology: Concepts of Altered Health States*, 8th edn. Philadelphia: Lippincott Williams & Wilkins.

Scottish Intercollegiate Guidelines Network (SIGN) (2007). *Management of Stable Angina*. Edinburgh: Scottish Intercollegiate Guidelines Network.

Tortora, G.J. and Derrickson, B. (2011). *Principles of Anatomy and Physiology*, 12th edn. New Jersey: John Wiley & Sons.

Waugh, A. and Grant, A. (2010). *Ross and Wilson: Anatomy and Physiology in Health and Illness*, 11th edn. Edinburgh: Churchill Livingstone.

6

The vascular system and associated disorders

Muralitharan Nair

Senior Lecturer, Department of Adult Nursing and Primary Care, School of Health and Social Work, University of Hertfordshire, Hatfield, Hertfordshire, UK

Contents

Fundamentals of Applied Pathophysiology: An Essential Guide for Nursing and Healthcare Students, Second Edition. Edited by Muralitharan Nair and Ian Peate.

Key words

- Arteries
- Arterioles
- Tunica media
- Vasodilatation
- Veins
- Venules
- Tunica intima
- Vasoconstriction
- Capillaries
- Tunica externa
- Aorta

Test your prior knowledge

- List three differences between arteries and veins.
- Can you name the arteries that transport oxygen-depleted blood and the veins that transport oxygen-rich blood?
- Which of arteries and veins has a greater volume of blood?
- List the physiological factors that affect blood pressure.
- Discuss the common disorders of the vascular system.

Learning outcomes

On completion of this section the reader will be able to:

- Describe the structures of the arteries, veins and capillaries.
- List some of the differences between an artery and a vein.
- Describe how venous valves function?
- Describe the factors controlling blood vessel diameter.
- Explain the microcirculation of the blood.

Don't forget to visit to the companion website for this book (www.wiley.com/ go/fundamentalsofappliedpathophsiology) where you can find self-assessment tests to check your progress, as well as lots of activities to practise your learning.

Introduction

Although the heart is the principle organ that pumps blood to the whole body, it is the blood vessels that transport blood throughout the system (Figure 6.1). As the blood flows through the arterial system, it transports nutrients and other substances essential for cellular metabolism and for homeostatic regulation. The waste products of metabolism are transported by the venous system for removal by the kidneys, lungs and skin. This chapter discusses the structure and functions of the blood vessels, factors affecting blood pressure, and vascular disorders and their related care. Where appropriate, the arteries and veins are collectively called blood vessels.

Overview of blood vessels

In the human body there are several kinds of blood vessels. Arteries and arterioles are the vessels that convey blood away from the heart. They transport oxygen-rich (oxygenated) blood except the pulmonary artery which carries oxygen-depleted blood. Veins and venules carry blood towards the heart and transport oxygen-depleted (deoxygenated) blood, except the pulmonary veins which carry oxygenated blood. Capillaries are the minute blood vessels where arteries terminate and veins begin. They form a delicate network of vessels and are in close proximity to most parts of the body tissues. Blood vessels can dilate, constrict, pulsate and form a closed delivery system for the blood which begins and ends at the heart.

Structure of the blood vessels

Blood vessels, with the exception of the capillaries, are composed of three distinct layers (Marieb and Hoehn, 2010) and a central lumen through which blood flows (Figure 6.2). The outer layer is called the tunica externa, formally known as the tunica adventitia. It is largely composed of collagen fibres that protect and support the blood vessels, and secure them to the surrounding tissues. The tunica externa is supplied with sympathetic nerve fibres and lymphatic vessels; the larger veins are also supplied with elastic fibres (Jenkins and Tortora, 2013). The tunica media is the middle layer and it contains smooth muscles and elastic tissue. The sympathetic nervous system (SNS) also innervates the smooth muscle layer and controls the diameter of the blood vessel (Marieb, 2011). As the blood vessels constrict or dilate the blood pressure increases or decreases, respectively. The inner layer is called the tunica interna and it is lined with endothelium. This lining makes the inner surface smooth, thus minimising friction as the blood flows through the vessel.

Although the role of the blood vessels is to transport blood, the tunica externa of the large blood vessels receives its blood supply via a network of blood vessels called the vasa vasorum. It provides nutrients to this part of the blood vessel. Vessels with thin walls receive oxygen and nutrients by diffusion from the blood passing through the lumen.

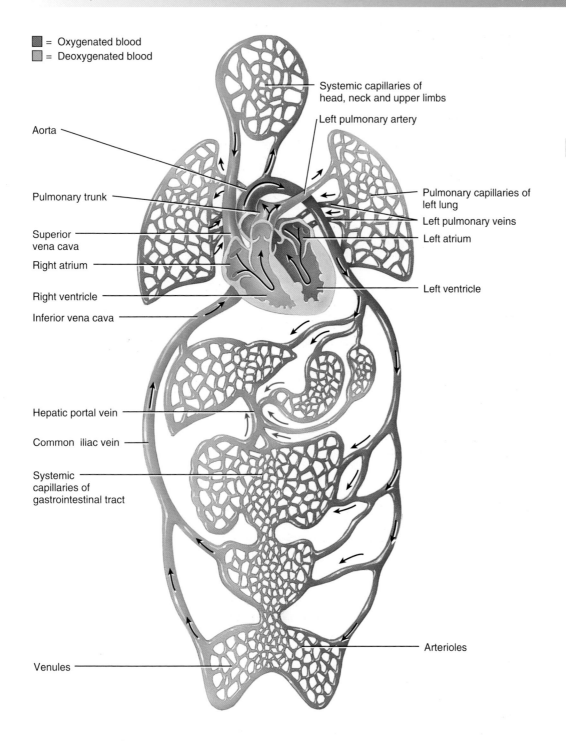

Figure 6.1   Blood flow.

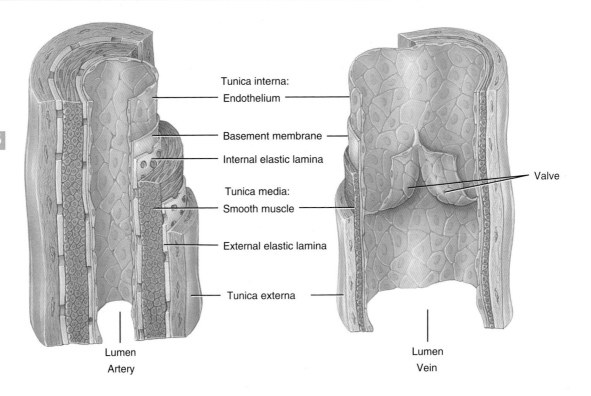

Tunica interna:
Endothelium

Basement membrane

Internal elastic lamina

Tunica media:
Smooth muscle

External elastic lamina

Tunica externa

Valve

Lumen
Artery

Lumen
Vein

Figure 6.2   Structures of an artery and a vein.

Arteries

Arteries can be subdivided into three groups – elastic arteries, muscular arteries and arterioles. Elastic arteries are thick-walled vessels found near the heart of which the aorta is the main artery. These vessels contain a high proportion of elastic fibres in the tunica media. Their larger lumen provides low resistance to blood flow, thus propelling blood onward (Figure 6.3). This ensures that the blood is moving forward even though the left ventricle is relaxed. As these arteries conduct blood from the left ventricle to the small arteries, they are sometimes referred to as conducting arteries.

From the elastic arteries the blood flows into the medium-sized arteries, called the muscular arteries. They contain more smooth muscles and fewer elastic fibres; therefore, they are capable of greater vasoconstriction and vasodilatation. Muscular arteries are also called distributing arteries because they distribute blood to specific organs and parts of the body. They include axillary, brachial, radial, splenic, femoral, popliteal and tibial arteries.

The muscular arteries then divide into smaller arteries called the arterioles and they play an important role in determining the amount of blood flowing into organs and tissues. Arterioles will branch into smaller arteries and direct the flow of blood into the capillaries (Figure 6.4). Larger arterioles have all the three layers, but the tunica media mainly consists of smooth muscle with a few elastic fibres, whilst the arterioles near the capillary end are composed of endothelial cells

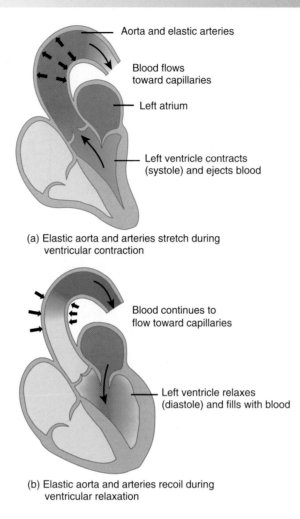

Aorta and elastic arteries

Blood flows
toward capillaries

Left atrium

Left ventricle contracts
(systole) and ejects blood

(a) Elastic aorta and arteries stretch during
ventricular contraction

Blood continues to
flow toward capillaries

Left ventricle relaxes
(diastole) and fills with blood

(b) Elastic aorta and arteries recoil during
ventricular relaxation

Figure 6.3   Elastic recoil of the aorta.

and an incomplete layer of smooth muscle (Jenkins and Tortora, 2013). Arterioles regulate the blood flow into the capillaries by altering the diameter of the capillaries. When they constrict, blood flow is diverted from the organs or tissue they supply. On the other hand, blood flow increases dramatically when the arterioles dilate.

Capillaries

Capillaries are the smallest network of blood vessels with walls mostly one-cell thick and they connect the arteriole to the venule (see Figure 6.1). The thin walls of the capillaries allow water, nutrients, gases and waste products of metabolism to move in and out of the blood and to nearby cells (Jenkins and Tortora, 2013). Capillaries are composed of a single layer of tunica intima and

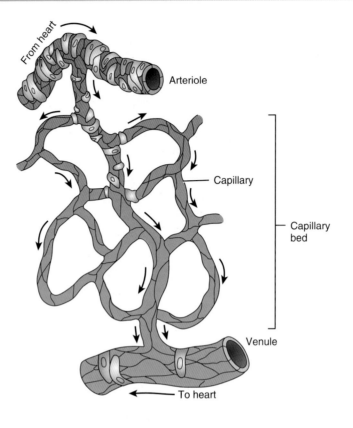

Figure 6.4   Capillaries.

they are found throughout the body except the epidermis of the skin and the cornea of the eye. Capillaries merge to form venules (see Figure 6.4).

Venules

Blood flows from the capillaries to the venules (see Figure 6.4). The smallest venules are mainly composed of endothelium and a few fibroblast cells. The venules are extremely porous and therefore will allow substance such as water, solutes and white blood cells to move in and out of the vessel into the extracellular fluid.

Veins

Venules unite to form veins and they contain the same three layers as the arteries. The walls of the veins, compared to the arteries, are thinner and contain less elastic and collagenous tissue and smooth muscle. The lumen of the veins is larger compared to the lumen of the arteries. Veins become larger and less branched as they move away from the capillaries and toward the heart. Some veins, most commonly those in the lower extremities, contain paired semilunar bicuspid

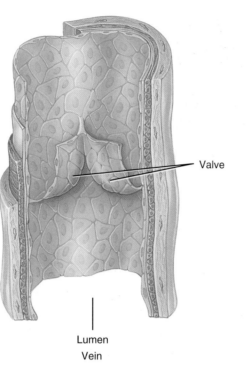

Valve

Lumen

Vein

Figure 6.5   Bicuspid valves of a vein.

valves (Figure 6.5) that allow blood flow towards the heart. Like arteries, veins receive their nour-ishment from tiny blood vessels called vasa vasorum (McCance *et al.*, 2010).

Blood pressure

Blood pressure (BP) refers to the force exerted by the circulating blood on the walls of the blood vessel. As the blood moves through the arteries, arterioles, capillaries, venules and veins, the blood pressure drops and thus the term 'blood pressure' refers to arterial blood pressure and it is usually measured in the larger arteries. BP fluctuates during the day and it depends on the state of health of the individual. The blood pressure is low when the person is sleeping at night and increases as the person wakes in the morning. There are three main factors that regulate blood pressure:

- neuronal regulation
- hormonal regulation
- autoregulation of blood pressure.

The neuronal regulation of BP is via a negative feedback system, which includes baroreceptors and chemoreceptors. The baroreceptors are located in the carotid sinus and the aortic arch, and they are sensitive to arterial blood pressure changes. The chemoreceptors are located in the aortic and carotid bodies. These bodies detect changes in oxygen, carbon dioxide and hydrogen ion concentrations. There are several hormones involved in the regulation of BP and they include the renin–angiotensin system, epinephrine (adrenaline) and norepinephrine (noradrenaline), antidiuretic hormone and atrial natriuretic peptide.

Factors that can affect blood pressure

Several factors affect blood pressure and they include:

- cardiac output
- circulating volume
- peripheral resistance
- blood viscosity
- hydrostatic pressure.

Other factors that can affect BP include age, gender, stress, hormones and drugs.

Diseases of the blood vessels

On completion of this section the reader will be able to:

- List some of the common diseases of the blood vessels and the risk factors associated with these diseases.
- Describe the pathophysiological responses associated with specific vascular health problems.
- List the possible investigations.
- Outline the care and management and interventions related to the disorders described.

Case study

Mrs Carly Symmons is a 66-year-old widow who lives in a first-floor flat. She used to work in the local supermarket as a cashier but is now retired. She suffers from type 2 diabetes, which is controlled by diet and tablets. She is overweight and smokes approximately 30 cigarettes per day but does not drink any alcohol.

Mrs Symmons has a small ulcer in her left ankle, which she cared for herself, but lately has noticed that the ulcer is weeping and she had pains in her left leg. Mrs Symmons made an appointment to see her GP. Her GP, after examining her foot, decided to refer her to the vascular surgeon at the local hospital.

Take some time to reflect on this case and then consider the following.

1. Discuss the possible causes of Mrs Symmons' leg ulcer.
2. Outline the assessments that you will carry out in order to plan her care.
3. Discuss the possible treatment of her leg ulcer.
4. Discuss the health education/promotion advice that you will give Mrs Symmons with before she is discharged from hospital.

Atherosclerosis/arteriosclerosis

Arteriosclerosis is the term describing arterial disorders in which degenerative changes result in decreased blood flow. Atherosclerosis is the most common form of arteriosclerosis where there is thickening and hardening of the vessel walls due to lipid accumulation. This condition is found mainly in the large- and medium-sized arteries, such as the aorta and its branches, the coronary arteries and the arteries that supply the brain, whereas arteriosclerosis mainly affects arterioles (Nowak and Handford, 2010).

Aetiology

The cause of atherosclerosis is not known, but certain risk factors have been identified:

- hypertension
- cigarette smoking (nicotine has a vasoconstricting effect)
- high lipid levels in the blood
- familial history
- obesity
- diabetes mellitus (high serum glucose levels cause vascular damage)
- lifestyle
- alcohol
- gender (men are at a higher risk than women).

Investigations

The following investigations may be done to confirm diagnosis:

- full blood chemistry
- Doppler ultrasound
- electrocardiogram
- arteriogram.

Pathophysiology of atherosclerosis

Atherosclerosis is a form of arteriosclerosis where the walls of the arteries are hard, thick and narrow as a result of lipid accumulation within the arterial walls. Lipids (low-density lipoproteins [LDL]) are deposited on the tunica intima of the damaged blood vessel where oxidation of LDL takes place. The oxidised LDL then enters the tunica intima of the arterial wall (Jowett and Thompson, 2007) where they are ingested by macrophages. The lipid-filled macrophages then become foam cells.

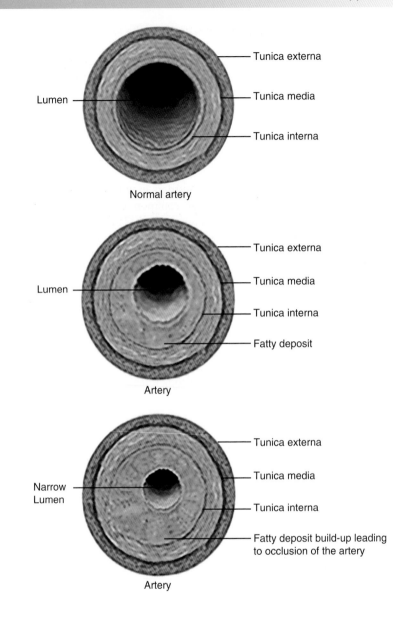

Normal artery

Tunica externa

Lumen

Tunica media

Tunica interna

Tunica externa

Lumen

Tunica media

Tunica interna

Fatty deposit

Artery

Tunica externa

Narrow Lumen

Tunica media

Tunica interna

Fatty deposit build-up leading to occlusion of the artery

Artery

Figure 6.6   Atheroma build-up in an artery.

Once the foam cells accumulate in significant numbers, they form a lesion called a fatty streak, which over time causes a bulge in the lumen of the blood vessel and this restricts blood flow. Affected blood vessels become hard, lose their elasticity, restrict blood flow and eventually occlude the artery (Figure 6.6). Greater blood pressure is needed to push the blood through these narrow blood vessels, which leads to hypertension. Although atherosclerosis can affect any organ or tissue, the arteries supplying the heart, brain, small intestines, kidneys and lower extremities are mostly affected. Table 6.1 lists the effects at the different affected sites.

Table 6.1   Effects of atherosclerosis on different sites.

Site	Effects
Abdominal aorta	Gangrene of toes and feet
	Aneurysms
Aorto-iliac and femoral arteries	Intermittent claudication
	Gangrene of toes and feet
	Aneurysms of iliac arteries
Coronary arteries	Myocardial infarction
	Angina pectoris
Carotid and vertebral arteries	Cerebrovascular accident
	Transient ischaemic attack
Renal arteries	Hypertension, renal ischaemia
Mesenteric arteries	Intestinal ischaemia

Adapted from Bullock and Henze (2010).

Signs and symptoms of atherosclerosis

- diminished or absent pulses
- skin is pallor or cyanosed
- pain
- muscle weakness

Care and management

A full care history is essential in order to provide high-quality care for patients with atherosclerosis. The assessment must include the identification of risk factors and symptoms of any cardiovascular disease. The care and management includes:

- Health promotion to prevent the disease must include advice on a healthy diet and regulating the lipid levels within normal range. Regular physical examination by a person's GP in order to monitor their blood pressure and cholesterol levels should be encouraged.
- Advice on the cessation of smoking and alcohol consumption should be offered as these are identified risk factors in atherosclerosis.
- Patients should be advised to lose weight if obesity is a problem (Caterson, 2005).
- Encourage the patient to undertake programmed exercise under the supervision of healthcare professionals. This will help in lowering their weight and cholesterol level, and in reducing their blood pressure and stress.

Pharmacological interventions for atherosclerosis

The aim of medications in the treatment of atherosclerosis is to restore blood flow and prevent the disease. The medications include:

- antihypertensives such as beta-blockers
- anticoagulant therapy with heparin
- lipid-lowering drugs such as simvastatin
- antiplatelet drugs.

In some patients, surgical procedures, such as balloon angioplasty, may be indicated to improve the blood flow through the vessel.

Hypertension

Hypertension refers to sustained elevation in systemic arterial blood pressure (McCance *et al.*, 2010). The elevation may be in either systolic or diastolic pressure, or in both. A normal upper limit for an adult is 130–139/85–89 mmHg (Alexander *et al.*, 2007) and any readings consistently above this are considered as hypertension. There are many classifications of hypertension, some of which are based on severity, e.g. mild or moderate. Types of hypertension include:

- Primary or essential hypertension.
- Secondary hypertension where there is an underlying cause, such as renal diseases or tumour of the adrenal medulla.
- Malignant hypertension occurs in the younger age groups with renal and collagen diseases.
- Isolated systolic hypertension mainly occurs when a combination of factors is seen in the elderly, and is due to increases in cardiac output, increased peripheral resistance and renal vascular resistance. Other possible causes include Paget's disease of the bone and beriberi (McCance *et al.*, 2010).

Note

Blood pressure = cardiac output × peripheral vascular resistance
(BP = CO × PVR)

Aetiology

Although the cause or causes of primary hypertension is unknown, several risk factors have been identified for its development:

- obesity
- stress
- cigarette smoking and alcohol consumption
- excessive intake of sodium causing fluid retention
- family history.

Secondary hypertension results from underlying causes such as:

- renal diseases
- Cushing's syndrome
- hypo/hyperthyroidism
- oral contraceptives
- excessive alcohol consumption
- coarctation (narrowing) of the aorta.

Investigations

These include:

- full blood chemistry
- physical examination
- electrocardiogram
- assessment of risk factors.

Common presenting symptoms

Many patients are unaware that they have hypertension and go untreated. They ignore symptoms such as headache, dizziness, nosebleed and fatigue. It is frequently identified through blood pressure screening or as a result of other diseases. Some patients have reported blurred vision and tinnitus, but usually when symptoms of hypertension do occur, the disease is at an advanced stage (Bullock and Henze, 2010).

Pathophysiology

Primary hypertension

Primary hypertension results from a combination of genetic and environmental factors which have an effect on renal and vascular functions; it accounts for 95% of cases. One of the possible causes of primary hypertension is a deficiency in the kidney's ability to excrete sodium, which increases extracellular fluid volume and cardiac output, resulting in an increase in blood flow to the tissues. The increased blood flow to the tissues results in arteriolar constriction and an increase in peripheral vascular resistance (PVR) and blood pressure (Nowak and Handford, 2010).

Secondary hypertension

Secondary hypertension accounts for 5% of cases and is caused by diseases of the organs resulting in a raised PVR and increased cardiac output. In most cases, the focus is on kidney diseases or excessive levels of hormones such as aldosterone and cortisol. These hormones stimulate the retention of sodium and water, resulting in increased blood volume and blood pressure. Once the underlying cause is treated, such as with the removal of the diseased organ, the blood pressure returns to normal.

Malignant hypertension

This is a rapidly progressive hypertension where the diastolic pressure is in excess of 120 mmHg (Waugh and Grant, 2010), which can result in encephalopathy, cerebral oedema and loss of consciousness. Malignant hypertension does not indicate that there is cellular injury, but because it is life-threatening, it is considered as an emergency. If untreated, cerebral oedema and cerebral dysfunction occur, leading to death of the individual. Malignant hypertension can cause a variety of complications, e.g. papilloedema, cardiac failure, cerebrovascular accident and retinopathy.

Isolated systolic hypertension

This is caused by an increase in cardiac output or PVR and has a higher incidence in the elderly. The rigidity of the vessels is often caused by atherosclerosis. The ageing process leads to hardening of the arteries, increased PVR and decreased baroreceptor sensitivity. In isolated systolic hypertension, the systolic blood pressure is over 140 mmHg and the diastolic pressure is less than 90 mmHg (Hogan and Hill, 2004). It is recognised as an important risk factor for cerebrovascular accident and cardiac failure, and thus should be treated as a medical emergency.

Non-pharmacological interventions

- A single recording of raised blood pressure does not indicate that the patient is suffering from hypertension. At least three recordings of raised blood pressure at different intervals are required to confirm hypertension. Some doctors will monitor patient's blood pressure using a 24-hour ambulatory monitoring device. This measurement is much more accurate than the blood pressure measurements done in the clinic.
- Advise the patient to restrict sodium intake as sodium promotes water retention, resulting in increased circulating volume and increased cardiac output, which lead to hypertension.
- Healthcare professionals need to advise the patient on the cessation of cigarette smoking and excessive alcohol consumption. Both are identified as risk factors for hypertension.
- In obese patients, weight reduction through exercise should be encouraged (BMI should be less than 25); this will lower cholesterol levels and help in the control of any underlying problems such as diabetes mellitus (National Institute for Health Clinical Excellence, 2010). Encourage patients to have their weight checked weekly.
- Dietary advice should be offered to the patient. A diet rich in fruit and vegetables and low in saturated fats can help in the reduction of blood pressure. Reduction of salt in cooking should be encouraged as excessive intake of salt promotes fluid retention, thus increasing circulating volume.
- Encourage patients to reduce their stress levels because relaxation aids in the reduction of blood pressure by decreasing the workload of the heart. Listening to music, gardening and going for walks have all been identified as helpful in the reduction of blood pressure.

Pharmacological interventions

In some patients, non-pharmacological interventions are sufficient in controlling their blood pressure while in others, combinations of both pharmacological and non-pharmacological methods are used in the treatment of hypertension. The medications include:

- Diuretics are prescribed to reduce fluid load, which leads to reduction in cardiac output, thus helping to reduce blood pressure.
- Medications, e.g. beta-blockers, calcium channel blockers and angiotensin-converting enzyme (ACE) inhibitors, are indicted for the treatment of hypertension (Jackson et al., 2005).

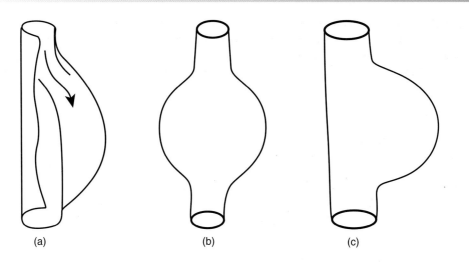

(a)   (b)   (c)

Figure 6.7   (a) A dissecting aneurysm; (b) a fusiform aneurysm; and (c) a saccular aneurysm.

Aneurysm

An aneurysm is a permanent dilatation of an artery or a chamber of the heart. Although it can occur in both arteries and veins, the aorta and the arteries at the base of the brain are the vessels most susceptible to aneurysms. It can occur in a localised part of the aorta or all along the vessel (Alexander *et al.*, 2007) because it is under constant pressure. The commonest cause of an aneurysm is atherosclerosis because the fatty deposits erode and weaken the vessel wall. Aneurysms can be classified according to their shape (Figures 6.7a–c) and they include:

- fusiform – involves the entire circumference of the vessel
- saccular – appears only on one part or side
- dissecting – a false aneurysm resulting from a tear in the tunica intima.

Aetiology

There are several causes and they include:

- Atherosclerosis – main cause of an aneurysm affecting the descending aorta.
- Infection – mainly due to syphilis affecting the ascending aorta.
- Hypertension – due to constant pressure, weakening of the vessel wall can occur in the elderly.
- Cystic medial degeneration – it mainly affects the thoracic aorta in a disorder called Marfan's syndrome. It affects the elastic fibres of the tunica media.

Investigations

These include:

- full blood chemistry
- angiography

- ultrasound
- chest X-ray.

Symptoms

Most aortic aneurysms are asymptomatic until they start to leak or rupture and the symptoms vary depending on the affected vessel. Symptoms may include:

- pain in the abdominal region or in the extremities due to compression of neighbouring organs
- dyspnoea (shortness of breath or difficulty in breathing) due to pressure on internal organs
- dysphagia (difficulty in swallowing)
- signs and symptoms of cerebrovascular accident occur if the cerebral arteries are affected.

Care and management

The main treatment for an aneurysm is surgery, and therefore it is vital that a full assessment of the patient is obtained. The surgery may include insertion of a graft (Figure 6.8). It is the healthcare professional's duty in the safe preparation of the patient for theatre to ensure all the relevant protocols of the individual hospital and the Nursing and Midwifery Council guidelines are adhered to. All care given should be documented in accordance with the Nursing and Midwifery Council guidelines (2009).

Postoperatively healthcare professionals should monitor the following:

- ABCDE – airway, breathing, circulation, disability and environment
- fluid and nutritional management
- elimination
- pain management
- wound management

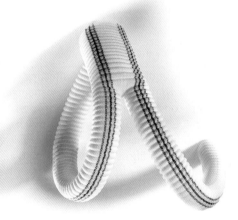

Figure 6.8   Dacron graft for an abdominal aortic aneurysm. Synthetic graft used for surgery. Reproduced with permission from Vascutek.

- detect early signs of postoperative complications of chest infection, deep vein thrombosis and wound infection
- communication
- documentation
- safe preparation of the patient for discharge.

Pharmacological interventions

The following medications may be prescribed for a patient with an aneurysm:

- antihypertensives
- anticoagulants
- antibiotics
- analgesics.

Case study

Mr Ah Peng Lee is a 55-year-old postman. He is married with two children. They live in a council house and his mother-in-law lives with them. Mr Lee smokes 40 cigarettes per day and drinks two cans of larger every day after work.

Lately his right leg has been aching so much that he has to stop during his delivery rounds to ease the pain and to catch his breath. Over a few weeks the pain has become more severe, so Mr Lee decided to see his GP to find out what is wrong with him and to get some pain killers. His GP examined Mr Lee and decided to refer him to the vascular surgeon at the local hospital.

Take some time to reflect on this case and then consider the following.

1. What is the possible diagnosis of Mr Lee? Explain your answer.
2. What questions will you ask Mr Lee that will assist diagnosis?
3. Can you explain, in physiological terms, why Mr Lee's aching leg was relieved by rest?
4. Mr Lee states that it is difficult for him to change his lifestyle. What role do you think health-care professionals can play in helping Mr Lee when he is discharged into the community?

Peripheral vascular disease

Peripheral vascular disease (PVD) is a condition where the blood flow is affected in both arteries and veins. The disorders include arterial occlusions due to arterial and venous insufficiency, varicose veins and Raynaud's disease.

Aetiology

The causes of PVD include:

- cardiovascular disease
- thrombi

- pulmonary disease
- prolonged standing.

Investigations

These include:

- Doppler ultrasound
- arteriogram/venogram
- full blood chemistry
- physical examination
- electrocardiogram.

Arterial insufficiency

Pathophysiology

If blood flows with reduced pressure, complications can result, such as formation of a thrombus which can occlude the flow of blood through that vessel. The lower limbs are most susceptible to arterial occlusion. The affected limbs are prone to arterial ulcers as a result of tissue hypoxia. A more severe blockage can lead to the development of gangrene, usually in the toe (Stubbling and Chesworth, 2010). Venous insufficiency may occur as the result of an obstruction in the veins by a thrombus or incompetent valves, which can lead to the formation of a venous ulcer as a result of poor circulation. There are distinct differences between arterial and venous insufficiency (Table 6.2).

Table 6.2   Comparison between an arterial and venous insufficiency.

	Arterial	Venous
Pain	Sudden severe pain, rest pain, intermittent claudication	Aching and cramp relieved by elevating the foot
Pulse	Diminished or absent	Present
Ulcer characteristics	Mainly in the toes, feet or other areas of the skin	Mainly over the inner or outer ankle
Skin characteristics	Shiny, cool or cold temperature; mild oedema if present	Thick and tough; skin normal colour; may have oedema, warm to touch
Complications	Gangrene	Poor healing
Blood flow	Doppler pressure readings lower below blockage	Normal pressure reading

Adapted from Hogan and Hill (2004).

Signs and symptoms

- intermittent claudication
- white, pale colour when legs are elevated
- leg ulcers (Table 6.2)
- absent pedal pulses
- numb and cold extremity
- thickened toenails.

Care and management

Pain control is paramount in patients with arterial insufficiency. If pain is caused by exercise, such as walking long distances, then the patient should be advised against it. However, light exercise that can be tolerated should be encouraged as it helps to improve circulation. Patients should be advised to keep themselves warm if they are affected by cold weather, but they should avoid the following:

- Tight fitting clothing as this restricts arterial blood flow.
- Cigarette smoking as it may cause vasoconstriction.
- Very cold temperatures as these may cause vasoconstriction.
- Hot baths or sitting near fires because of the risk of burns with decreased sensation to the limbs
- Cutting toenails as soft tissue damage may be slow to heal because of poor peripheral circulation. Toenails should be cut by a chiropodist.
- Sitting cross-legged for too long as this will restrict blood flow to the lower limbs.

A well-balanced healthy diet high in fruit, fibre and vegetables and low in saturated fat should be encouraged. Fluid intake of 2.5–3 L should be encouraged as dehydration causes increased blood viscosity and thus increases the risk of clot formation.

Some patients may require bypass surgery to treat the condition, which involves using a vein or Dacron graft (Figure 6.9). It is the healthcare professional's duty to prepare the patient safely for theatre and to monitor their postoperative recovery. Postoperative complications should be reported and treated immediately to prevent undue harm to the patient.

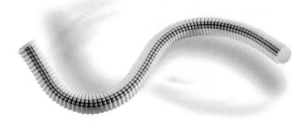

Figure 6.9   Dacron graft for peripheral vascular disease. Synthetic graft used for surgery. Reproduced with permission from Vascutek.

Pharmacological interventions

Patients with PVD may be given the following medications:

- vasodilators
- anticoagulants
- antiplatelet drugs.

Venous insufficiency/varicose veins

Varicose veins are vessels that have become dilated and tortuous due to incompetent valves, which allow back flow and pooling of blood in the veins. This mainly happens in the saphenous veins of the leg, deep communicating veins and superficial veins (Figure 6.10). One cause of venous distension is prolonged standing, which diminishes the action of the calf-muscle pump (Figure 6.11) (Vowden and Vowden, 2010). The calf-muscle pump aids venous return to the heart.

People who are susceptible to varicose veins are pregnant women, the obese, those who have to stand for long periods because of the nature of their occupation, e.g. theatre nurses, and the older age group. There is no conclusive evidence to suggest that varicosity is hereditary.

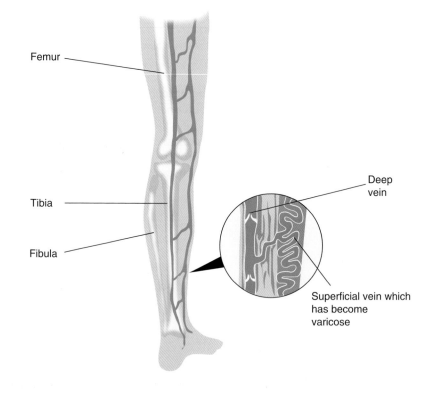

Figure 6.10   Varicose veins.

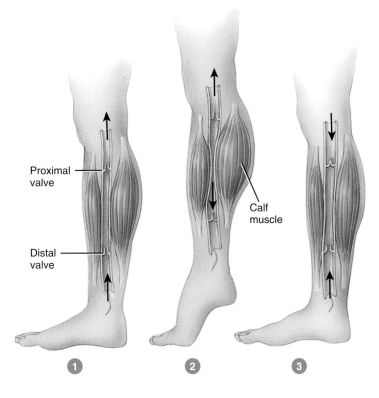

Proximal
valve

Distal
valve

Calf
muscle

① ② ③

Figure 6.11   Calf-muscle pump.

Veins affected with varicosity

Any vein in the leg can develop varicosity (Figure 6.12); however, the common veins are the:

- long saphenous veins
- short saphenous veins
- perforating veins.

Signs and symptoms

- swelling of the lower extremities
- distended and tortuous veins
- dull aching in the leg
- ulcers (rare)
- leg fatigue and heaviness

Complications

Complications such as venous ulcers, venous eczema, lipodermatosclerosis and skin pigmentation (Figure 6.13a–c) are seen in some patients with varicose veins. Untreated tissue necrosis and infection can occur.

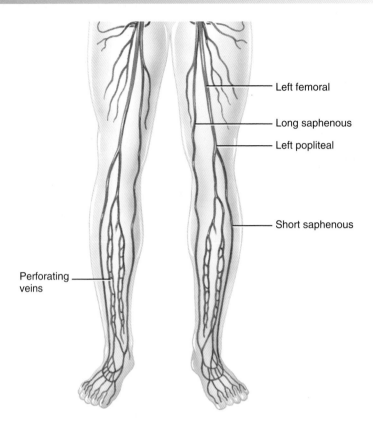

Left femoral

Long saphenous

Left popliteal

Short saphenous

Perforating veins

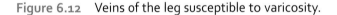

Figure 6.12   Veins of the leg susceptible to varicosity.

Care and management

In the UK, stripping and ligation of varicose veins are not routinely undertaken in the NHS unless the veins present a health risk; however, varicose veins can be treated privately. After surgery most patients return to their normal routine within 1–3 weeks. Postoperative care includes apply-ing pressure bandages for about 6 weeks, elevating the foot and gradually increasing ambulation (LeMone *et al.*, 2011). The surgical treatment is successful; however, 20–30% of the patients may require repeat surgery.

Pain should be managed by bed rest and elevation of the feet, which improves venous return. Prolonged standing in one position should be discouraged and walking (2–3 miles per day) should be encouraged to activate the calf-muscle pump, which helps in venous flow (see Figure 6.10) and to reduce oedema and complications such as deep vein thrombosis. Supportive anti-embolism stockings should be worn to reduce swelling in the leg and to provide support to the veins.

- Encourage patients to stop smoking as the nicotine may cause vascular damage.
- Encourage adequate fluid intake of 2–3 L per day and a healthy diet for tissue healing.
- Avoid unnecessary trauma to the feet.

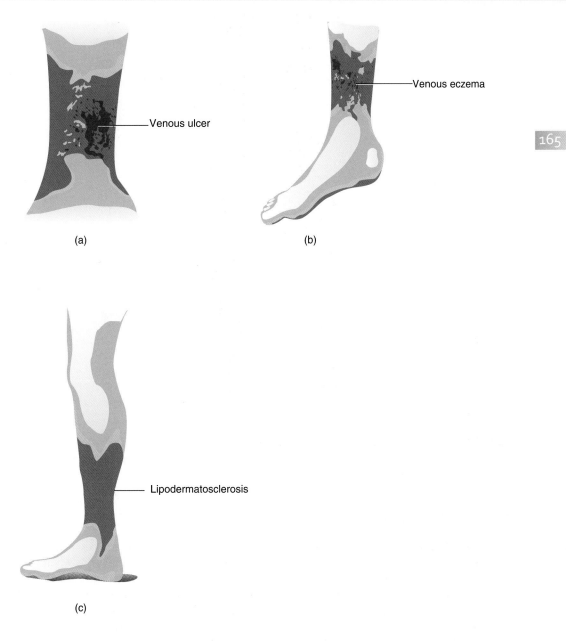

Venous ulcer

Venous eczema

Lipodermatosclerosis

Figure 6.13   (a) Venous ulcer; (b) venous eczema; and (c) lipodermatosclerois.

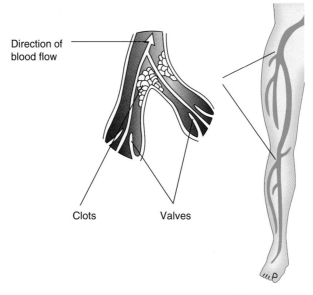

Figure 6.14   Formation of thrombosis.

- Inform patients not to cross their leg when seated as this restricts blood return.
- Educate patients in the benefits of regular exercise.
- Encourage all patients to maintain normal weight for their height.

Deep vein thrombosis

Deep vein thrombosis (DVT) is the formation of a thrombus (clot) in the veins when the flow of blood is reduced. It primarily occurs in the veins of the lower extremity (Figure 6.14), such as the femoral, popliteal and the deep veins of the pelvis (Porth, 2010).

Aetiology

DVT is associated with:

- Stasis of blood in the veins, which can result from immobility after surgery.
- Obstruction to the flow of blood in the veins as a result of trauma.
- Hypercoagulability of blood due to dehydration, hormone replacement therapy and oral contraceptive pills.
- Use of intravenous cannulae may cause damage to the tunica intima, resulting in the formation of clots.

Other factors include age (people over the age of 40 years are at greater risk), obesity, pregnancy, varicose veins and smoking.

Pathophysiology

A thrombus can develop in the superficial or deep veins of the legs. The blood flow is sluggish in the affected vessels and the clotting cascade takes place. Platelets aggregate at the site of injury to the vessel wall or where there is venous stasis (LeMone *et al.*, 2011). Platelet aggregation occurs because platelets are exposed to collagen (a protein in the connective tissue, which is found in the inner surface of the blood vessel). When platelets come into contact with the exposed collagen, they release adenosine diphosphate and thromboxane. These substances make the surface of the platelets sticky and as they adhere to each other, a platelet plug is formed (Figure 6.15). Other cells such as the red blood cells are trapped in the fibrin mesh (Figure 6.16) and the thrombus grows.

The thrombus triggers the inflammatory response, causing tenderness, swelling and erythema at the affected site. Initially the thrombus stays within the affected area; however, fragments of the thrombus may become loose and travel through the circulation as an embolus, which may lodge in the lungs and cause a pulmonary embolism.

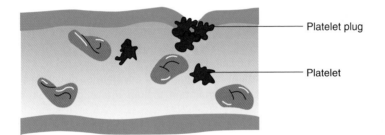

Figure 6.15   Formation of a platelet plug.

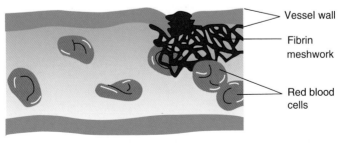

Formation of a clot

Figure 6.16   Formation of a clot.

Signs and symptoms

The signs and symptoms of DVT are:

- usually asymptomatic
- dull aching pain in the affected limb, especially when walking
- oedema of the affected leg
- cyanosis of the affected leg
- redness and warmth on the affected part
- dilatation of the surface vein.

Care and management

- Maintain the patient on bed rest until mobilisation is encouraged.
- Monitor the vital signs (temperature, pulse, respiration and blood pressure) of the patient 1–2 hourly to prevent complications such as pulmonary embolism.
- Observe the calf muscle for swelling. Measure the circumference 10–20 cm above and below the knee. Measurements should be accurately recorded as changes will allow prompt interventions.
- Elevate the foot to promote venous return and to reduce oedema.
- The patient should be advised not to massage the affected calf muscle so as not to dislodge the clot.
- The assessment of pain includes testing for Homan's sign – the patient lies flat with their legs straight and dorsiflexes the foot quickly (Alexander *et al.*, 2007). The test is positive if the patient complains of pain in the calf.
- Check every 4 hours if the patient is experiencing any pain or discomfort in the affected leg.
- The patient should be advised to maintain a fluid intake of 2–2.5 L per day to prevent dehydration.
- Check to ensure that compression stockings are fitted correctly.

Pharmacological interventions

The following medications may be prescribed for the patient with DVT:

- anticoagulants such as low-molecular-weight heparin
- antiplatelet drugs
- anti-inflammatory drugs
- thrombolytic drugs.

Conclusion

The overall aim of this chapter was to provide the learner with an understanding of the vascular system and its related disorders. In order to care for the patient with vascular dysfunction, health-care professionals need to understand the normal physiology of the vascular system. There are numerous diseases related to the vascular system; however, it is not the remit of this chapter to cover all them. Some of the main diseases are discussed with their related care and management. The key role of the healthcare professional is to provide comfort, offer advice and prevent complications that could be detrimental to the patient's health. Caring for patients with vascular disorders requires skilled management, which incorporates ongoing assessment, and implementing and evaluating the care.

Test your knowledge

- Describe the process of atherosclerotic occlusion of a vessel.
- List the possible causes of PVD.
- Describe the pathophysiology of hypertension.
- Briefly describe the pathophysiology of an aneurysm.
- Discuss the care and management of the patient with varicose veins.

Activities

 Here are some activities and exercises to help test your learning. For the answers to these exercises, as well as further self-testing activities, visit our website at www.wiley.com/go/fundamentalsofappliedpathophysiology

Fill in the blanks

Peripheral vascular disease (PVD) occurs when there is significant narrowing of _____ distal to the arch of the aorta, most often due to _____. Symptoms vary from _____ pain on exercise (intermittent claudication) to rest pain (critical limb ischaemia), skin ulceration and _____. If left untreated, _____ of the _____ may eventually be necessary. If the narrowing of the arteries is severe, the pain may start after _____ only a few metres. The _____, vice-like leg pain forces the patient to rest until it passes.
PVD usually develops when _____ build up on the _____ of the arteries. The fatty deposits cause your arteries to _____. This means that the supply of _____ to the _____ and _____ is reduced. The patient may feel pain when they start to _____, because the muscles in the leg cannot get enough _____.

Choose from:
Cramping; Walls; Narrow; Arteries; Atherosclerosis; Oxygen; Exercise; Fatty deposits; Amputation; Calf; Walking; Gangrene; Limb; Blood; Tissues; Muscles

Label the diagram

Using the list of words supplied, label the diagram.

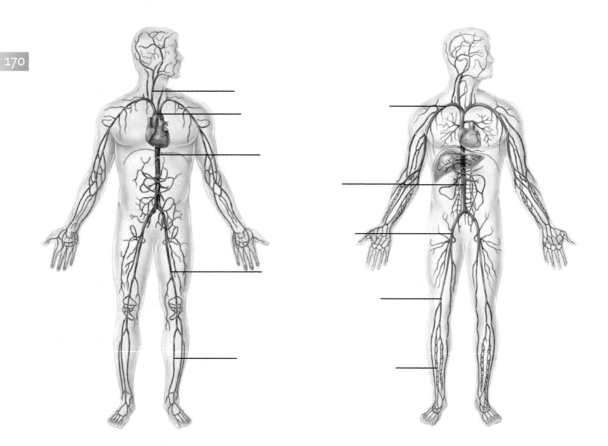

Right common carotid; Right subclavian vein; Arch of aorta; Inferior vena cava; Thoracic aorta; Left femoral artery; Right external iliac vein; Left posterior tibial; Right popliteal vein; Right anterio tibial

Word search

V	A	C	Y	N	E	T	M	N	H	C	E	T	L	R
O	U	A	R	N	X	B	C	O	A	E	O	S	S	M
E	S	S	L	O	L	I	A	P	L	V	S	N	U	O
B	R	C	L	O	T	T	I	N	G	E	T	P	O	S
C	O	A	O	P	T	L	D	S	E	N	T	B	M	M
E	T	D	O	U	L	E	T	S	E	U	E	O	A	S
E	P	E	N	A	B	E	R	M	E	L	R	Y	U	C
I	E	I	R	E	A	S	U	Y	S	E	U	Y	Q	D
Q	C	I	R	U	C	L	C	E	T	S	V	N	S	S
A	E	N	A	X	O	B	M	O	R	H	T	R	E	M
S	R	O	T	P	E	C	E	R	O	M	E	H	C	V
N	O	I	S	N	E	T	R	E	P	Y	H	M	E	V
N	M	A	C	R	O	P	H	A	G	E	S	T	A	C
L	S	S	O	O	T	I	S	Y	O	T	A	L	L	G
Q	O	X	I	D	A	T	I	O	N	R	L	O	D	O

Capillaries	Oxidation	Cascade
Hypertension	Thromboxane	Squamous
Erythema	Venules	Optic
Clotting	Aneurysm	Tunica
Lumen	Chemoreceptors	Venules
Macrophages	Osmoreceptors	Blood

Further resources

Patient UK

http://www.patient.co.uk/doctor/Peripheral-Vascular-Disease.htm
This is a comprehensive health information website that GPs and nurses use during consultations. Students should access this website as there is much useful information that can be shared with patients to promote health.

Scottish Intercollegiate Guidelines (SIGN)

http://www.sign.ac.uk/pdf/sign89.pdf
The SIGN website provides guidelines relating to the diagnosis and management of peripheral arterial disease.

National Institute for Health and Clinical Excellence (NICE)

http://www.nice.org.uk/CG034
This link takes you to the NICE website. This section of the NICE website recommends endovascular stent-grafts as a possible treatment for people with abdominal aortic aneurysms. Students accessing this link should bear in mind that every trust will have its own local policies and guidelines.

Department of Health (DH)

http://www.dh.gov.uk/en/Publicationsandstatistics/index.htm
All healthcare professionals should access this government website. It provides DH publications, including statistical reports, surveys, press releases, circulars and legislation.

British Hypertension Society

http://www.bhsoc.org/
The British Hypertension Society provides a medical and scientific research forum to enable the sharing of cutting-edge research into the origin of high blood pressure so as to improve its treatment. This site provides useful information not otherwise found in textbooks.

British Heart Foundation

http://www.americanheart.org/presenter.jhtml?identifier=4692
This useful website provides information on different vascular diseases and the roles of anticoagulants and aspirin.

Glossary of terms

Adenosine diphosphate:	found inside cells, it helps to produce ATP during reactions that produce cellular energy and is itself formed from ATP at a later stage. It is this continual synthesis and breaking down of ADP and ATP that produces the energy.
Aneurysm:	a localised dilatation of a blood vessel, usually the aorta or the arteries at the base of the brain.
Aorta:	first major blood vessel of the arterial circulation. Emerges from the left ventricle of the heart.
Artery:	a blood vessel that carries blood away from the heart.
Arteriole:	a small artery.
Arteriosclerosis:	a condition in which there is thickening, hardening, loss of elasticity of the vessel wall leading to narrowing of the artery.
Baroreceptor:	a neuron sensing changes in fluid, air and blood pressures.
Blood pressure:	the force exerted by the blood against the walls of the blood vessel due to the contraction of the heart.
Capillary:	a small blood vessel where exchanges between blood and tissue cells take place.
Chemoreceptor:	a sensory receptor that detects the presence of a specific chemical.
Clotting cascade:	a series of steps in the clotting process of the blood.
Collagen fibre:	the most abundant of the three fibre types found in the connective tissues.
Endothelium:	a single layer of simple squamous cells found in the heart, blood vessels and lymphatic vessels.
Erythema:	a superficial redness of the skin.
Extracellular fluid:	the fluid that surrounds and bathes the body's cells.
Fibroblast cells:	the most common connective tissue cells and only found in the tendons. It is responsible for the production and secretion of extracellular matrix materials.
Hypertension:	raised blood pressure.
Lumen:	the inside spaceof a tubular structure.
Macrophage:	a phagocyte produced from monocytes that engulfs and digests cellular debris, microbes and foreign matter.

Oxidation:	a chemical reaction where electrons are lost.
Paget's disease:	a disorder of the bone. Excessive remodelling of the bone causes enlarged and deformed bones and weakening of the bones, leading to bone pain and fractures.
Papilloedema:	a swelling of the optic disc in the eye.
Thromboxane:	a compound synthesised in platelets from prostaglandin. It acts to aggregate platelets.
Tunica externa:	the membranous outer layer of the blood vessel.
Tunica intima:	the inner lining of a blood vessel.
Tunica media:	the middle muscle layer of the blood vessel.
Vasoconstriction:	a decrease in the diameter of a blood vessel due to the relaxation of smooth muscle in the vessel wall; may occur as a result of hormones or after stimulation of the vasomotor centre leading to increased peripheral resistance.
Vasodilatation:	an increase in the diameter of a blood vessel due to relaxation of smooth muscle in the vessel wall; may occur as a result of hormones or after decreased stimulation of the vasomotor centre leading to decreased peripheral resistance.
Vein:	a blood vessel that carries blood to the heart.
Venule:	a small vein.

References

Alexander, M.F., Fawcett, J.N. and Runciman, P.J. (eds) (2007). *Nursing Practice: Hospital and Home: The Adult*, 3rd edn. Edinburgh: Churchill Livingstone.

Bullock, B.A. and Henze, R.L. (2010). *Focus on Pathophysiology*. Philadelphia: Lippincott.

Caterson, I.D. (2005). Obesity in 2005 and in DOM. *Diabetes, Obesity and Metabolism.* 7(3): 209–210.

Hogan, M.A. and Hill, K. (2004). *Pathophysiology – Reviews and Rationales*. New Jersey: Prentice Hall.

Jackson, S., Bereznicki, L. and Peterson, G. (2005). Under-use of ACE-inhibitor and beta blocker therapies in congestive heart failure. *Australian Pharmacist.* 24(12): 936.

Jenkins, G.W. and Tortora, G.J. (2013). *Anatomy and Physiology*. New Jersey: John Wiley & Sons.

Jowett, N.I. and Thompson, D.R. (2007). *Comprehensive Coronary Care*, 4th edn. London: Baillere Tindall.

LeMone, P., Burke, K. and Bauldoff, G. (2011). *Medical – Surgical Nursing; Critical Thinking in Client Care*, 4th edn. New Jersey: Pearson.

Marieb, E.N. (2011). *Essentials of Human Anatomy and Physiology*, 9th edn. San Francisco: Pearson Benjamin Cummings.

Marieb, E.N. and Hoehn, K. (2010). *Human Anatomy and Physiology*, 8th edn. San Francisco: Pearson Benjamin Cummings.

McCance, K.L., Huether, S.E., Brashers, V.L. and Rote, N.S. (2010). *Pathophysiology: The Biologic Basis for Disease in Adults and Children*, 6th edn. St. Louis: Mosby

National Institute for Health Clinical Excellence (2010). *Management of Type 2 Diabetes: Management of Blood Glucose*. London: NICE.

Nowak, J. and Handford, A.G. (2010). *Essentials of Pathophysiology: Concepts and Applications for Health Care Professionals*, 3rd edn. Boston: McGraw-Hill.

Nursing and Midwifery Council (2009). *Record Keeping: Guidance for Nurses and Midwives*. London: Nursing and Midwifery Council.

Porth, C.M. (2010). *Pathophysiology: Concepts of Altered Health States*, 8th edn. Philadelphia: Lippincott Williams & Wilkins.

Stubbling, N. and Chesworth, J. (2010). Assessment of patients with vascular disease. In: Murray, S. (ed.) *Vascular Disease: Nursing and Management*. London: Whurr.

Vowden, K. and Vowden, P. (2010). Venous disorder. In: Murray, S. (ed) *Vascular Disease: Nursing and Management*. London: Whurr.

Waugh, A. and Grant, A. (2010). *Ross and Wilson: Anatomy and Physiology in Health and Illness*, 11th edn. Edinburgh: Churchill Livingstone.

7

The blood and associated disorders

Muralitharan Nair

Senior Lecturer, Department of Adult Nursing and Primary Care, School of Health and Social Work, University of Hertfordshire, Hatfield, Hertfordshire, UK

Contents

Fundamentals of Applied Pathophysiology: An Essential Guide for Nursing and Healthcare Students, Second Edition. Edited by Muralitharan Nair and Ian Peate.
© 2013 John Wiley & Sons, Ltd. Published 2013 by John Wiley & Sons, Ltd.

Key words

- Erythrocytes
- Platelets
- Haemostasis
- Antigens
- Plasma
- Haemoglobin
- Coagulation
- Agglutination
- White blood cells
- Erythropoietin
- Blood groups
- Haematocrit

Test your prior knowledge

- What is the function of the red blood cell?
- How many types of white blood cells are there? Can you name them?
- Why does the arterial blood look bright red?
- What do you understand by the term blood doping?

Learning outcomes

On completion of this section the reader will be able to:

- Describe the normal composition of blood.
- List the functions of the red blood cells, white blood cells and platelets.
- Explain the life cycle of the red blood cells and the white blood cells.
- Discuss the factors affecting coagulation.
- Explain the ABO and Rh systems of blood typing.

Don't forget to visit to the companion website for this book (www.wiley.com/go/ fundamentalsofappliedpathophysiology) where you can find self-assessment tests to check your progress, as well as lots of activities to practise your learning.

Introduction

Blood is a type of connective tissue consisting of cells and cell fragments. It does not connect or give mechanical support. It is called a connective tissue because it develops from mesenchyme and consists of blood cells which are surrounded by non-living fluid called plasma. The cells and the cell fragments are formed elements of the blood and the liquid part is called the plasma. The formed elements are made up of red blood cells (erythrocytes), which account for 45% of the blood. Plasma makes up 55% of the total blood volume (Stanfield, 2011). The remaining 1% consists of white blood cells and platelets (Figure 7.1). The percentage of the formed elements constitutes the haematocrit or packed cell volume. The volume of blood is constant in a healthy person unless the person has physiological problems. This chapter focuses on the composition, structure and functions of various blood cells and their related disorders.

Composition of blood

Blood is composed of plasma, a yellowish liquid containing nutrients, hormones, minerals and various cells, mainly red blood cells, white blood cells and platelets (Figure 7.2). Both the formed elements and the plasma play an important role in homeostasis.

Properties of blood

In a healthy person, blood forms about 7–9% of total body weight. A man has 5–6 L of blood, while a woman has 4–5 L. Blood is thicker, denser and flows much slower than water due to the red blood cells and proteins, such as albumin and fibrinogen. It has a high viscosity which offers resistance to blood flow. The red blood cells and proteins contribute to the viscosity of blood,

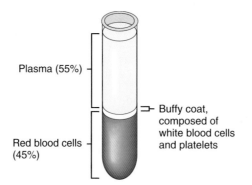

Figure 7.1   Components of blood.

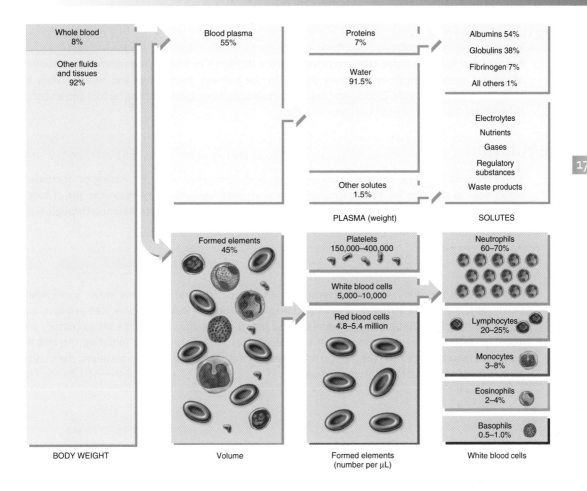

Figure 7.2   Cells of the blood.

which ranges from 3.5 to 5.5 compared with 1.0 for water. The more red blood cells and plasma proteins in blood, the higher the viscosity and the slower the flow of blood. The specific gravity (density) of blood is 1.045–1.065 compared with 1.000 for water, and the pH of blood ranges from 7.35 to 7.45.

Functions of blood

Overall, there are three categories of blood function:

- transportation
- regulation
- protection.

Transportation

Red blood cells in the blood transport oxygen from the lungs to body tissues and waste products of cellular metabolism from the body tissues to the kidneys, liver, lungs and sweat glands for elimination from the body. Blood also transports nutrients, hormones, clotting factors and enzymes throughout the body to maintain homeostasis.

Regulation

Blood regulates blood clotting to stop bleeding; body temperature by increasing or decreasing blood flow to the skin for heat exchange; and acid–base balance to maintain the pH of blood within a normal range (7.35–7.45). It also regulates fluid and electrolyte balance through renal function.

Protection

Blood defends the body against bacteria and viruses (pathogens) in several ways. Some white blood cells, e.g. the neutrophils, engulf and destroy pathogens while lymphocytes produce and secrete antibodies into blood. Antibodies in the blood play a vital role in the inflammatory and immune response. These responses prevent blood loss after an injury by initiating the clotting mechanisms, without which the person will bleed to death. Clotting involves platelets, the plasma protein fibrinogen and the clotting factors.

Plasma

Plasma is the liquid part of the blood and is composed of water (91%), proteins (8%; albumin, globulin, prothrombin and fibrinogen), salts (0.9%; sodium chloride, sodium bicarbonate and others) and the remaining 0.1% is made up of organic materials, e.g. fats, glucose, urea, uric acid, cholesterol and amino acids (Mader, 2011). The blood cells are composed of erythrocytes (red blood cells), leucocytes (white blood cells) and thrombocytes (platelets). These substances give plasma greater density and viscosity than water.

Water in plasma

The water in plasma is available to cells, tissues and extracellular fluid of the body to maintain homeostasis. It is a solvent where chemical reactions between intracellular and extracellular reactions occur. Water contains solutes, e.g. electrolytes, whose concentrations change to meet the body's needs.

Plasma proteins

Plasma contains three principal types of protein:

- albumins
- globulins
- fibrinogen.

Plasma proteins make up 7% of the plasma and these proteins stay in the blood vessel as they are too large to diffuse through capillaries and are responsible for creating the osmotic pressure of blood. When plasma proteins are lost in patients who suffer from burns, fluid moves into tissues, causing oedema by a process called osmosis.

Albumin

Albumin is the most abundant plasma protein (about 60%). It is synthesised in the liver and its main function is to maintain plasma osmotic pressure. Albumins also act as carrier molecules for other substances, such as hormones and lipids (Waugh and Grant, 2010).

Globulins

The next most abundant plasma proteins are globulins (about 36%). They are synthesised from the liver and B lymphocytes. They are divided into three groups based on their structure and function:

- alpha globulin
- beta globulin
- gamma globulin.

The alpha and beta globulins are produced by the liver and they transport lipids and fat-soluble vitamins. Gamma globulins are immunoglobulins, which are complex proteins produced by lymphocytes, and have a vital role in immunity. They prevent diseases such as measles and tetanus (Waugh and Grant, 2010).

Fibrinogen

Fibrinogen, which is synthesized in the liver, forms approximately 4% of the plasma proteins and is essential for blood clotting. When fibrinogen and several other proteins involved in clotting are removed, the remaining fluid is called serum.

Plasma electrolytes

Electrolytes are inorganic molecules that separate into ions when dissolved in water. They are involved in muscle contraction and transmission of nerve impulses, and play a role in maintaining the pH of blood. The ions are either positively charged (cations) or negatively charged (anions). The principal plasma cation is sodium (Na^+) and the principal anion is chloride (Cl^-).

Gases

Oxygen, carbon dioxide and nitrogen are the principal gases dissolved in plasma. Oxygen is transported by haemoglobin in red blood cells and some is dissolved in plasma. Most of the carbon dioxide is transported by bicarbonate ions in plasma.

Nutrients and waste products of metabolism

Nutrients such as amino acids, fatty acids and glycerol are obtained from the digestion of food in the gastrointestinal tract. They are vital to cellular function. Waste products of protein

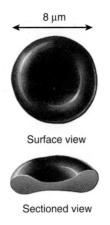

Surface view

Sectioned view

Figure 7.3   Red blood cell.

metabolism, such as urea, creatinine and uric acid, are transported in the blood to the kidneys for elimination (Mader, 2011).

Formed elements of blood

The formed elements of the blood consist of:

- Red blood cells
- White blood cells
- Platelets.

Red blood cells

Red blood cells are also known as erythrocytes and are small biconcave discs (Figure 7.3). The biconcave shape is maintained by a network of protein called spectrin, which also allows the red blood cells to change shape as they are transported through the blood vessel. There are approximately 4–5.5 million red blood cells in each cubic millimetre of blood (Marieb and Hoehn, 2010). They are a pale buff colour that is lighter in the centre. Young red blood cells contain a nucleus; however, the nucleus is absent in mature red blood cells, as are any organelles such as mitochondria.

The main function of the red blood cell is to transport the respiratory gases oxygen and carbon dioxide (approximately 20%). As red blood cells lack mitochondria to produce energy (adenosine triphosphate), they utilise anaerobic respiration to produce energy and do not use any of the oxygen they are transporting.

Haemoglobin

Haemoglobin is composed of the protein called globin bound to the iron-containing pigment called haem. Each globin molecule has four polypeptide chains consisting of two alpha and two beta

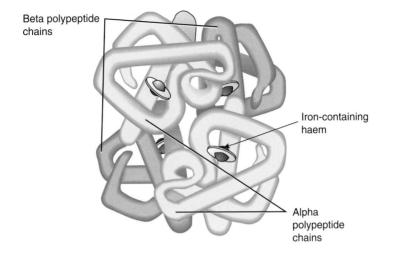

Beta polypeptide chains

Iron-containing haem

Alpha polypeptide chains

Figure 7.4   Haemoglobin molecule.

chains (Figure 7.4). Each haemoglobin molecule has four atoms of iron and each atom of iron will transport one molecule of oxygen; therefore, one molecule of haemoglobin will transport four molecules of oxygen. There are approximately 250 million haemoglobin molecules in one red blood cell and therefore one red blood cell will transport a billion molecules of oxygen.

Formation of red blood cells

Red blood cells are formed from the stem cells in the red bone marrow. In the bone marrow, the multipotent stem cells divide to produce myeloid stem cells which divide to produce erythroblasts (Figure 7.5). Erythroblasts develop in the red bone marrow to form red blood cells. During maturation, red blood cells lose their nucleus and organelles, and gain more haemoglobin molecules, thus increasing the amount of oxygen they can transport. As mature red blood cells do not have a nucleus, their lifespan is approximately 120 days. It is estimated that approximately 2 million red blood cells are destroyed per second (Mader, 2011); however, these are replaced with an equal number to maintain the balance.

The production of red blood cells is controlled by the hormone erythropoietin (Marieb and Hoehn, 2010) and the essential components for the synthesis of red blood cells are:

- iron
- folic acid
- vitamin B$_{12}$.

Transport of respiratory gases

The major role of red blood cells is to transport oxygen from the lungs to the tissues. The oxygen in the alveoli (air sacs) of the lungs combines with iron molecules in the haemoglobin to form oxyhaemoglobin. This is then transported by the blood to the tissues. As the oxygen level in the

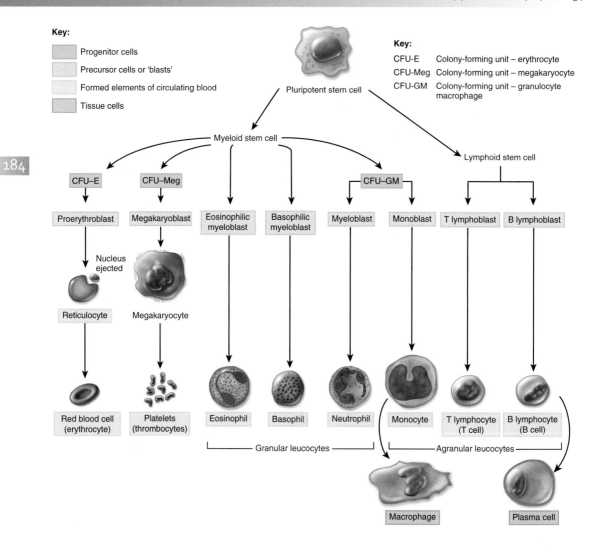

Key:

Progenitor cells

Precursor cells or 'blasts'

Formed elements of circulating blood

Tissue cells

Key:

CFU-E   Colony-forming unit – erythrocyte
CFU-Meg Colony-forming unit – megakaryocyte
CFU-GM   Colony-forming unit – granulocyte
               macrophage

Pluripotent stem cell

Myeloid stem cell

Lymphoid stem cell

CFU–E   CFU–Meg   CFU–GM

Proerythroblast   Megakaryoblast   Eosinophilic   Basophilic   Myeloblast   Monoblast   T lymphoblast   B lymphoblast
                                     myeloblast   myeloblast

Nucleus ejected

Reticulocyte   Megakaryocyte

Red blood cell   Platelets   Eosinophil   Basophil   Neutrophil   Monocyte   T lymphocyte   B lymphocyte
(erythrocyte)   (thrombocytes)   (T cell)   (B cell)

—————— Granular leucocytes ——————   —————— Agranular leucocytes ——————

Macrophage   Plasma cell

Figure 7.5   Formation of blood cells.

red blood cell increases, it becomes bright red, and when the level of oxygen content drops, the colour changes to a dark bluish red (Waugh and Grant, 2010).

In addition to transporting oxygen from the lungs to the body tissues, red blood cells transport carbon dioxide from the tissues to the lungs. Carbon dioxide is transported in three ways:

- 10% is dissolved in the plasma.
- 20% combines with the haemoglobin of the red blood cell to form carbaminohaemoglobin.
- 70% with water to form carbonic acid which is converted to bicarbonate and hydrogen ions.

$$CO_2 + H_2O \xleftarrow{\text{carbonic anhydrase}} \underset{\text{carbonic acid}}{H_2CO_3} \leftrightarrow \underset{\text{bicarbonate ion}}{HCO_3^-} + \underset{\text{hydrogen ion}}{H^+}$$

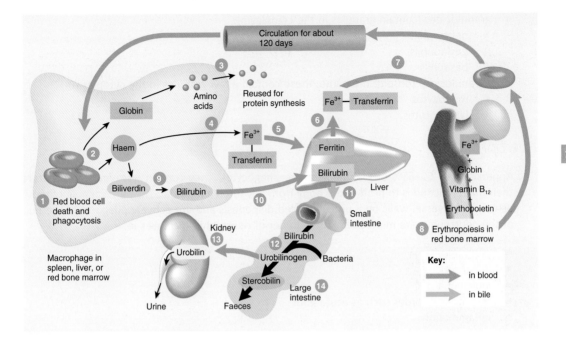

Figure 7.6   Haemolysis of red blood cells.

The reaction occurs primarily in red blood cells which contain large amounts of carbonic anhydrase (an enzyme that facilitates the reaction). Once the bicarbonate ions are formed, they move out of the red blood cells into the plasma.

Destruction of red blood cells

Haemolysis (breakdown) is carried out by macrophages in the spleen, liver and bone marrow (Figure 7.6). As red blood cells age, they are susceptible to haemolysis; haem and globin are separated. The globin is broken down into amino acids and used for protein synthesis. Iron is separated from haem and is stored in the muscle and the liver, and reused in the bone marrow to manufacture new red blood cells. Haem is the portion of the haemoglobin that is converted to bilirubin and is transported by plasma albumin to the liver and eventually secreted in bile.

White blood cells

White blood cells are also known as leucocytes. There are approximately 5000–10 000 white blood cells in every cubic millimetre of blood. The number may increase in infections to approximately 25 000 per cubic millimetre of blood. An increase in white blood cells is called leucocytosis and an abnormally low level of white blood cell is called leucopenia. Unlike red blood cells, white blood cells do have nuclei and they are able to move across blood vessel walls into the tissues. White blood cells are able to produce a continuous supply of energy, unlike the red blood cells. They are able to synthesise proteins and thus their lifespan can be from a few days to years. There are two main types of white blood cells:

- granulocytes (contain granules in the cytoplasm):
  - neutrophils
  - eosinophils
  - basophils
- agranulocytes (despite the name, these contain a few granules in the cytoplasm)
  - monocytes
  - lymphocytes.

Neutrophils

Approximately 60–65% of granulocytes are phagocytes. They contain lysozymes and therefore their main function is to protect the body from any foreign material. They are capable of moving across blood vessel walls by a process called diapedesis and are actively phagocytic. The nuclei of the neutrophils are multilobed. The number of neutrophils increases in:

- pregnancy
- infection
- leukaemia
- metabolic disorder such as acute gout
- inflammation
- myocardial infarction.

Eosinophils

These form approximately 2–4% of granulocytes and have B-shaped nuclei. Like neutrophils, they too migrate from blood vessels. They are phagocytes; however, they are not as active as neutrophils. They contain lysosomal enzymes and peroxidase in their granules, which are toxic to parasites, resulting in the destruction of the organisms. Numbers increase in allergy, such as hay fever and asthma, and parasitic infection, e.g. tapeworm infection.

Basophils

Basophils account for approximately 1% of granulocytes and contain elongated lobed nuclei. In inflamed tissue they become mast cells and secrete granules containing heparin, histamine and other proteins that promote inflammation. Basophils play an important role in providing immunity against parasites.

Monocytes

Monocytes account for 5% of the agranulocytes and they are circulating leucocytes. Monocytes develop in the bone marrow. Some of the monocytes migrate into the tissue where they develop into macrophages and engulf pathogens or foreign proteins. Macrophages play a vital role in immunity and inflammation by destroying specific antigens.

Lymphocytes

Lymphocytes account for 25% of the leucocytes and most are found in the lymphatic tissue such as the lymph nodes and the spleen. They get their name from the fluid that transports them – the lymph. They can leave and re-enter the circulatory system. Their lifespan ranges from a few hours to years. The main difference between lymphocytes and other white blood cells is that lymphocytes are not phagocytes. Two types of lymphocytes are identified – T and B lymphocytes. T lymphocytes originate from the thymus gland, while B lymphocytes originate in the bone marrow, hence their names. T lymphocytes mediate the cellular immune response, which is part of the body's own defence. The B lymphocytes, on the other hand, become large plasma cells and produce antibodies which attach to antigens.

Platelets

Platelets are small blood cells consisting of some cytoplasm surrounded by a plasma membrane. They are produced in the bone marrow from megakaryocytes (see Figure 7.5) and fragments of megakaryocytes break off to form platelets. Their lifespan is approximately 5–9 days (Stanfield, 2011). The surface of platelets contains proteins and glycoproteins that allow them to adhere to other proteins such as collagen in the connective tissues. Platelets play a vital role in blood loss by the formation of platelet plugs (see Figure 6.15), which seal the holes in the blood vessels.

Haemostasis

Haemostasis plays an important part in maintaining homeostasis and it consists of three main components:

- vasoconstriction
- platelet aggregation
- coagulation.

Vasoconstriction

- results from contraction of the smooth muscle of the vessel wall
- constriction blocks small blood vessels, thus preventing blood flow through them
- the action of the sympathetic nervous system is to cause vasoconstriction
- platelets release thromboxanes

Platelet aggregation

- platelets contain contractile proteins called actin and myosin
- platelet adhesion occurs when platelets are exposed to collagen in the blood vessels
- platelets release adenosine diphosphate, thromboxane and other chemicals

Coagulation

If blood vessel damage is so extensive that platelet aggregation and vasoconstriction cannot stop the bleeding, the complicated process of coagulation (blood clotting) will begin. The clotting phase involves several clotting factors (Table 7.1). Most of the clotting factors are synthesised in the liver.

A simplified clotting cascade involves the following stages:

1. Thromboplastinogenase, an enzyme released by the blood platelets, combines with antihaemophilic factor to convert the plasma protein thromboplastinogen into thromboplastin.

Table 7.1   Blood clotting factors.

I	Fibrinogen
II	Prothrombin
III	Thromboplastin
IV	Calcium
V	Proaccelerin, labile factor
VII	Serum prothrombin conversion accelerator
VIII	Antihaemophilic factor
IX	Christmas factor, plasma thromboplastin component
X	Stuart–Power factor
XI	Plasma thromboplastin antecedent
XII	Hageman factor
XIII	Fibrin-stabilising factor

2. Thromboplastin combines with calcium ions to convert the inactive plasma protein pro-thrombin into thrombin.
3. Thrombin acts as a catalyst to convert the soluble plasma protein fibrinogen into the insoluble plasma protein fibrin.
4. The fibrin threads trap blood cells to form a clot.
5. Once the clot is formed, the damaged blood vessel heals and this restores the integrity of the blood vessel.

Two pathways have been identified in triggering a blood clot – the intrinsic and extrinsic pathways. The extrinsic pathway is a rapid clotting system activated when the blood vessels are ruptured and tissue damage takes place. The intrinsic pathway is slower than the extrinsic pathway and it is activated when the inner walls of the blood vessels are damaged.

Blood groups

The surface of the red blood cell contains molecules called antigens and in the plasma there are molecules called antibodies. The antibodies are specific to certain antigens. When an antibody combines with the specific antigen on the red blood cell, they form a link to connect other red blood cells to it. As a result, clumping or agglutination of the red blood cells occurs.

The antigens on the red blood cells have been categorised into blood groups. Although numerous blood groups have been identified, ABO (Figure 7.7) and rhesus (Rh) blood groups are the most important in blood transfusion.

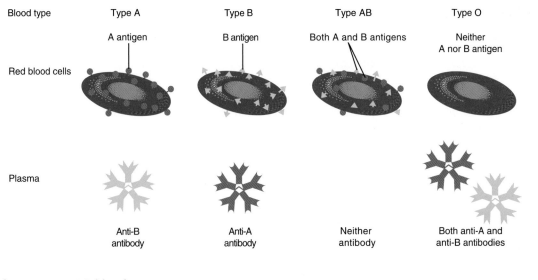

Figure 7.7   ABO blood groups.

Table 7.2   Blood groups.

Blood type	Antigens	Antibodies	Can donate blood to	Can receive blood from
A	Antigen A	Anti-B	A, AB	A, O
B	Antigen B	Anti-A	B, AB	B, O
AB	Antigen A	None	AB	A, B, AB, O
	Antigen B			
O	None	Anti-A	A, B, AB, O	O
		Anti-B		

Type A blood group has type A antigen on its surface and anti-B antibody in the plasma; type B blood group has type B antigen on its surface and anti-A antibody in the plasma; type AB blood group has both antigens A and B on its surface but does not contain either antibodies in the plasma; and type O blood group has neither antigens A nor B on its surface but contains both anti-A and anti-B antibodies in the plasma. About 45% of the population in the UK is blood group O and 55% of the population is either blood group A, B or AB (Waugh and Grant, 2010). People with blood group O are known as universal donors as their red blood cells do not have either A or B antigens on their surface. Conversely, people with blood group AB are known as universal recipients as their red blood cells contain A and B antigens on their surface (Table 7.2).

Rhesus factor

The rhesus factor (Rh) is another important antigen identified on the surface of red blood cells. The rhesus factor is so called because it was first identified in rhesus monkeys. In the UK, approximately 85% of the population is rhesus positive, i.e. they possess factor D on their red blood cells. The remaining 15% of the population is rhesus negative as their red blood cells do not have factor D. It is important to consider the rhesus factor when cross-matching and transfusing blood to patients to avoid unnecessary complications such as agglutination.

Diseases of the blood

Learning outcomes

On completion of this section the reader will be able to:

- List some of the common diseases of blood and identify risk factors associated with the diseases.

- Describe the pathophysiological processes related to specific blood disorders.

- Outline the care and management and interventions related to the disorders described.

Case study

Mrs Martha Sinclare is a 48-year-old second-year student nurse. She is very happy that she can finally achieve something for herself. Mrs Sinclare is keen to finish her studies and earn some money so that she can help her husband financially. Lately, Mrs Sinclare has been complaining of tiredness, breathlessness and that her ankles are slightly swollen. She does suffer from gastritis and over 5 years ago half of her stomach was removed because of cancer. Mrs Sinclare does drink alcohol but not excessively. Her husband persuaded her to go and see her GP to get some advice and treatment.

Take some time to reflect on this case and then consider the following.

1. Which type of anaemia is Mrs Sinclare suffering from?
2. Discuss the possible investigations that may be carried out to confirm diagnosis.
3. List the medications the GP may prescribe to treat her illness.
4. What advice will you give Mrs Sinclare with regards her diet and life style?

Anaemia

Anaemia, from the Greek word meaning 'without blood', refers to a reduction in red blood cells and/or haemoglobin. This results in a reduced ability of the blood to transport oxygen to the tissues, causing hypoxia. The normal level of haemoglobin in an adult male is approximately 13–17 g/100 mL of blood and in an adult female it is approximately 12–16 g/100t#>mL of blood (Porth, 2010). Anaemia can result from:

- excessive loss of blood through haemorrhage
- destruction of red blood cells (haemolysis)
- deficient red blood cell production due to red bone marrow failure
- infections such as malaria
- lack of intake of iron, folic acid and vitamin B_{12}
- pregnancy.

There are three major types of anaemia:

- microcytic anaemia (small red blood cells)
- macrocytic anaemia (large blood cells)
- normocytic anaemia (normal-sized red blood cells).

Microcytic anaemia

Microcytic anaemia is characterised by small red blood cells. There are several types of microcytic anaemia of which iron deficiency anaemia is the most common cause of anaemia in the UK. Iron is essential for the production of young red blood cells. As iron is a component of haem, a deficiency of iron leads to decreased haemoglobin synthesis, resulting in impairment of oxygen transport. In iron deficiency anaemia, the red blood cells are small (microcytic) and pale (hypochromic).

Iron deficiency anaemia

Aetiology
Iron deficiency anaemia results from:

- dietary deficiency of iron
- loss of iron through haemorrhage
- poor absorption of iron from the gastrointestinal tract after gastrectomy
- increased demands such as growth and pregnancy.

Investigations
The following investigations may be carried out to confirm diagnosis:

- full blood count (red blood cells, white blood cells, haemoglobin concentration, mean corpuscular volume, haematrocrit)
- test for levels of ferritin, serum iron, transferring, folate, vitamin B_{12}
- bone marrow examination
- physical examination.

Pathophysiology
Iron deficiency anaemia is present when the demand for iron in the body exceeds supply; anaemia develops slowly in three stages:

- The body's iron stores are depleted; however, erythropoiesis continues normally.
- Iron transportation to bone marrow is diminished, resulting in deficiency in red cell production.
- The number of microcytic red blood cells increases in the circulation, replacing the normal mature red blood cells.

Iron is constantly used in the production of young red blood cells. Iron is obtained from food sources and absorbed from the gastrointestinal tract. Excess iron is stored in the liver and muscle cells and is readily available for the production of red blood cells.

Some inflammatory disorders such as Crohn's disease will affect the absorption of iron from the gastrointestinal tract, affecting the synthesis of red bloods cells. In some instances, substantial segments of bowel are surgically removed, due to carcinoma of the bowel, again affecting the absorption of iron from the gastrointestinal tract. Inadequate dietary intake also contributes to iron deficiency anaemia in the older adult. Limited access to transportation may make it difficult for the patient to eat a healthy diet rich in meat, fruit and vegetables. Iron deficiency can produce significant gastrointestinal abnormalities such as angular stomatitis and glossitis. Other diseases include peptic ulcer where the condition produces gastrointestinal bleeding and iron deficiency. The organs affected are the stomach and the duodenum where there is inflammation and erosion of the membrane.

Signs and symptoms

Patients suffering from iron deficiency anaemia may experience:

- brittle nails
- spoon-shaped nails (koilonychias)
- atrophy of the papillae of the tongue
- brittle hair
- cheilosis (cracks at the corners of the mouth)
- dizziness – due to lack of oxygen supply to the brain
- hypoxia
- pica (craving to eat unusual substances such as clay, starch and coal)
- breathlessness – physiological compensation resulting from the lack of oxygen
- loss of appetite, which may be due to a sore mouth.

Care and management

The care and management of the patient with iron deficiency anaemia will include a full assessment, including a comprehensive risk assessment to prevent injuries from falls, before planning the appropriate care. The care planned should consider a holistic approach, which includes physical, psychological and social aspects of care.

Patients with iron deficiency anaemia may require blood transfusion. It is the healthcare professional's duty to ensure that the transfusion is administered without complications from transfusion, such as reactions from incompatible blood and hypertension. The patient's vital signs, e.g. temperature, blood pressure, heart rate and respirations should be monitored every 15 minutes for the first hour as transfusion reactions are likely to occur in the first 15 minutes. Any change in the vital signs should be reported immediately to the nurse in charge and documented in the nursing notes in accordance with the Nursing and Midwifery Council (2009) guidelines and local policies.

Patients may be concerned about the risk of contracting HIV or hepatitis C through blood transfusion, and therefore it is the healthcare professional's duty to explain the screening procedures undertaken on donor's blood (Alexander *et al.*, 2007) and the low risk associated with blood transfusion.

Dietary advice on foods rich in iron, such as red meat, liver and vegetables, should be encouraged as iron is an essential component for the production of red blood cells.

Advice on oral hygiene should include the use of a soft-toothed toothbrush, care of dentures and the use of suitable ointments to prevent cracked lips (Jamieson *et al.*, 2007).

Anaemic patients should be advised not to change position suddenly, e.g. standing up quickly from a sitting position, to avoid falling and injuring themselves as a result of dizziness.

Pharmacological interventions

Patients with iron deficiency anaemia may be prescribed an iron supplement, e.g. ferrous sulphate. Patients should be advised about the side effects, which include constipation, nausea and even diarrhoea. They should be advised to drink 2–3 L of fluid per day to prevent constipation.

Macrocytic anaemia

Macrocytic anaemia is also termed megaloblastic anaemia. It is characterised by defective deoxyribonucleic acid (DNA) synthesis resulting in the production of unusually large stem cells (macrocytes) in the circulation. In addition to an increase in diameter, the thickness and volume of the cell also increases.

Aetiology

Macrocytic anaemia results from:

- folate deficiency
- vitamin B_{12} deficiency.

Both these coenzymes are essential for DNA maturation. Vegans and vegetarians are at risk of developing macrocytic anaemia due to a lack of vitamin B_{12} which is found in most meat products.

Folate deficiency

Folic acid (folate) is an essential vitamin for the production and maturation of red blood cells. Folate is obtained from the diet and is absorbed from the jejunum and stored in the liver. It is found in leafy vegetables, fruit, cereals and meat; most of it is lost in cooking.

Aetiology

Deficiency in folate can result from:

- malnutrition
- malabsorption from the jejunum caused by diseases such as coeliac disease
- medications that inhibit absorption from the jejunum, e.g. oral contraceptives and anticonvulsants such as phenytoin
- alcohol abuse – alcohol interferes with folate metabolism in the liver
- anorexia.

Symptoms

- fatigue
- palpitations
- shortness of breath
- diarrhoea
- progressive weakness
- pallor

Vitamin B_{12} deficiency

The most common type of megaloblastic anaemia is pernicious anaemia (PA) resulting from vitamin B_{12} deficiency. Vitamin B_{12} is essential for the synthesis of DNA and a deficiency impairs cellular division and maturation, especially in rapidly proliferating red blood cells. The absorption of vitamin B_{12} in the intestine requires the presence of intrinsic factor (IF), which is produced by the gastric mucosa. IF binds to vitamin B_{12} in food, protecting it from gastrointestinal enzymes and facilitating its absorption. Lack of vitamin B_{12} alters the structure and disrupts the function of the peripheral nerves, spinal cord and brain.

Aetiology

Deficiency in vitamin B_{12} can result from:

- total gastrectomy, partial gastrectomy or gastrojejunostomy
- gastric lesions
- carcinoma of the stomach
- alcohol abuse
- malabsorption due to inflammatory disease such as Crohn's disease.

Symptoms

- pallor
- slight jaundice
- smooth sore tongue
- diarrhoea
- paresthesias – numbness and tingling in the extremities
- impaired proprioception (ability to identify one's position in space)
- problems with balance

Care and management of macrocytic anaemia

Care and management of the patient with macrocytic anaemia is similar to that described earlier for iron deficiency anaemia. A full assessment is essential for planning high-quality care. Most patients with folate deficiency are cared for in the community by their general practice. Patients with folate deficiency anaemia will need dietary advice on which foods contain folic acid and how to avoid destroying it in cooking (Alexander *et al.*, 2007). Advice on folic acid supplements and how to take them should be offered to patients.

Some patients with vitamin B_{12} deficiency may be admitted to hospital for their treatment. The treatment for those patients lacking in IF includes the injection of cyanocobalamin, initiallyweekly until vitamin B_{12} deficiency is corrected, then monthly. Patients should be advised to eat foods that contain vitamin B_{12} such as eggs, meat and dairy products. PA as a result of vitamin B_{12} deficiency cannot be cured, so the treatment is lifelong. Some patients may need a blood transfusion if they develop complications such as heart failure.

Normocytic anaemia

Normocytic anaemia is characterised by red blood cells that are relatively normal in size and in haemoglobin content, but insufficient in number. It is less common than microcytic and macrocytic anaemias. Normocytic anaemias include:

- aplastic anaemia
- haemolytic anaemia
- sickle cell anaemia.

Aplastic anaemia

Aplastic anaemia (AA) is a serious condition affecting the bone marrow. It is characterised by a reduction of all the blood cells, i.e. the red blood cells, white blood cells and platelets. When all three types of blood cells are low the condition is termed pancytopenia.

Aetiology

The condition is idiopathic; however, the condition has been associated with:

- viral diseases, e.g. hepatitis and HIV
- ionising radiation
- metastases of the bone
- cytotoxic drugs
- chemical compounds, e.g. benzene.

Pathophysiology

AA occurs as a result of reduced bone marrow function, resulting in low numbers of blood cells. Fat cells proliferate to replace stem cells. The formed red blood cells are immature and the transportation of oxygen is affected. As a result of a shortened lifespan of platelets and white blood cells, patients are prone to infections and bleeding. The most common causes of death are severe haemorrhage, infections and septic shock (Bullock and Henze, 2010). In severe cases, mortality can be high and thus requires prompt intervention.

Symptoms

The initial presenting symptoms include:

- weakness
- fatigue
- pallor caused by anaemia
- petechiae – small haemorrhages under the skin
- ecchymoses – bruises on the skin

- bleeding from mucous membranes of the nose, gums, vagina and gastrointestinal tract may occur as a result of decreased platelet level
- prone to infections as a result of a low neutrophil count.

Care and management

AA can result in life-threatening complications, such as septic shock, which requires prompt intervention. Specific therapy is determined by the underlying cause of the disorder. The management will include treatment with medications, dietary modifications and blood transfusion if necessary. The healthcare professional's role will include:

- early detection and treatment of the disease
- prevention of infections and providing care for septic patients
- early detection and management of bleeding.

Blood transfusion may be indicated to replace the blood lost, and discontinued as soon as the bone marrow commences the synthesis of blood cells. Healthcare professionals need to be aware of blood transfusion complications such as:

- hypertension as a result of fluid overload from transfusion
- transfusion reaction such as rashes and bronchial wheezing
- electrolyte imbalance
- incompatibility between a patient's blood and the donor's blood, e.g. back pain, dyspnoea, cyanosis and tachycardia.

As the risk of adverse reaction is high when the blood is transfused, patient's vital signs must be monitored every 15 minutes for the first hour as many reactions are evident within 15 minutes of transfusion (Kozier et al., 2008).

Care and management in the prevention of AA includes teaching good dietary habits, such as having a diet high in iron, folate and vitamin B_{12}, as these are essential in the synthesis of red blood cells. Vegetarians should be encouraged to ingest food rich in vitamin C as it enhances the absorption of iron from grains and other sources.

Pharmacological interventions

Patients with AA may be prescribed:

- iron supplement
- folic acid supplement
- vitamin B_{12} supplement.

Haemolytic anaemia

Haemolytic anaemia results from the premature destruction of red blood cells, leading to the retention of iron and other products of red blood cell destruction. This rare condition is either acquired or inherited. In haemolytic anaemia, the synthesis of red blood cells in the bone marrow is increased to match the number of red blood cells destroyed.

Aetiology

The causes of haemolytic anaemia can be either inherited or acquired and they include:

- spherocytosis – fragility of the red blood cell membrane
- haemoglobin defects – thalassaemia and sickle cell disease
- mismatched blood transfusion
- direct cell injury from drugs, e.g. sodium chlorate
- disseminated intravascular coagulation
- haemoglobinopathies – abnormalities in haemoglobin structure.

Pathophysiology

The lifespan of red blood cells in haemolytic anaemia is much shorter than the normal lifespan of 120 days. The cell membrane is fragile, resulting in the excessive destruction of the red blood cells; this in turn causes a reduction in the number of red blood cells available for the transportation of oxygen, which leads to hypoxia in the tissues. In response to the excessive destruction, the bone marrow becomes hyperactive and produces more red blood cells by erythropoiesis. In haemolytic anaemia, red blood cell destruction can occur in the vascular system or by phagocytosis by the reticuloendothelial system (Porth, 2010). As a result of the increased destruction of the red blood cells, there is an increased level of bilirubin and urobilinogen.

Signs and symptoms

The presence of signs and symptoms depends on the severity of the disease. Some of the clinical manifestations are:

- jaundice, if red blood cell destruction exceeds the liver's ability to conjugate and excrete bilirubin
- fatigue
- hypoxia from impaired oxygen transport
- dyspnoea
- the spleen may become enlarged in patients with congenital haemolytic disorders.

Care and management

Care and management of the patient with haemolytic anaemia will include advice on diet as for other forms of anaemia, relieving anxiety in patients and their relatives, management of blood transfusion and administration of prescribed medication (see aplastic anaemia). If patients are breathless, they must be nursed upright, supported by pillows, and oxygen administered as prescribed.

Sickle cell anaemia

Sickle cell anaemia is a hereditary, chronic haemolytic anaemia characterised by the presence of an abnormal haemoglobin (HbS) molecule (Figure 7.8). This abnormality occurs as a result of a genetic mutation in which one amino acid (valine) replaces another amino acid (glutamic acid). The haemoglobin forms a sickle shape when oxygen is removed from it (Mehta and Hoffbrand, 2009).

In heterozygous twins, if one child inherits the abnormal haemoglobin gene from one parent and a normal haemoglobin (HbA) from the other parent. The child develops the sickle cell trait

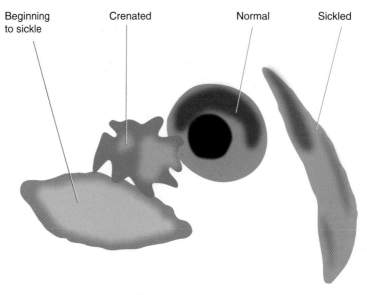

Red blood cells

Figure 7.8   Sickled red blood cell.

and is unaware of this until exposed to hypoxic conditions. The trait is passed on to any child. In homozygous twins, the child inherits the abnormal gene from both parents and will suffer from sickle cell anaemia.

Pathophysiology

The cause of the sickle shape is the deoxygenation of the haemoglobin. When the haemoglobin is fully saturated with oxygen, the red blood cell has the normal shape but this changes to the sickle shape as the oxygen content is reduced. Sickled red blood cells are stiff and cannot change shape as normal red blood cells do when they pass through capillaries (Figure 7.9). As a result, the sickled red blood cells obstruct blood flow, causing vascular obstruction, pain and tissue ischaemia.

Sickling is not permanent; most sickled red blood cells regain their normal shape once they are saturated with oxygen. However, repeated sickling causes loss of elasticity of the cell membrane and over time the cells fail to return to the normal shape when oxygen concentration increases. The weakened red blood cells are haemolysed and removed from the circulation.

Symptoms

Common presenting symptoms include:

- pain and swelling caused by occluded blood vessels affecting the hands and feet
- priapism – persistent painful erection of the penis
- abdominal pain if the abdominal blood vessels are occluded

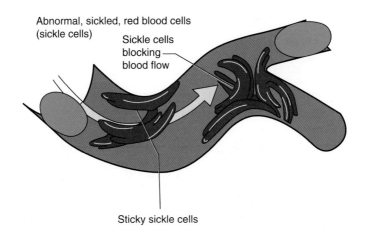

Figure 7.9   Sickle cell in microcirculation.

- increased incidence of infection such as osteomyelitis
- pulmonary hypertension
- tachycardia
- may present with haematuria (blood in the urine)
- may develop stasis ulcers of the hands, ankles and feet
- white blood cells and platelets are often elevated, thus contributing to vaso-occlusion.

Care and management

There is no known cure for sickle cell anaemia. Care and management of the patient will include alleviation of symptoms and promoting a good quality of life. The care will include:

- Pain management – patients with sickle cell disease may have intensely painful episodes called vaso-occlusive crises. Pain management will require opioid analgesia until pain has settled. For patients with milder levels of pain, non-steroidal anti-inflammatory drugs such as diclofenac could be the drugs of choice. For more severe pain crises, most patients will require admission to hospital for intravenous opioids or patient-controlled analgesia to control their pain level. Treatment for patients experiencing pain crises also includes rest, oxygen therapy, analgesia and hydration.
- Patients will need advice on the avoidance of situations that may trigger a crisis. Risk factors include emotional stress, extreme fatigue and infection.
- Early treatment of infection with antibiotics is important to prevent a crisis occurring. Patients' vital signs should be monitored 2–4 hourly to detect infection in order to commence treatment with antibiotics.
- Blood transfusion is indicated for patients who are breathless as a result of severe hypoxia.
- Genetic counselling should be offered to patients and their families to inform them about the disorder, its inheritance and its consequences.
- During a crisis, fluid therapy is essential to improve blood flow, reduce pain and prevent renal damage and dehydration.

Leukaemia

Case study

Mr John Tate is a 44-year-old policeman. He is married to Sarah and they have two sons aged 11 and 13 years. His wife is a teacher who is often busy with her work. Mr Tate enjoys socialising, keep-fit and reading.

Over the past 2–3 months Mr Tate has been feeling excessively tired. Although he sleeps well at night, he does not feel rested in the morning. Over the past 2 weeks, Mr Tate has been complaining of a sore throat, persistent colds and mouth ulcers. At first he attributed these symptoms to being tired and run down. His wife persuaded him to see his GP. After a thorough physical examination, it was decided that Mr Tate should be seen by a specialist at the hospital.

Mr Tate is seen by the haematology consultant at the local hospital and after some blood tests and investigations a provisional diagnosis of acute myeloid leukaemia is made. The consultant decided to admit Mr Tate for further investigations and treatment.

Take some time to reflect on this case and then consider the following.

1. Discuss the possible tests that may be done to confirm diagnosis.
2. What are the risk factors associated with acute myeloid leukaemia?
3. What advice would you give Mr Tate if he is to commence chemotherapy?
4. Outline Mr Tate's care during his stay in hospital.

Leukaemia is a malignant disorder where there is an abnormal or excessive proliferation of immature white blood cells. In the UK, leukaemia is the 12th most common cancer in adults, affecting more men than women. There are two principal types – acute and chronic leukaemia. Each of these is further subdivided:

*   acute myeloid leukaemia (AML)
*   acute lymphoblastic leukaemia (ALL)
*   chronic myeloid leukaemia (CML)
*   chronic lymphoblastic leukaemia (CLL).

Aetiology

The risk factors include:

*   exposure to radiation
*   exposure to benzene (one of the chemicals used in petrol and a solvent used in the rubber and plastic industry)
*   certain genetic conditions such as Down's syndrome
*   smoking
*   age – chronic leukaemia is more common over the age of 40 years
*   previous cancer treatments
*   diseases that affect the immune system such as HIV.

Pathophysiology

White blood cells are produced by the bone marrow. They then pass from the bone marrow into the bloodstream and the lymphatic system. White blood cells are involved in various functions of the body's immune system, which protects the body against infections.

Acute leukaemia is more aggressive and develops rapidly. It is more common in the younger age group and the symptoms develop quickly; if untreated, it becomes life-threatening. Leukaemic cells are immature and poorly differentiated; they proliferate rapidly, have a long lifespan and do not function normally. AML is overproduction of immature myeloid white blood cells and ALL is the overproduction of immature myeloid lymphocytes, called lymphoblasts. In acute leukaemia, the cells reproduce very quickly and do not become mature enough to carry out their role in the immune system.

CLL is more common in men and occurs most frequently between the ages of 50 and 70 years. In CLL, abnormal lymphocytes proliferate, accumulate in the blood and spread to the lymphatic tissue. Patients affected may live with symptoms for several years. CML has a gradual onset, occurring primarily between the ages 30 and 50 years, and the incidence is slightly higher in men. In CML, there is uncontrolled production of myeloid cells. These cells are abnormal and are not able to carry out the normal functions of white blood cells, such as fighting infections. Their lifespan is long, so over a period of time they replace normal functioning cells (red and white blood cells, and platelets) in the bone marrow (Blows, 2005). This is a slow process and progressively gets worse over time.

Symptoms

Common presenting symptoms include:

- tiredness, breathlessness and pale skin (due to anaemia and reduction in red blood cells)
- abnormal bleeding from the gums and epistaxis
- bone pain
- abdominal pain due to an enlarged spleen and/or liver
- swollen lymph glands in the groin, neck and under the arms
- weight loss.

Care and management

Patients suffering from leukaemia will need an accurate and full assessment of pain level, activity tolerance, vital signs, nutrition and signs of bleeding or infection in order to plan high-quality care.

- Advice on preventative measures for bleeding should be offered, i.e. the use of a soft-bristled toothbrush, safety in the use razors and measures to prevent falls.
- Patients will need advice on measures to maintain hydration and nutrition. Weight is monitored weekly in order to assess weight loss.
- Encourage patients and their relatives to discuss concerns and fears (which may include bone marrow and stem cell transplants).
- Stomatitis (inflammation of the mouth) is a common occurrence and therefore daily oral hygiene should be encouraged.
- Fatigue as a result of anaemia may be a problem and therefore patients should be advised to take frequent rest periods and not to over-exert themselves.

- Patients should be protected from infections, e.g. washing hands before and after attending to them and discouraging unnecessary visitation by relatives.

Pharmacological and non-pharmacological interventions

Medications and other treatments of leukaemia include:

- chemotherapy (use of cytotoxic drugs)
- radiotherapy
- stem cell and bone marrow transplants
- monoclonal antibodies
- ATRA (all trans-retinoic acid) is given alongside chemotherapy
- opioid drugs to control pain.

Thrombocytopenia

Thrombocytopenia is the term for a reduced platelet count. It occurs when platelets are lost from circulation faster than they are produced in the bone marrow. Haemorrhage from trauma or spontaneous bleeding may occur when the platelet count is below 20 000 per cubic millimetre of blood.

Aetiology

Many disease processes can cause thrombocytopenia:

- anaemia as a result of vitamin B_{12} or folic acid deficiency
- systemic lupus erythematous
- sepsis, systemic viral or bacterial infections
- chemotherapy
- radiation
- heparin-induced thrombocytopenia (white clot syndrome)
- HIV.

Pathophysiology

The pathophysiology is related to three basic mechanisms:

- accelerated platelet destruction
- defective platelet production
- disordered platelet distribution.

Three distinct types have been identified:

- idiopathic thrombocytopenic purpura (acute and chronic) (ITP)
- thrombotic thrombocytopenic purpura (TTP)
- haemolytic–uremic syndrome (HUS).

ITP is a disease in which antibodies form and destroy the body's platelets. As the destruction is believed to be caused by the body's immune system, it is classified as an autoimmune disorder.

Although the bone marrow increases the synthesis of platelets, it cannot keep up with the demand. Acute ITP is more common in children, while chronic ITP is more common in adults. Platelets become coated with antibodies as a result of the autoimmune response mediated by B lymphocytes. Although the platelets function normally, the spleen identifies them as foreign protein and destroys them.

TTP is a rare disease in which small blood clots form suddenly throughout the body. The numerous blood clots result in a high level of platelet usage in clotting, which reduces their number.

HUS is a rare disorder related to TTP in which the number of platelets decreases and there is reduction in the number of red blood cells. HUS can also occur with intestinal infections with *Escherichia coli* and with the use of some drugs such as cyclosporine.

Signs and symptoms

Patients with thrombocytopenia may experience:

- unexpected bruising
- petechiae (small red spots under the skin)
- bleeding from the gastrointestinal tract
- epistaxis (bleeding from the nose)
- pain in the joints and muscles
- heavier than usual menstrual periods in women.

Care and management

As a result of a low level of platelets, the patient is at risk of bleeding, especially from the gums. Early identification of bleeding is important in order to prevent blood loss.

- Monitor vital signs – heart rate, respiratory rate and blood pressure – every 4 hours. Observe for bleeding from other parts of the body, such as in the urine (haematuria), gastrointestinal tract, nasal membrane and vagina.
- Observe the skin for petechiae.
- Advise the patient about the use of safety measures to minimise the risk of bleeding, such as use of a soft-bristled toothbrush and an electric razor for shaving. Hard bristles may abrade the oral mucosa, causing bleeding, and increase the risk of infection.
- Encourage the patient to rinse the mouth with salt solution every 2–4 hours to maintain oral hygiene.
- Advise the patient to take 2–2.5 L of fluid over 24 hours to prevent dehydration and infection.
- Advise the patient to avoid medications that interfere with platelet function such as aspirin.
- A healthy diet high in fibre should be encouraged to prevent constipation. Straining to have a bowel movement could increase the risk of internal bleeding from the gastrointestinal tract.

Pharmacological and non-pharmacological interventions

- Platelet transfusion may be required to treat acute bleeding.
- Oral glucocorticoids such a prednisolone may be prescribed to suppress the autoimmune response.
- Splenectomy may be performed in patients with ITP.

Conclusion

This chapter has discussed some of the common disorders of blood the learner might encounter. Healthcare professionals need to have a good knowledge about the physiology of blood in order to understand the pathophysiology of blood disorders and to provide appropriate care. Patients are often frightened when they are informed that they have a certain blood disorder. It is the healthcare professionals' duty to ensure that the patient receives accurate information relating to their disease and to provide the necessary care.

Test your knowledge

- List the functions of blood.
- Explain the clotting process.
- Explain what would happen if a patient receives mismatched blood.
- Where is most of the body's blood found?
- If the blood in the veins is dark red, why does it appear bright red when the vein is cut and bleeding?

Activities

Here are some activities and exercises to help test your learning. For the answers to these exercises, as well as further self-testing activities, visit our website at www.wiley.com/go/fundamentalsofappliedpathophysiology

Fill in the blanks

The _____ of the _____ is to pump blood around the _____. The heart is a hollow, muscular _____ divided by a vertical _____ called the _____. These two _____ are further divided into the thin walled _____ above, and a thick walled _____ below, making four chambers. Between each pair of chambers are _____ preventing any back flow of _____. Blood vessels leaving the heart generally carry _____ blood through vessels known as _____. These are large, hollow, elastic tubes with thick muscular _____ that are designed to withstand the high pressure with the blood leaving the heart. Their size gradually _____ as they spread throughout the body, ultimately reaching fine, hair-like vessels known as _____. Blood vessels that return blood to the heart are known as _____ which carry _____ blood to the heart. They are elastic tubes containing valves to help prevent _____ of blood. Blood is forced through arteries by the pressure from the heart whereas venous flow is aided by muscular _____.

Choose from:
Valves; Arteries; Walls; Capillaries; Septum; Body; Heart; Veins; Back flow; Blood; Ventricle; Chambers; Oxygenated; Function; Wall; Diminishes; Atrium; Organ; Contraction; De-oxygenated

Label the diagram

Using the list of words supplied, label the diagram.

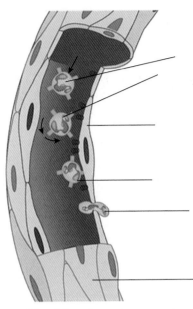

Blood flow through a vessel

Neutrophil; Endothelial cell; Sticking; Rolling; Blood vessel; Squeezing through endothelial cells

Word search

P	A	T	H	O	G	E	N	S	G	N	S	I	Y	A
I	I	T	A	H	A	B	A	M	E	U	N	I	M	N
N	T	M	E	O	M	A	I	G	E	L	O	D	O	T
E	I	I	M	I	E	N	I	L	I	H	I	I	T	I
L	R	C	O	U	E	T	C	M	E	S	T	O	C	B
O	C	G	S	L	N	U	N	I	L	A	A	P	E	O
N	O	I	T	A	N	I	T	U	L	G	G	A	R	D
I	T	N	A	A	N	D	T	U	S	T	E	T	T	I
N	A	M	S	A	I	E	G	Y	A	A	R	H	S	E
O	M	H	I	E	R	A	S	C	P	I	G	I	A	S
G	E	R	S	N	O	E	O	P	O	L	G	C	G	U
L	A	O	T	C	A	T	E	L	E	T	A	L	P	S
A	H	A	E	M	O	G	L	O	B	I	N	S	S	S
B	I	L	I	R	U	B	I	N	I	G	S	T	M	E
S	I	S	O	M	S	O	I	E	T	L	N	E	T	A

Antibodies	Coagulation	Haemoglobin
Agglutination	Gastrectomy	Osmosis
Aggregation	Haematocrit	Plasma
Antigen	Idiopathic	Platelet
Bile	Immunity	Pathogens
Bilirubin	Haemostasis	Nucleus

Further resources

Contact a Family

http://www.cafamily.org.uk/about.html
Students will find this website a useful source of information on leukaemia. Contact a Family provides support, advice and information for families with disabled children, no matter what their condition or disability. Patients can be referred to this website for support.

National Institute for Health and Clinical Excellence (NICE) – Treatment for chronic myeloid leukaemia

http://www.hc2d.co.uk/content.php?contentId=18399
In this press release article you can read about NICE's decision regarding commonly used expensive drugs for leukaemia. 'NICE has not been able to recommend dasatinib, high-dose imatinib or nilotinib for the treatment of CML (chronic myeloid leukaemia) that is resistant to standard-dose imatinib.'

National Institute for Health and Clinical Excellence (NICE) – Treatment of anaemia in patients with chronic kidney disease

http://www.nice.org.uk/newsroom/pressreleases/anaemiamanagementinckd.jsp
This link gives NICE guidance on how to treat anaemia in people with chronic kidney disease. It is a useful link for your studies of blood disorders.

Sheffield NHS

http://www.sheffield.nhs.uk/library/resources/ebpnews/ebpnewsnov10.pdf

This news bulletin summarises recent developments in evidence-based practice. It contains news items taken from the *Daily Health Bulletin* and contents listings of new issues of evidence-based practice journals held in the Health Library. Students will find a variety of web links to various healthcare issues.

Biomedical Central

http://www.biomedcentral.com/bmcblooddisord/
BMC Blood Disorders is an open access journal publishing original peer-reviewed research articles in all aspects of the prevention, diagnosis and management of blood disorders, as well as related molecular genetics, pathophysiology and epidemiology. Students may find this website too high powered, but nevertheless a useful site for reference.

National Heart, Lung and Blood Institute

http://www.nhlbi.nih.gov/health/dci/Diseases/bmsct/bmsct_whatis.html
This is a good web link to find out about bone marrow stem cell transplant in patients with blood disorders. This link provides an overview of the type of patients who may need a stem cell transplant and some of the issues before and after the treatment.

Glossary of terms

Adenosine triphosphate (ATP):	a compound of an adenosine molecule with three attached phosphoric acid molecules. Essential for the production of cellular energy.
Agglutination:	a process by which red blood cells adhere to one another.
Antibody:	a protein in the blood that binds specifically to a particular foreign substance (its antigen). It is a major part of the immune system.
Antigen:	a foreign substance (e.g. an infecting micro-organism) that can be recognised by the immune system and generates an antibody response.
Bile:	an alkaline fluid secreted by the liver that aids digestion of lipids.
Bilirubin:	a pigment found in bile resulting from the destruction of red blood cells.

Blood groups:	the classification of blood based on the type of antigen found on the surface of the red blood cell.
B lymphocyte:	a type of lymphocyte that produces specific antibodies.
Coagulation:	the process of transforming a liquid into a solid (especially a blood clot) or the hardening of tissue by physical means.
Coenzyme:	a molecule that binds to an enzyme and is essential for its activity, but is not permanently altered by the reaction.
Connective tissue:	a primary tissue characterised by cells separated by a matrix; supports and binds other body tissue.
Epistaxis:	bleeding from the nose.
Erythrocyte:	another name for a red blood cell.
Erythropoietin:	a hormone produced by the kidneys that regulates the production of red blood cells.
Gastrectomy:	excision of part or the whole of the stomach.
Haematocrit:	the percentage of blood volume occupied by erythrocytes.
Haemoglobin:	a protein consisting of globin and four haem groups that is found within erythrocytes (red blood cells). Responsible for the transport of oxygen.
Haemostasis:	the stoppage of bleeding.
Homeostasis:	maintenance of relatively constant conditions within the body's internal environment despite external environment changes.
Idiopathic:	without a known cause.
Immunity:	a protective mechanism that forms antibodies to help protect the body against foreign substances.
Immunoglobulin:	another name for antibody. Antibodies are opsonins that are manufactured by the B lymphocytes and help the phagocytic cells to destroy invading micro-organisms in the immune response.
Intrinsic factor:	a protein secreted by the parietal cells of the gastric glands and essential for the absorption of vitamin B_{12}.
Lysozyme:	a bacteria-destroying enzyme found in lysosomes, sweat, tears, saliva and other bodily secretions..
Mesenchyme:	the embryonic mesoderm that develops into connective tissue.
Mitochondria:	cytoplasmic organelles responsible for ATP production.

Molecule:	a particle containing two or more atoms joined together by chemical bonds.
Nucleus:	a large organelle that contains genetic information and acts as the control centre of the cell.
Organelle:	a structural and functional part of a cell that acts like a human organ to fulfil all the needs of the cell so that it can grow, reproduce and carry out its functions.
Osmosis:	the passive movement of water through a selectively permeable membrane from an area of high concentration of a chemical to an area of low concentration.
Pathogen:	a micro-organism that causes problems – is 'infectious'.
Phagocyte:	white blood cell that engulfs and destroys micro-organism.
Plasma:	the fluid component of the blood.
Platelet:	a type of blood cell important in blood clotting.
Polypeptide:	a chain of amino acids.
Urobilinogen:	a product of bilirubin breakdown.
White blood cell:	a leucocyte.

References

Alexander, M.F., Fawcett, J. and Runciman, P.J. (2007). *Nursing Practice – Hospitals and Home*, 3rd edn. Edinburgh: Churchill Livingstone.

Blows, W.T. (2005). *The Biological Basis of Nursing: Cancer*. London: Routledge.

Bullock, B.A. and Henze, R.L. (2010). *Focus on Pathophysiology*. Philadelphia: Lippincott.

Jamieson, E.M., McCall, J.M. and Whyte, C.A. (2007). *Clinical Nursing Practice*, 5th edn. Edinburgh: Churchill Livingstone.

Kozier, B., Erb, G., Berman, A., Snyder, S.J., Lake, R. and Harvey, S. (2008). *Fundamentals of Nursing. Concepts, Processes and Practice*. Harlow: Pearson Education.

Mader, S.S. (2011). *Understanding Human Anatomy and Physiology*. Boston: McGraw Hill.

Marieb, E.N. and Hoehn, K. (2010). *Human Anatomy and Physiology*, 8th edn. San Francisco: Pearson Benjamin Cummings.

Mehta, A. and Hoffbrand, V. (2009). *Haematology at a Glance*. Oxford: Blackwell.

Nursing and Midwifery Council (2009). *Record Keeping: Guidance for Nurses and Midwives*. London: Nursing and Midwifery Council.

Porth, C.M. (2010). *Pathophysiology: Concepts of Altered Health States*, 8th edn. Philadelphia: Lippincott Williams & Wilkins.

Stanfield, C.L. (2011). *Principles of Human Physiology*, 4th edn. Boston: Benjamin Cummings.

Waugh, A. and Grant, A. (2010). *Ross and Wilson: Anatomy and Physiology in Health and Illness*, 11th edn. Edinburgh: Churchill Livingstone.

8

The renal system and associated disorders

Muralitharan Nair

Senior Lecturer, Department of Adult Nursing and Primary Care, School of Health and Social Work, University of Hertfordshire, Hatfield, Hertfordshire, UK

Contents

Fundamentals of Applied Pathophysiology: An Essential Guide for Nursing and Healthcare Students, Second Edition. Edited by Muralitharan Nair and Ian Peate.
© 2013 John Wiley & Sons, Ltd. Published 2013 by John Wiley & Sons, Ltd.

Key words

- Kidneys
- Hilus
- Renal artery
- Nephron
- Ureter
- Renal medulla
- Renal vein
- Glomerulus
- Urethra
- Renal cortex
- Renal pelvis
- Filtration

Test your prior knowledge

- Name four functions of the kidneys.
- Which substances are reabsorbed and which are excreted by the kidneys?
- List the composition of urine.
- What is the colour of urine? Think about the destruction of the red blood cells.

Learning outcomes

On completion of this section the reader will be able to:

- Describe the structure and function of the kidney.
- Describe the microscopic structure of the kidney.
- Explain glomerular filtration.
- List the chemical composition of urine.

Don't forget to log on to the companion website for this book (www.wiley.com/go/ fundamentalsofappliedpathophysiology) where you can find self-assessment tests to check your progress, as well as lots of activities to practise your learning.

Introduction

The kidneys play an important role in maintaining homeostasis. They remove waste products through the production and excretion of urine, and regulate fluid balance in the body. As part of their function, the kidneys filter essential substances such as sodium and potassium from the blood and selectively reabsorb substances essential to maintain homeostasis. Any substances that are not essential are excreted in the urine. The formation of urine is achieved through the processes of filtration, selective reabsorption and excretion. The kidneys also have an endocrine function, secreting hormones such as renin and erythropoietin. This chapter discusses the structure and functions of the renal system. It also describes some common disorders and their related care, management and treatment.

The renal system

The renal system, also known as the urinary system (Figure 8.1) consists of the:

- kidneys
- ureters
- urinary bladder
- urethra.

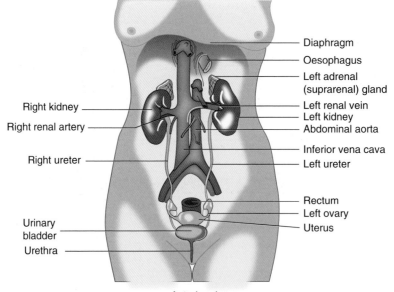

Anterior view

Figure 8.1   Renal system.

The organs of the renal system ensure that a stable internal environment is maintained for the survival of cells and tissues in the body – homeostasis.

Kidneys

External structures

There are two kidneys, one on each side of the spinal column. They are approximately 11 cm long, 5–6 cm wide and 3–4 cm thick (Marieb and Hoehn, 2010). They are bean-shaped organs where the outer border is convex; the inner border is known as the hilum (also known as the hilus), and it is from here that the renal arteries, renal veins, nerves and ureters enter and leave the kidneys. The right kidney is in contact with the liver's large right lobe and hence the right kidney is approximately 2–4 cm lower than the left kidney.

Three layers cover and support the kidneys (Figure 8.2):

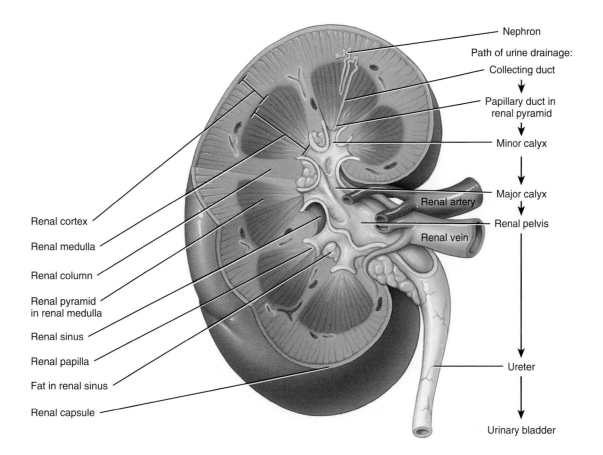

Figure 8.2   External layers of the kidney.

- renal fascia – outer layer
- adipose tissue – middle layer
- renal capsule – inner layer.

Internal structures

There are three distinct regions inside a kidney (Figure 8.3):

- renal cortex
- renal medulla
- renal pelvis.

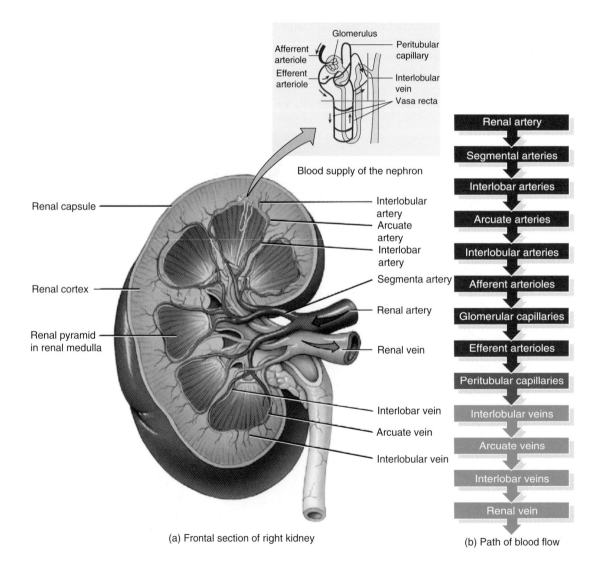

(a) Frontal section of right kidney

(b) Path of blood flow

Figure 8.3   Internal structures showing blood vessels.

The renal cortex is the outermost part of the kidney. It is reddish brown and has a granular appearance, which is due to the capillaries and the structures of the nephron. The medulla is lighter in colour and has an abundance of blood vessels and tubules of the nephron (Figure 8.3). The medulla consists of approximately 8–12 renal pyramids (Figure 8.3). The renal pelvis is formed from the expanded upper portion of the ureter and is funnel shaped. It collects urine from the calyces (Figure 8.2) and transports it to the urinary bladder.

Nephrons

These are small structures found in the kidney. There are over one million nephrons per kidney and it is in these structures that urine is formed (Figure 8.4). The nephrons:

- filter blood
- perform selective reabsorption
- excrete unwanted waste products from the filtered blood.

The nephron is divided into several sections and each section performs a different function (Figure 8.4).

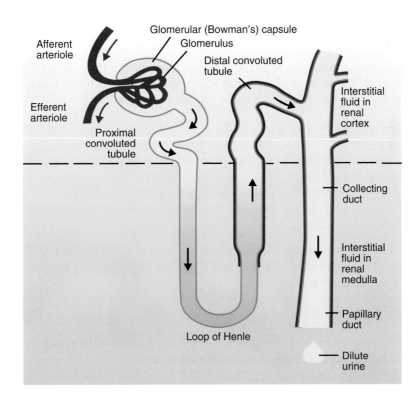

Figure 8.4 Nephron.

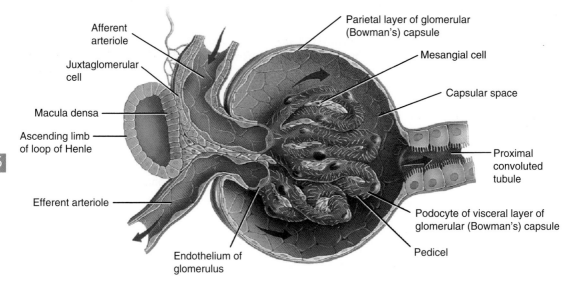

Figure 8.5　Bowman's capsule.

Bowman's capsule

Also known as the glomerular capsule, this is the first portion of the nephron (Figure 8.5). It is in this section that the network of capillaries, called the glomerulus (Marieb and Hoehn 2010), is found. Filtration of blood takes place in this portion of the nephron.

Proximal convoluted tubule

From the Bowman's capsule, the filtrate drains into the proximal convoluted tubule (Figure 8.4). The cells lining this portion of the tubule actively reabsorb water, nutrients and ions into the peritubular fluid (the interstitial fluid surrounding the renal tubule).

Loop of Henle

The proximal convoluted tubule then bends into the loop of Henle (Figure 8.4). The loop of Henle is divided into the descending and ascending loop. The ascending loop of Henle is much thicker than the descending portion.

Distal convoluted tubule

The thick ascending portion of the loop of Henle leads into the distal convoluted tubule (Figure 8.4). The distal convoluted tubule is an important site for:

- active secretion of ions and acids
- selective reabsorption of sodium and calcium ions
- selective reabsorption of water.

Collecting ducts

The distal convoluted tubule then drains into the collecting ducts (Figure 8.4). Several collecting ducts converge and drain into a larger system called the papillary ducts, which in turn empties into the minor calyx (plural – calyces). From here the filtrate, now called urine, drains into the renal pelvis.

Functions of the kidney

The kidneys maintain fluid, electrolyte and acid–base balance of the blood. Functions of the kidney can be summarized as:

- filtration
- regulation of blood volume
- regulation of osmolarity
- secretion of renin and erythropoietin
- maintenance of acid–base balance
- synthesis of vitamin D
- detoxification of free radicals and drugs
- gluconeogenesis.

Blood supply

Approximately 1200 mL of blood flows through the kidney each minute. Each kidney receives its blood supply directly from the aorta via the renal artery (Figure 8.2) which divides into the anterior and posterior renal arteries. Two large veins emerge from the hilus and empty into the inferior vena cava.

Urine formation

Three processes are involved in the formation of urine:

- filtration
- selective reabsorption
- secretion.

Filtration

Filtration takes place in the glomerulus, which lies in the Bowman's capsule. The blood for filtration is supplied by the renal artery. In the kidney, the renal artery divides into smaller arterioles. The arteriole entering the Bowman's capsule is called the afferent arteriole, which further subdivides into a cluster of capillaries called the glomerulus. The fluid from the filtered blood is protein free but contains electrolytes such as sodium chloride, potassium chloride and waste products of cellular metabolism, e.g. urea, uric acid and creatinine (McCance et al., 2010). The filtered blood then returns to the circulation via the efferent arteriole and finally the renal vein.

Selective reabsorption

Selective reabsorption processes ensure that any substances in the filtrate that are essential for body function are reabsorbed into the plasma. Substances such as sodium, calcium, potassium and chloride are reabsorbed to maintain the fluid and electrolyte balance and the pH of blood. However, if these substances are in excess of body requirements, they are excreted in the urine.

Secretion

Any substances not removed through filtration are secreted into the renal tubules from the peritubular capillaries (Figure 8.6) of the nephron (Waugh and Grant, 2010); these include drugs and hydrogen ions.

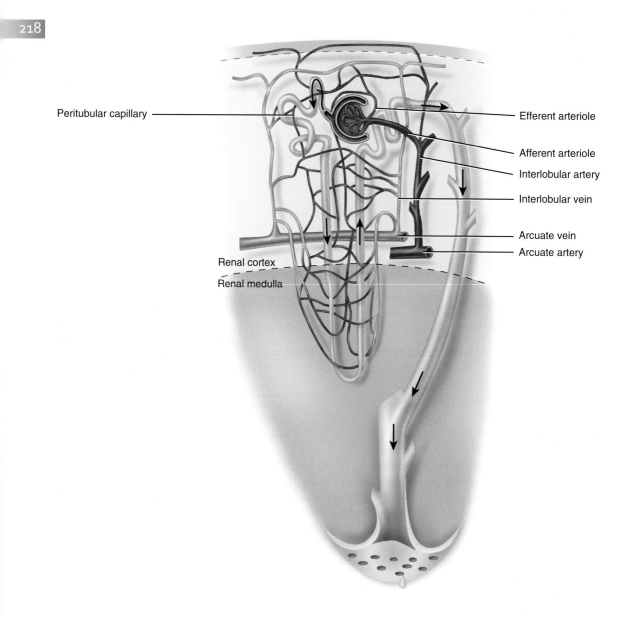

Figure 8.6   Nephron with capillaries.

Table 8.1 Summary of the solutes of the kidney.

Inorganic solutes	Organic solutes
Sodium	Urea
Potassium	Creatinine
Calcium	Uric acid
Magnesium	
Iron	
Chloride	
Sulphate	
Phosphate	
Bicarbonate	
Ammonia	

Adapted from Mader (2011).

Composition of urine

Urine is a sterile and clear fluid containing nitrogenous waste and salts. It is transparent with an amber or light yellow colour. It is slightly acidic and the pH may range from 4.5 to 8. The pH is affected by an individual's dietary intake. Diet that is high in animal protein tends to make the urine more acidic, while a vegetarian diet may make the urine more alkaline.

Urine is 96% water and approximately 4% solutes. The solutes include organic and inorganic waste products (Table 8.1).

Ureters

The ureters are approximately 25–30 cm in length and 5 mm in diameter (Mader, 2011) and they extend from the kidney to the bladder. The ureters terminate at the bladder and enter obliquely through the muscle wall of the bladder. They pass over the pelvic brim at the bifurcation of the common iliac arteries (Figure 8.7).

The ureters have three layers:

- transitional epithelial mucosa (inner layer)
- smooth muscle layer (middle layer)
- fibrous connective tissue (outer layer).

Urine is propelled from the kidney to the bladder by peristaltic contraction of the ureters.

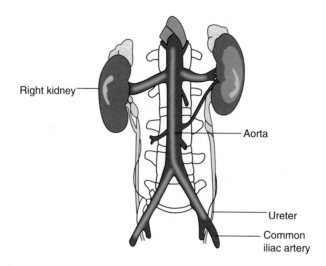

Figure 8.7   Common iliac vessels and ureter.

Urinary bladder

The urinary bladder is located in the pelvic cavity posterior to the symphysis pubis. In the male, the bladder lies anterior to the rectum and in the female, it lies anterior to the vagina and inferior to the uterus (Mader, 2011); it is a smooth muscular sac which stores urine. As urine accumulates, the bladder expands without a significant rise in the internal pressure of the bladder. The bladder normally distends and holds approximately 350 mL of urine.

The urinary bladder has three layers (Figure 8.8):

- transitional epithelial mucosa
- a thick muscular layer
- a fibrous outer layer.

Urethra

The urethra is a muscular tube that drains urine from the bladder and conveys it out of the body. The urethra varies in length in both males and females. Sphincters keep the urethra closed when urine is not being passed. The internal urethral sphincter is under involuntary control and lies at the bladder–urethra junction. The external urethral sphincter is under voluntary control.

The male urethra passes through three different regions:

- prostatic region – passes through the prostate gland
- membranous portion – passes through the pelvic diaphragm
- penile region – extends the length of the penis.

The female urethra is bound to the anterior vaginal wall. The external opening of the urethra is anterior to the vagina and posterior to the clitoris (Figure 8.9).

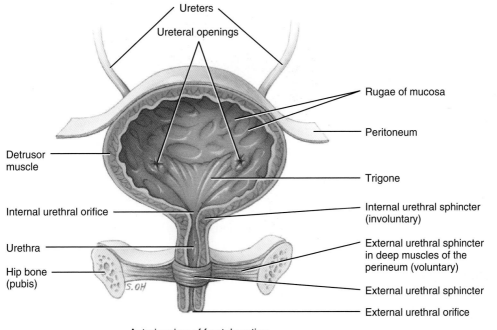

Ureters

Ureteral openings

Rugae of mucosa

Peritoneum

Detrusor
muscle

Trigone

Internal urethral orifice

Internal urethral sphincter
(involuntary)

Urethra

External urethral sphincter
in deep muscles of the
perineum (voluntary)

Hip bone
(pubis)

External urethral sphincter

External urethral orifice

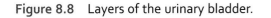
Anterior view of frontal section

Figure 8.8   Layers of the urinary bladder.

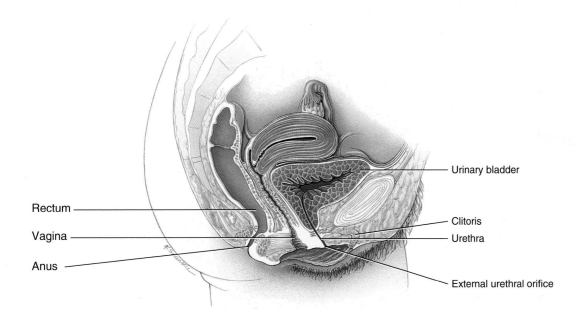

Urinary bladder

Rectum

Vagina

Clitoris

Urethra

Anus

External urethral orifice

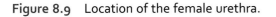
Figure 8.9   Location of the female urethra.

Disorders of the renal system

Learning outcomes

On completion of this section the reader will be able to:

* List some of the common diseases of the renal system and identify risk factors associated with the diseases.

* Describe the pathophysiological processes related to specific renal disorders.

* List the possible investigations.

* Outline the care, management and interventions related to the disorders described.

Case study

Mrs Goldstein Spears is a 32-year-old woman who presents with a 48-hour history of needing to urinate frequently, and it hurts when she does. Mrs Spears also thinks she may have seen blood in her urine but is not sure. She says that she has never had a urinary tract infection (UTI) as an adult, but had a UTI as a child. She has some back and loin pain, but no vaginal irritation or discharge. She takes the oral contraceptive pill and tells you it is extremely unlikely she is pregnant as she had her period last week.

Take some time to reflect on this case and then consider the following.

1. What other information about her clinical history would you like to know?
2. You have been asked to do Mrs Spears' urinalysis. Explain why you are doing the urinalysis and explain any abnormal findings.
3. What advice would you offer Mrs Spears to prevent reoccurrence of her UTI?
4. Outline a plan of care for Mrs Spears.

Pyelonephritis

Pyelonephritis is inflammation of the renal pelvis and the functional units of the kidney (nephrons). It involves the cortex and the medulla, which is called the parenchyma of the kidney. The incidence is higher in women than in men. There are two main types – acute and chronic pyelonephritis.

Acute pyelonephritis

In acute pyelonephritis, there is sudden or severe infection of the kidney by Gram-negative bacteria such as *Escherichia coli* and *Proteus mirabilis*. Gram-negative bacteria are those that do not retain crystal violet dye after an alcohol wash. They may have a red or pink colouration when another dye such as safranin is added to the slide. Gram-positive bacteria will retain the dye and have a purple colouration. They usually ascend from the lower urinary tract (urethra and urinary bladder). In men, prostatitis and prostatic hypertrophy causing urethral obstruction predispose to bacterial infection. Acute pyelonephritis can be caused by blood infection such as septicaemia.

Signs and symptoms

Patients with acute pyelonephritis may present with the following signs and symptoms:

- sudden onset of fever
- chills
- nausea
- vomiting
- groin pain
- haematuria
- dysuria
- rigor.

Investigations

The following may be carried out to confirm diagnosis:

- midstream specimen or catheter specimen of urine to identify causative organism
- full blood count – raised white blood cells may indicate urine infection
- intravenous pyelogram to identify any obstruction in the urinary tract
- full nursing and medical history to identify any previous urinary tract infection and kidney stones.

Care and management

Patients with acute pyelonephritis should be encouraged to be on bed rest until symptoms of pyrexia and the severe groin pain subside. It is important to observe for and report signs of pain, such as restlessness, tachycardia and sweating, in order to take prompt action.

Intravenous fluid therapy may be commenced in the early stages if the patient is unable to take oral fluids due to nausea and vomiting. When able to take oral fluids, the patient should be encouraged to take 2.5–3 L (Thomas, 2008) of fluid per day to increase urine production and lessen the irritation of urethral mucosa on micturition.

LeMone et al. (2011) report that the female patient should be instructed in proper cleansing of the perineal region. They should be instructed to wipe front to back after voiding urine or defecating, and advised to void urine before and after sexual intercourse in an attempt to flush out bacteria that may have been introduced into the urethra and the bladder.

Vital signs such as temperature, heart rate and respiratory rate should be monitored hourly for the first 24–48 hours to check the effect of treatment.

Patients will need psychological support and reassurance during the course of the illness and should have the opportunity to ask questions and voice their anxiety (Alexander et al., 2007). Patients will need information on how to recognise the signs and symptoms of urinary tract infection and to take preventative measures.

Pharmacological interventions

The following medications may be prescribed to treat acute pyelonephritis:

- analgesics for pain management
- antibiotics to treat the infection
- anti-emetics for nausea and vomiting
- antipyretics to treat the pyrexia.

Chronic pyelonephritis

Chronic pyelonephritis progresses from acute pyelonephritis. The calyces and the renal pelvis of the kidney are affected. Chronic pyelonephritis can begin in childhood. Repeated urinary tract infections can lead to scaring and fibrosis of the kidney destroys the parenchyma. Over a period of time, the kidneys become small and irregular in shape, resulting in renal failure.

Signs and symptoms

This condition may be asymptomatic in the early stages and until the patient presents with renal failure. The patient may present with:

- fever
- abdominal and groin pain
- hypertension
- dysuria
- uraemia
- proteinuria.

Investigations

The investigations are the same as those for acute pyelonephritis.

Care and management

The care and management of the patient with chronic pyelonephritis is the same as for acute pyelonephritis. However, patients who have recurrence of urinary tract infection may require long-term antibiotic therapy. In the event of renal failure as a result of kidney damage, the patient may need kidney dialysis. Healthcare professional should prepare and educate the patient in lifestyle changes resulting from kidney dialysis, such as diet and fluid intake.

Cystitis

Cystitis is the inflammation of the urinary bladder and the inflamed bladder may haemorrhage. Cystitis is the most common form of urinary tract infection and affects women more than men. The bacteria responsible for the infection are *E. coli*, which is found in the lower gastrointestinal tract, and *P. mirabilis*. In women, the bacteria gain entry into the urinary bladder through the short female urethra. Cystitis can also result from non-bacterial irritation, such as from clothing that is made from synthetic fibres, hygiene sprays and talcum powder.

Aetiology

There are several causes:

- bacterial infection
- sexual intercourse
- pregnancy
- rectal intercourse
- urinary tract obstruction as a result of an enlarged prostate gland
- chemicals in washing powder
- nylon underwear
- talcum powder
- stress.

Investigations

Midstream specimen urine should be cultured to identify the organism.

- sometimes a flexible cystoscopy may be carried out to detect abnormalities
- urine cytology to rule out renal cancer.

Signs and symptoms

The patient may present with the following signs and symptoms:

- dysuria
- urgency
- pyuria
- haematuria
- abdominal discomfort
- nocturia
- urinary incontinence.

Care and management

The main objective is to identify the cause of cystitis in order to offer the correct treatment; cystitis may not be the result of bacterial contamination. The patient will need reassurance, psychological support and health education. With recurrent urinary tract infection, the patient may need long-term antibiotic therapy. The patient should be advised on the importance of taking the prescribed medication. Information on side effects of antibiotics, such as diarrhoea, vomiting and allergic reactions, should be provided by the nurses.

Unless contraindicated, the patient should be advised to take 2.5–3 L of fluid per day (Thomas, 2008). This helps with the production of urine and to flush out any bacteria in the renal tract. Measurements of vital signs, e.g. temperature and pulse, should be recorded every 4 hours until symptoms of cystitis subside or as the patient's condition dictates. Health education is the same as for the patient with acute pyelonephritis. Unless contraindicated, advise the patient to drink two glasses of cranberry or blueberry juice per day to maintain an acidic urine (LeMone et al., 2011). These fruit juices contain benzoic acid, which coats the lining of the bladder wall and prevents bacteria from infiltrating into the bladder wall. Advise the patient to avoid materials or chemicals that may cause bladder irritation, such as underwear made from synthetic material, the use of hygiene sprays or bubble bath.

Acute kidney injury and chronic kidney disease

Acute kidney injury (AKI), previously known as acute renal failure (ARF), is a condition in which the kidneys are unable to remove accumulated metabolites from the blood, leading to altered fluid, electrolyte and acid–base balance. The cause may be a primary kidney disorder, or renal failure may be secondary to a systemic disease or other urological defects. AKI may be either acute or chronic.

Chronic kidney disease (CKD), previously known as chronic renal failure (CRF), is a silent disease, developing slowly and insidiously, with few symptoms until the kidneys are severely damaged and unable to meet the excretory needs of the body.

Both forms are characterized by azotemia – increased levels of nitrogenous waste in the blood.

Acute kidney injury

AKI is the acute decline in renal function leading to azotemia (accumulation of nitrogenous waste in the blood), and fluid and electrolyte imbalance. AKI has an abrupt onset and with prompt intervention is often reversible; if left untreated it leads to permanent renal damage.

Pathophysiology

The causes of AKI can be categorised into prerenal, intrarenal and postrenal (Table 8.2). Prerenal AKI is the most common, accounting for about 55% of the total. In prerenal AKI, hypoperfusion leads to AKI without directly affecting the integrity of the kidney tissue. Intrinsic (or intrarenal) AKI, due to direct damage to the functional kidney tissue, is responsible for another 40%. Urinary tract obstruction with resulting kidney damage is the precipitating factor for postrenal AKI, the least common form.

Prerenal

Prerenal causes include insufficient blood flow to the kidneys, resulting in reduced cardiac output as a result of heart failure, hypovolaemia resulting from haemorrhage and shock. The kidneys receive 20–25% of cardiac output to maintain glomerular filtration (LeMone *et al.*, 2011). With a

Table 8.2 Summary of aetiology of acute kidney injury.

Prerenal	Intrarenal	Postrenal
Haemorrhage	Glomerulonephritis	Ureteric calculi
Low cardiac output	Hypertension	Neoplasm
Myocardial disease	Nephrotoxic drugs	Prostatic hyperplasia
Shock	Bacterial toxins	Phimosis
Heart failure	Chemicals	Urethral stricture
Liver failure		
Severe dehydration		

Adapted from Bullock and Henze (2010).

reduction in renal blood flow, glomerular filtration is affected and this causes ischaemic changes to the renal tissues.

Intrarenal

Intrarenal failure results from conditions that impair renal function. The renal parenchyma and nephrons are damaged, leading to renal failure. Glomerulonephritis, hypertension, chemicals such as ethyl glycol and drugs, e.g. antibiotics, can all affect renal function.

The nephrons of the kidneys are susceptible to trauma from poor renal blood flow, hypertension and shock. The cell membranes of the nephrons are damaged as a result of the trauma. The renal tubules become blocked with debris, thus increasing tubular pressure, resulting in poor elimination of sodium, water and metabolic waste.

Nephrotoxic drugs such as aminoglycoside antibiotics, non-steroidal anti-inflammatory drugs and toxins from bacteria destroy tubular cells. The damaged tubular cells become permeable to water, sodium and metabolic waste.

Postrenal

Postrenal failure results from obstruction along the ureters, urinary bladder and urethra. Obstruction resulting from stones in the ureters, prostatic hyperplasia and urethral stricture could restrict urine flow, leading to postrenal failure.

Investigations

The following investigations may be carried out:

- full blood count may indicate reduced red blood cell count, anaemia
- urea and electrolyte studies may indicate an increase in urea level and electrolyte imbalance, such as hyperkalemia and hyponatraemia
- urinalysis may indicate proteinuria, haematuria and increased cell casts
- intravenous pyelogram is carried out to evaluate renal function
- abdominal X-ray may be performed to identify obstructions
- renal biopsy may be necessary to differentiate between acute kidney injury and chronic kidney disease
- ultrasound may be carried out to identify the cause of renal failure
- arterial blood gases may indicate metabolic acidosis.

Signs and symptoms

- sudden onset
- oliguria to anuria
- nausea
- vomiting
- hyperkalaemia

Stages

AKI progresses through three phases – anuric, oliguric and diuretic.

The anuric phase can last from hours to days. During this period, kidney function is suppressed. The patient is oliguric or anuric during this phase. Haemorrhage may be a problem if there is tubular damage.

During the oliguric phase, which can last from 1 to 2 weeks, urine output is minimal (Alexander *et al.*, 2007). Fluid and electrolyte imbalance occurs during this phase and the specific gravity of urine is the same as plasma. Serum creatinine and blood urea and nitrogen (BUN) levels are elevated.

The final stage is the diuretic phase. During this phase, kidney function returns and urine production increases (diuresis). Diuresis can last for 24 hours and the patient may pass approximately 4–6 L of urine per day. Although a large volume of urine is produced, full renal function is still impaired. Dehydration is a problem as a result of increased fluid loss and the inability of the kidneys to perform selective reabsorption.

Care and management

A full nursing assessment of vital signs, weight, fluid intake and output, nursing history and assessment of the patient's knowledge of the disease process should all be carried out in order to provide high-quality care.

It is important to alleviate patient's and relatives' worries and anxieties. Healthcare professionals should give the patient time to ask questions, and should respond appropriately. Psychological care is important in the care and management of the patient with AKI.

An accurate fluid intake and output should be maintained to prevent fluid overload in the early stages of the disease and dehydration in the diuretic phase.

Strict nutritional status should be maintained. Protein intake should be limited to minimise the increase in nitrogenous compounds. Carbohydrate should be increased to provide energy (LeMone *et al.*, 2011).

A patient's vital signs should be monitored hourly to 2 hourly in the initial stages of the disease. Any changes should be reported immediately in order to allow prompt action to be taken.

Healthcare professionals should educate the patient in monitoring weight, vital signs and fluid intake.

Pharmacological interventions

The patient may be prescribed the following medications:

- furosemide to induce diuresis
- antihypertensives, such as angiotensin converting enzyme (ACE) inhibitors, for the patient's hypertension
- antacids to prevent gastric ulcers
- analgesia for pain.

It is the healthcare professional's duty to educate the patient to recognise side effects of the prescribed medications.

Chronic kidney disease

Chronic kidney disease (CKD) is defined as the progressive reduction in renal function over months to years. The condition is irreversible and eventually affects all the organs of the body. The parenchyma and the nephrons are destroyed and the renal function progressively diminishes.

Aetiology

There are many causes for CKD, including (Alexander *et al.*, 2007):

- renal disease such as polycystic disease
- arteriosclerosis
- chronic glomerulonephritis
- chronic pyelonephritis
- tuberculosis of the kidneys
- diabetes nephropathy
- hypertension
- renal calculi
- prostatic hypertrophy.

Investigations

- urinalysis to detect abnormalities and specific gravity
- BUN and electrolyte levels are carried out to determine renal function
- urine culture to identify urinary tract infection
- renal biopsy to detect kidney diseases
- full blood count to identify the extent of anaemia
- renal ultrasound to determine the size of the kidney.

Signs and symptoms

In the early stages of the disease the patient may be asymptomatic. As the disease progresses the patient may present with the following symptoms:

- lethargy
- headache
- breathlessness
- proteinuria
- haematuria
- oliguria, anuria
- symptoms of anaemia
- hypertension
- pallor.

Pathophysiology

The pathophysiology of CKD involves the gradual loss of nephrons and the renal mass progressively gets smaller. There are three phases to CKD – early phase, second phase and third phase. In the early phase, the BUN levels are elevated (2–5 mg/mL) and the glomerular filtration rate is greatly reduced. During this phase, the unaffected nephrons compensate until they are damaged. The patient may be asymptomatic.

In the second phase, the BUN levels are above 10 mg/mL and creatinine is above 0.4 mg/mL. The glomerular filtration rate is greatly reduced. The patient may present with symptoms such as nocturia and anaemia.

In the third phase, the BUN levels are above 20 mg/mL and the creatinine is above 0.5 mg/mL. The glomerular filtration rate is greatly reduced and most of the nephrons are damaged. The patient may present with symptoms of CKD (see earlier for signs and symptoms).

Care and management

The patient and their relatives will require support to come to terms with the disease. The disease is not curable and can lead to death. The healthcare professional should encourage the patient to express their feelings or concerns and assist the patient with coping strategies. If necessary, the patient should be referred to specialist nurses such as the palliative care team.

A full nursing assessment of the patient is important in order to plan and implement high-quality care. The assessment should include the general condition of the patient, vital signs and the patient's knowledge of the disease and support systems.

Vital signs should be monitored and recorded every 2–4 hours and any changes reported immediately in order to allow prompt action to be taken. Fluid intake and output should be monitored to prevent fluid depletion or fluid overload.

Assistance should be provided in maintaining personal hygiene, such as oral hygiene, washing and dressing.

A diet should be recommended that is low in sodium and protein, and high in carbohydrate.

The patient with CKD may need dialysis and it is the healthcare professional's duty to ensure that safety is maintained at all times. Strict asepsis should be adhered to when the patient is receiving dialysis. Whether the patient has an arteriovenous fistula or peritoneal dialysis, the wound site should be observed for any signs of infection, such as pyrexia, tachycardia and inflammation. This should be reported immediately to allow prompt action to be taken. All care given should be documented in accordance with the Nursing and Midwifery Council guidelines (Nursing and Midwifery Council, 2010). The effects and side effects of prescribed medications should be documented (Nursing and Midwifery Council, 2009).

Pharmacological interventions

The following medications may be prescribed for CKD:

- diuretics such furosemide to decrease fluid load
- antihypertensive, e.g. ACE inhibitors
- iron and folic acid for the treatment of anaemia
- analgesia if the patient is in pain.

Case study

Mr Lee Hong is a 38-year-old owner of a small restaurant. He lives with his wife and their two children. One day while at work, Mr Hong collapsed with severe pain around his kidney region. His wife, who was at work with him, called for an ambulance and Mr Hong was rushed to the local hospital. On arrival at the accident and emergency department, Mr Hong was still in a lot of pain and asked the student nurse for a urinal to pass some urine. He passed approximately 100 ml of urine and gave it to the student nurse. The student nurse observed that Mr Hong had blood in his urine. Mr Hong was examined by the duty doctor and a provisional diagnosis of renal colic was made.

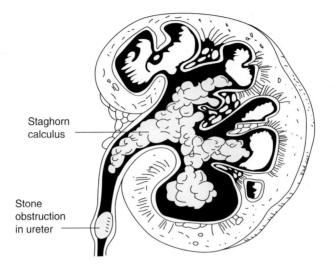

Staghorn calculus

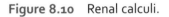

Stone obstruction in ureter

Figure 8.10   Renal calculi.

Take some time to reflect on this case and then consider the following.

1. Discuss the possible medications that may be prescribed for Mr Hong.
2. Explain the role of the drugs you have identified.
3. What advice would you offer Mr Hong regarding his fluid and dietary intake.
4. What advice would you give Mr Hong to prevent a future reoccurrence of his problem?

Renal calculi

Renal calculi are stones in the urinary tract and are the most common cause of upper urinary tract obstruction (Figure 8.10) (Porth, 2010). Men are more at risk than women. Stones may develop and obstruct any part of the urinary tract.

Aetiology

Some of the causes include:

- dehydration
- immobility
- carcinoma of the bone
- urinary tract infection
- excessive dietary intake of calcium
- excessive dietary intake of vitamin D
- excessive dietary intake of protein

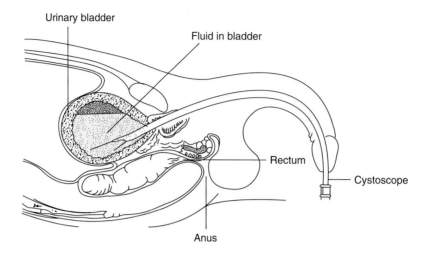

Figure 8.11   Cystoscopy.

- gout
- hyperparathyroidism
- family history of kidney stones increases the risk of developing kidney stones.

Investigations

- urinalysis to detect urinary tract infection and haematuria
- abdominal X-ray to identify urinary obstruction
- ultrasound to determine urinary obstruction
- intravenous pyelogram to show position of stone
- full blood count
- urea and electrolytes to detect electrolyte imbalance
- cystoscopy (Figure 8.11)

Signs and symptoms

In the early stages, the condition may be asymptomatic. The presenting symptoms depend on the location of the renal stone. Stones forming in the kidney may go undetected for years until identified by routine abdominal X-ray. The patient with stones obstructing the ureters may present with colicky pain, haematuria, nausea and vomiting. Stones in the urinary bladder may not have any symptoms except for a dull pain in the suprapubic region after voiding urine.

Care and management

Full nursing assessment should be carried out to establish the cause of renal calculi. The care, management and treatment will depend on the identified risk factors.

Dietary modification should be encouraged if the renal calculi are the result of excessive intake of calcium, protein, oxalate or vitamin D. Food rich in oxalate includes chocolate, rhubarb and nuts.

The patient should be encouraged to drink 2.5–3 L of fluid per day to flush the kidneys of any bacteria that may cause a urinary tract infection and to prevent dehydration. The patient should be taught how to recognise the signs and symptoms of urinary tract infection and to take preventative measures.

The patient should be encouraged to undertake exercise, such as walking, swimming or running, to prevent urinary stasis. Exercise improves heart rate and circulation. It also improves blood flow to the kidneys, resulting in good urine output.

The patient should be instructed to take medications as prescribed and educated in the importance of this. The patient should be taught to recognise any side effects of the prescribed medications.

The patient should be taught to test and strain their urine for stones, saving any passed stone for analysis. The patient should be advised to pass all urine into a urinal as small stones can be passed in the urine unobserved by the patient. Kumar and Clark (2009) report that stones less than 0.5 cm in diameter may be passed in the urine without any intervention.

Some patients will require surgery to remove the stones. Approximately one in five stones will not pass spontaneously and may require surgical intervention. If the stone is small, shock-wave lithotripsy may be used to break the stone into smaller pieces; larger stones may be removed using ureteroscopy (Parmar, 2004).

The healthcare professional should provide psychological support to reduce anxiety by actively listening to the patient and relatives and offer information about the prevention of renal calculi.

Pharmacological interventions

The following medications may be prescribed for patients with renal calculi:

- analgesia for persistent pain
- antibiotics if the patient presents with urinary tract infection.

Conclusion

The renal system consists of the kidneys, ureters, urinary bladder and urethra. This chapter has provided the reader with an overview of the renal system and has discussed some of the disease processes related to the system. It is not the remit of this chapter to discuss all the diseases of the renal system. Healthcare professionals play a vital role in caring for the patient with renal disorders. In order to deliver high-quality care, they need a sound understanding of the anatomy and physiology of the renal system. Apart from the physical aspects, they need to consider the psychosocial aspects of care.

Patients and their relatives will need advice and support to come to terms with the disease, particularly CKD which is not curable and can lead to death. Often nurses are good at providing the physical aspects of care for the patient but fail to include the relatives when planning the patient's care. Chronic renal conditions may lead to lifestyle changes for the patient and their relatives, and Healthcare professionals are in the forefront to offer support and guidance to the patient and their relatives.

Test your knowledge

- What happens to the urine output in a patient who is hypovolaemic?

- What happens to the urine output if you eat large quantities of salty potato crisps?

- List the functions of the kidney.

- Explain the effect of alcohol on urine production.

- Are males or females more prone to cystitis? Explain.

Activities

Here are some activities and exercises to help test your learning. For the answers to these exercises, as well as further self-testing activities, visit our website at www.wiley.com/go/fundamentalsofappliedpathophysiology

Fill in the blanks

The urinary system may also be called the _____ system. Some textbooks even refer to the _____ system. This is because the organs of the urinary system are located in close proximity to those of the _____ system.

In the _____ and _____ of each kidney are more than _____ microscopic structures called _____. The nephron function is to _____ the _____ so as to regulate the amount of water, _____ and waste products circulating the body. The filtrate that is produced is _____, which flows down the _____ to the urinary _____.

Each nephron is composed of a Bowman's capsule, _____, proximal convoluted tubule, loop of _____ and _____ convoluted tubule. The renal corpuscle includes the _____ capsule and the glomerulus. The renal tubule is the part of the nephron that directs the _____ away from the glomerular capsule. The collecting duct is not considered part of the nephron as many nephrons drain into one collecting duct.

Choose from:
Distal; Bladder; Reproductive; Ureters; Blood; Urine; Filtrate; Nephrons; Renal; Henle; Glomerulus; Filter; Medulla; Glomerular; Cortex; Electrolytes; One million; Genito-urinary

Label the diagram

Using the list of words supplied, label the diagram.

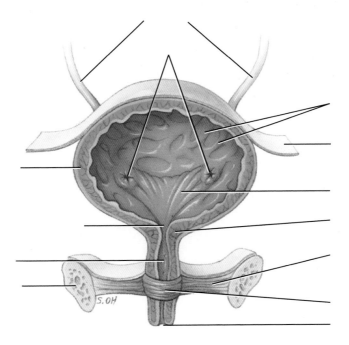

Ureters; Ureteral openings; Trigone; Peritoneum; Rugae of mucosa; Internal uretheral sphincter; External uretheral sphincter; External uretheral sphincter in the urogenital diaphragm; External uretheral orifice; Hip bone; Urethra; Internal uretheral orifice; Detrusor muscle

Word search

G	A	I	L	E	E	O	S	N	A	Y	D	C	T
G	L	N	A	P	R	R	O	S	C	P	O	U	H
N	F	O	E	A	Y	I	A	N	U	R	I	A	R
R	B	I	M	P	T	U	E	U	T	L	R	M	F
M	U	L	B	E	H	G	R	E	P	M	O	I	A
C	R	U	R	R	R	R	X	I	A	R	I	B	E
C	U	C	D	U	O	M	O	T	A	H	R	R	K
I	X	L	Y	R	P	S	U	N	I	P	E	I	I
E	X	A	S	A	O	R	I	L	R	O	T	P	D
E	P	C	U	R	I	E	U	S	U	I	N	S	N
R	M	A	R	A	E	S	T	A	G	S	A	E	E
H	F	F	I	L	T	R	A	T	I	O	N	A	Y
R	G	H	A	O	I	F	C	A	L	Y	C	E	S
I	L	O	O	O	N	E	T	D	O	E	E	O	I

Anterior	Excretion	Kidneys
Anuria	Fibrosis	Nephron
Calculi	Filtration	Oliguria
Calyces	Glomermulus	Cortex
Dysuria	Harmaturia	Urgency
Erythropoietin	Hilus	Pyuria

Further resources

National Institute for Health and Clinical Excellence (NICE)

http://www.nice.org.uk/CG73
This link provides NICE guidance on chronic kidney disease. Whether your study is in renal nursing or general field study, this link provides information with regard to treatment and care.

Department of Health (DH) – Renal dialysis

http://www.dh.gov.uk/en/Publicationsandstatistics/Publications/PublicationsPolicyAnd
Guidance/DH_4005752
Here you will find DH guidelines on good practice for renal dialysis. These guidelines highlight
potential hazards for dialysis patients in the renal unit and the measures that can be taken to
prevent any blood-borne infection during dialysis.

British Journal of Renal Medicine

http://www.bjrm.co.uk/bjrm/
This journal will be a valuable resource for students, whether you are a specialist nurse in the
renal unit or a nursing student. Here you will find current issues in the care and treatment of renal
patients. The articles date back to 1998.

Journal of Renal Nursing

http://www.internurse.com/cgi-bin/go.pl/library/issues.html?journal_uid=45
This is a valuable journal for students. Here you will find excellence in clinical practice and provide
up-to-date accessible, practical and information. From the articles written by experts, you should
gain a good knowledge base and learn about evidence-based practice in renal nursing.

The Renal Association

http://www.renal.org/Clinical/GuidelinesSection/AcuteKidneyInjury.aspx
This link is a valuable source for students who would like to research acute kidney injury. Here
you will find information on prevention, treatment and management of patients with acute kidney
injury.

Department of Health – National Service Framework

http://www.dh.gov.uk/en/Publicationsandstatistics/Publications/PublicationsPolicyAnd
Guidance/DH_4101902
This link provides information on the National Service Framework for Renal Service. Students
should find this site very useful as it gives 23 markers of good practice in the prevention of chronic
kidney diseases.

Glossary of terms

Anterior:	front.
Anuria:	absence of urine.
Bifurcation:	dividing into two branches.
Calculus:	a stone.
Calyces:	a small funnel-shaped cavity formed from the renal pelvis.

Diuresis:	excess urine production.
Dysuria:	painful urination.
Erythropoietin:	a hormone produced by the kidneys that regulates red blood cell production.
Excretion:	the elimination of waste products of metabolism.
Fibrosis:	growth of fibrous connective tissue.
Filtration:	a passive transport system.
Glomerulus:	a network of capillaries found in the Bowman's capsule.
Haematuria:	blood in the urine.
Hilus:	the small indented part of the kidney.
Hyperkalemia:	a high potassium level in the blood.
Hyponatremia:	a low sodium level in the blood.
Involuntary:	cannot be controlled.
Kidney:	an organ situated in the posterior wall of the abdominal cavity.
Micturition:	the act of voiding urine.
Nephron:	the functional unit of the kidney.
Nocturia:	excessive urination at night.
Oliguria:	diminished urine output; deficient secretion of urine; less than 30 mL per hour.
Osmolarity:	the osmotic pressure of a fluid.
Parenchyma:	the soft tissue of the kidney involving the cortex and the medulla.
Posterior:	behind.
Proteinuria:	protein in the urine.
Pyrexia:	elevated temperature associated with fever.
Pyuria:	presence of white blood cells in the urine.
Renal artery:	a blood vessel that takes blood to the kidney.
Renal cortex:	the outermost part of the kidney.
Renal medulla:	the middle layer of the kidney.
Renal pelvis:	the funnel-shaped section of the kidney.
Renal pyramid:	a cone-shaped structure of the medulla.
Renal vein:	the blood vessel that returns filtered blood into the circulation.

Renin:	a renal hormone that alters systemic blood pressure.
Specific gravity:	density.
Sphincter:	a ring-like muscle fibre that can constrict.
Ureter:	a membranous tube that drains urine from the kidneys to the bladder.
Urethra:	a muscular tube that drains urine from the bladder.
Urgency:	a feeling of the need to void urine immediately.
Voluntary:	can be controlled.

References

Alexander, M.F., Fawcett, J. and Runciman, P.J. (2007). *Nursing Practice – Hospitals and Home*, 3rd edn. Edinburgh: Churchill Livingstone.

Bullock, B.A. and Henze, R.L. (2010). *Focus on Pathophysiology*. Philadelphia: Lippincott.

Kumar, P. and Clark, M. (2009). *Clinical Medicine*, 7th edn. Edinburgh: WB Saunders.

LeMone, P., Burke, K. and Bauldoff, G. (2011). *Medical – Surgical Nursing; Critical Thinking in Client Care*, 4rd edn. New Jersey: Pearson.

Mader, S.S. (2011). *Understanding Human Anatomy and Physiology*. Boston: McGraw Hill.

Marieb, E.N. and Hoehn, K. (2010). *Human Anatomy and Physiology*, 8th edn. San Francisco: Pearson Benjamin Cummings.

McCance, K.L., Huether, S.E., Brashers, V.L. and Rote, N.S. (2010). *Pathophysiology: The Biologic Basis for Disease in Adults and Children*, 6th edn. St. Louis: Mosby

Nursing and Midwifery Council (2008). *Standards for Medicines Management*. London: NMC.

Nursing and Midwifery Council (2009). *Record Keeping: Guidance for Nurses and Midwives*. London: Nursing and Midwifery Council.

Parmar, M.S. (2004). Kidney stones. *British Medical Journal*. 328(7453): 1420–1424.

Porth, C.M. (2010). *Pathophysiology: Concepts of Altered Health States*, 8th edn. Philadelphia: Lippincott Williams & Wilkins.

Thomas, N. (ed) (2008). *Renal Nursing*, 3rd edn. London: Bailliere Tindall.

Waugh, A. and Grant, A. (2010). *Ross and Wilson: Anatomy and Physiology in Health and Illness*, 11th edn. Edinburgh: Churchill Livingstone.

9

The respiratory system and associated disorders

Anthony Wheeldon

Senior Lecturer, Department of Adult Health and Primary Care, School of Health and Social Work, University of Hertfordshire, Hatfield, Hertfordshire, UK

Contents

Fundamentals of Applied Pathophysiology: An Essential Guide for Nursing and Healthcare Students, Second Edition. Edited by Muralitharan Nair and Ian Peate.
© 2013 John Wiley & Sons, Ltd. Published 2013 by John Wiley & Sons, Ltd.

Key words

- Carbon dioxide (CO_2)
- External respiration
- Hypoxaemia
- Oxygen (O_2)
- Dyspnoea
- Haemoglobin (Hb)
- Hypercapnia
- Respiration
- Expiration
- Hypoxia
- Inspiration
- Respiratory failure

Test your prior knowledge

- Name five major anatomical structures of the lower respiratory tract.
- What is the main function of the respiratory system?
- What physiological observations would you use to assess a patient's respiratory status?

Learning outcomes

On completion of this section the reader will be able to:

- List the main anatomical structures of both the upper and the lower respiratory tracts.
- Describe the process of pulmonary ventilation.
- Discuss the principles of external respiration.
- Explain how the body is able to control the rate and depth of breathing.

Don't forget to visit to the companion website for this book (www.wiley.com/go/ fundamentalsofappliedpathophysiology) where you can find self-assessment tests to check your progress, as well as lots of activities to practise your learning.

Introduction

All human cells require a continuous supply of oxygen; indeed, cells will only survive for a few minutes without it. Fortunately, around 21% of the air within our atmosphere is oxygen, providing a plentiful supply. As cells use oxygen, the waste gas (carbon dioxide) is produced. If allowed to build up, carbon dioxide can disrupt cellular activity and homeostasis. The principal function of the respiratory system, therefore, is to ensure that the body extracts enough oxygen from the atmosphere whilst disposing of excess carbon dioxide. The collection of oxygen and removal of carbon dioxide is referred to as respiration. Respiration involves four distinct processes – pulmonary ventilation, external respiration, transport of gases and internal respiration. Although all four are examined in this chapter, only pulmonary ventilation and external respiration are the sole responsibility of the respiratory system. As oxygen and carbon dioxide are transported around the body in blood, effective respiration is also reliant upon a fully functioning cardiovascular system.

The respiratory system is divided into the upper and lower respiratory tracts. It is within the lower respiratory tract that external respiration occurs and the structures involved are microscopic, very fragile and easily damaged by infection. For this reason, both the upper and the lower respiratory tracts are equipped to fight off any invading airborne pathogens.

The air we breathe is contaminated by a wide variety of pollutants (e.g. exhaust fumes, industrial gases, cigarette smoke) and as a result respiratory diseases are highly prevalent throughout the world. Respiratory disease accounts for 20% of all deaths in the UK, more than coronary heart disease. The most common respiratory diseases include lung cancer, asthma, chronic obstructive pulmonary disease (COPD), pneumonia and tuberculosis (TB). Together they place a heavy burden on the NHS, costing an estimated £3 billion pounds a year. Every year in the UK, one in every five men and one in every four women consults their GP regarding a respiratory complaint, resulting in around 62 million prescriptions (British Thoracic Society, 2006).

Anatomy and physiology

The upper respiratory tract

The upper respiratory tract consists of the oral cavity (mouth), the nasal cavity (the nose), the pharynx and the larynx (Figure 9.1). As well as providing smell and speech, the upper respiratory tract ensures that the air entering the lower respiratory tract is warm, damp and clean. First and foremost, the spaces just inside the nostrils are lined with course hairs that filter incoming air, ensuring that large dust particles do not enter the airways. The nasal cavity is also lined with a mucous membrane made from pseudostratified ciliated columnar epithelium, which contains a network of capillaries and a plentiful supply of mucus-secreting goblet cells. The blood flowing through the capillaries warms the passing air, while the mucus moistens it and traps any passing dust particles. The mucus-covered dust particles are then propelled by the cilia towards the pharynx where they can be swallowed or expectorated. To add further protection, the upper respiratory tract is lined with irritant receptors, which when stimulated by invading particles (e.g. dust or pollen) force a sneeze, ensuring the offending material is ejected through the nose or mouth.

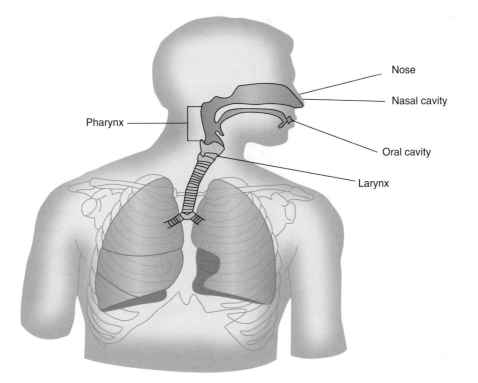

Nose

Nasal cavity

Pharynx

Oral cavity

Larynx

Figure 9.1   The main structures of the upper respiratory tract.

Unlike the nasal cavity and larynx, the pharynx acts as a passage for food as well as air. The pharynx also contains five tonsils. The two tonsils visible when the mouth is open are the palatine tonsils; behind the tongue lie the lingual tonsils and the pharyngeal tonsil or adenoid sits on the upper back wall of the pharynx. Tonsils are lymph nodules and part of the body's defence system. The epithelial lining of their surface has deep folds, called crypts. Inhaled bacteria or particles become entangled within the crypts and are then engulfed and destroyed.

The larynx (voice box) also provides a degree of protection, this time from food. The larynx occupies the space between the pharynx and the trachea – the first section of the lower respiratory tract. Also nearby is the oesophagus, which propels food towards the stomach. Attached to the top of the larynx is a leaf-shaped piece of epithelial-covered elastic cartilage, called the epiglottis. On swallowing, the epiglottis blocks entry to the larynx and food and liquid are diverted towards the oesophagus. Inhalation of solid or liquid substances can block the lower respiratory tract and cut off the body's supply of oxygen – this medical emergency is referred to as aspiration and necessitates the swift removal of the offending substance.

The lower respiratory tract

The lower respiratory tract includes the trachea, the right and left primary bronchi, and the constituents of both lungs (Figure 9.2). The trachea (or windpipe) is a tubular vessel that carries air

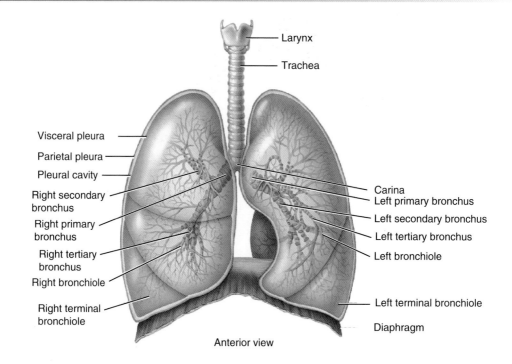

Larynx

Trachea

Visceral pleura

Parietal pleura

Pleural cavity

Right secondary
bronchus

Right primary
bronchus

Right tertiary
bronchus

Right bronchiole

Right terminal
bronchiole

Carina
Left primary bronchus

Left secondary bronchus

Left tertiary bronchus

Left bronchiole

Left terminal bronchiole

Diaphragm

Anterior view

Figure 9.2 Gross anatomy of the lower respiratory tract.

from the larynx down towards the lungs. The trachea is also lined with pseudostratified ciliated columnar epithelium so that any inhaled debris are trapped and propelled upwards towards the oesophagus and pharynx to be swallowed or expectorated. The trachea and the bronchi also contain irritant receptors, which stimulate coughs that force larger invading particles upwards. The outermost layer of the trachea contains connective tissue that is reinforced by a series of 16–20 C-shaped cartilage rings. The rings prevent the trachea from collapsing despite the pressure changes that occur during an active breathing cycle. If any obstruction occurs above the larynx, be it a foreign object, inflammation or trauma, a hole or stoma may be created in the trachea and a small tube inserted. This procedure is called a tracheostomy and can ensure that the blocked portion of the upper airway is bypassed, enabling the patient to breathe (Paul, 2010).

The lungs are two cone-shaped organs that almost fill the thorax. They are protected by a framework of bones, the thoracic cage, which consists of the ribs, sternum (breast bone) and vertebrae (spine). The tip of each lung, the apex, extends just above the clavicle (collar bone) and their wider bases sit just above a concave muscle called the diaphragm. The lungs are divided into distinct regions called lobes. There are three lobes in the right lung and two in the left. The heart along with its major blood vessels sits in a space between the two lungs called the cardiac notch. Each lung is surrounded by two thin protective membranes called the parietal and visceral pleura (Figure 9.2). The parietal pleura lines the walls of the thorax, whereas the visceral pleura lines the lungs themselves. The space between the two pleura, the pleural space, is minute and contains a thin film of lubricating fluid. This reduces friction between the two pleura, allowing both layers to slide over one another during breathing. The fluid also helps the visceral and

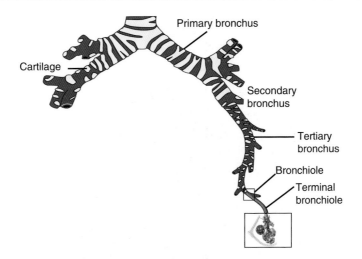

Figure 9.3   The bronchial tree.

parietal pleura to adhere to one another, in the same way two pieces of glass stick together when wet.

The airways of the lower respiratory tract divide into branches; for this reason they are often called the bronchial tree. Within the lungs, the primary bronchi divide into the secondary bronchi, each serving a lobe (three secondary bronchi on the right and two on the left). The secondary bronchi split into tertiary bronchi (Figures 9.2 and 9.3) of which there are 10 in each lung. Tertiary bronchi continue to divide into a network of bronchioles, which eventually lead to a terminal bronchiole. The section of the lung supplied by a terminal bronchiole is referred to as a lobule and each lobule has its own arterial blood supply and lymph vessels. The bronchial tree continues to subdivide with the terminal bronchiole leading to a series of respiratory bronchioles which in turn generate several alveolar ducts. The airways terminate with numerous sphere-like structures called alveoli, which are clustered together to form alveolar sacs (Figure 9.4). There are approximately 490 million alveoli in the lungs (Ochs *et al.*, 2004).

Pulmonary ventilation

Pulmonary ventilation describes the process more commonly known as breathing. The way gases behave helps explain how air flows in and out of the lungs. For instance, gases always flow from an area of high pressure to one of low pressure. All the gases that constitute air collectively exert atmospheric pressure. Air within the lungs also exerts a pressure known as alveolar pressure (Patel *et al.*, 2007). During inspiration, the thorax expands and alveolar pressure falls below atmospheric pressure. Because alveolar pressure is now less than atmospheric pressure, air will naturally move into the airways until the pressure difference no longer exists. This phenomenon is explained by Boyle's law which states that at a constant temperature, the pressure of gas in the lungs is inversely proportional to their size. In other words, as the size of the thorax increases,

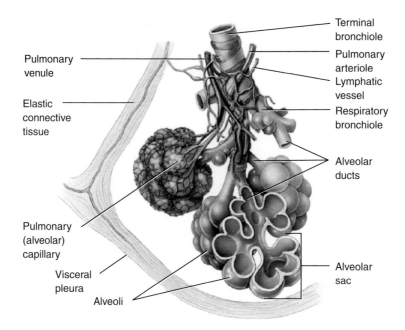

Figure 9.4   Microscopic anatomy of a lobule.

the pressure inside falls as the gas molecules have more room to circulate (Martini and Nath, 2009).

A range of respiratory muscles are used to achieve thoracic expansion during inspiration (Figure 9.5). The rib cage is pulled outwards and upwards by the external intercostal muscles, whilst the diaphragm contracts downwards, pulling the lungs with it. Expiration is a more passive process. The external intercostal muscles and the diaphragm relax, allowing the natural elastic recoil of the lung tissue to spring it back into shape, forcing air back into the atmosphere (Figure 9.6). Other respiratory muscles can also be utilised. The abdominal wall muscles and internal intercostal muscles, for instance, are utilised to force air out beyond a normal breath, e.g. when playing a musical instrument or blowing out candles on a birthday cake. Muscles such as the sternocleido-mastoids, the scalenes and the pectoralis can also be used to produce a deep forceful inspiration. These muscles are referred to as accessory muscles, so called because they are rarely used in normal quiet breathing (Wheeldon, 2011).

External respiration

External respiration only occurs beyond the respiratory bronchioles. For this reason, the end portion of the bronchial tree is called the respiratory zone. The remainder of the bronchial tree from the trachea down to the terminal bronchioles is the conducting zone. Because the air

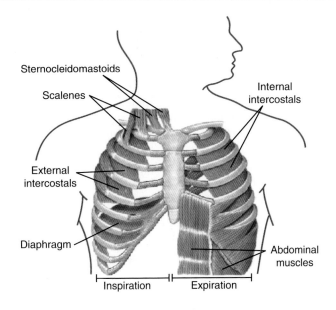

Figure 9.5 Muscles involved in pulmonary ventilation.

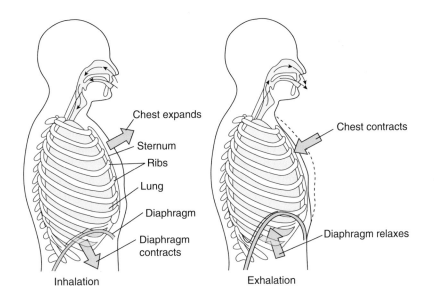

Figure 9.6 Movements of inspiration and expiration.

present in the conducting zone plays no part in supplying the body with oxygen, it is also referred to as the anatomical dead space. External respiration is the diffusion of oxygen from the alveoli into the pulmonary circulation (blood flow through the lungs) and the diffusion of carbon dioxide in the opposite direction. Diffusion occurs because gas molecules always move from areas of high concentration to ones of low concentration. Each lobule of the lung has its own arterial blood supply; this blood supply originates from the pulmonary artery, which stems from the right ventricle of the heart. The blood present in the pulmonary artery has been collected from the systemic circulation and is therefore low in oxygen and relatively high in carbon dioxide. The amount (and therefore concentration) of oxygen in the alveoli is far greater than in the passing arterial blood supply. Oxygen therefore moves passively out of the alveoli, into the pulmonary circulation and on towards the left-hand side of the heart. Because there is less carbon dioxide in the alveoli than in pulmonary circulation, carbon dioxide transfers into the alveoli ready to be exhaled (Figure 9.7).

Transport of gases and internal respiration

Blood transports oxygen and carbon dioxide between the lungs and all the tissue cells of the body. Cells utilise oxygen when manufacturing their prime energy source, adenosine triphosphate (ATP). In addition to ATP, the cells also produce water and carbon dioxide. Internal respiration describes the exchange of oxygen and carbon dioxide between blood and tissue cells, a phenomenon governed by the same principles as for external respiration. Because cells are continually using oxygen, its concentration within tissue is always lower than within blood. Likewise, the continual use of oxygen ensures that the level of carbon dioxide within tissue is always higher than within blood. As blood flows through the capillaries, oxygen and carbon dioxide follow their concentration gradients and continually diffuse between blood and tissue (Figure 9.7).

Control of breathing

Respiratory centres within the medulla oblongata and pons are responsible for controlling the rate and depth of breathing (Figure 9.8). Within the medulla oblongata there are chemoreceptors, which continually analyse carbon dioxide levels within the cerebrospinal fluid. As levels of carbon dioxide rise, messages are sent via the phrenic and intercostal nerves to the diaphragm and intercostal muscles, instructing them to contract. Another set of chemoreceptors found in the aorta and carotid arteries analyses levels of oxygen as well as carbon dioxide. If oxygen falls or carbon dioxide rises, messages are sent to the respiratory centres via the glossopharyngeal nerve and vagus nerve, stimulating further contraction (Figure 9.9). Throughout the day, whether at work, rest or play, respiration rate changes in order to meet the body's oxygen demands.

Although breathing is essentially a subconscious activity, its rate and depth can be controlled voluntarily or even stopped altogether, e.g. when swimming under water. However, this voluntary control is limited as the respiratory centres have a strong urge to ensure breathing is continuous. Breathing can also be influenced by state of mind. The inspiratory area of the respiratory centres (Figure 9.8) can be stimulated by both the limbic system and hypothalamus, two areas of the brain responsible for processing emotions. Fear, anxiety or even the anticipation of stressful activities can cause an involuntary increase in the rate and depth of breathing. Other factors that can affect breathing include pyrexia and pain. Because breathing is largely beyond an individual's control, any changes in respiration rate are clinically significant (Table 9.1).

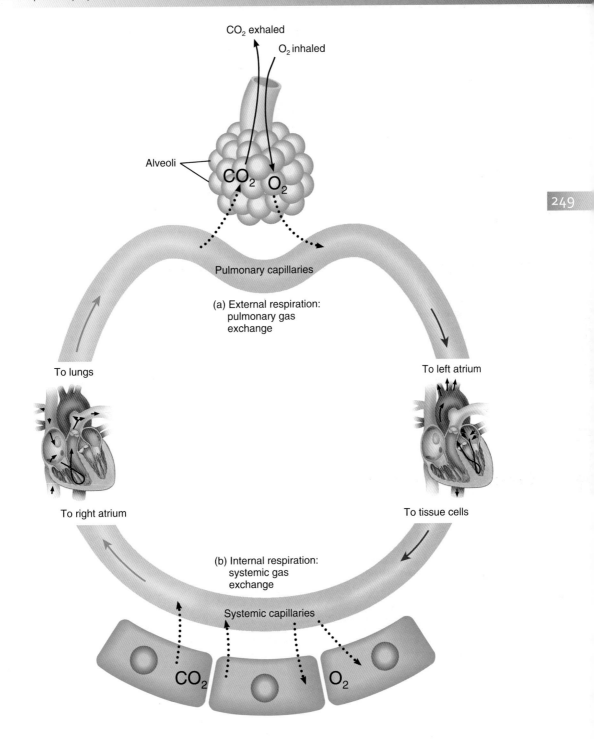

Figure 9.7 External and internal respiration.

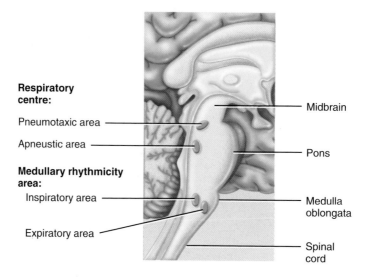

Respiratory
centre:

Pneumotaxic area

Apneustic area

Medullary rhythmicity
area:
Inspiratory area

Expiratory area

Midbrain

Pons

Medulla
oblongata

Spinal
cord

Figure 9.8   The respiratory centres of the brainstem.

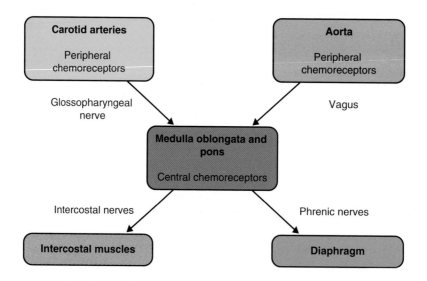

Figure 9.9   Actions of the central and peripheral chemoreceptors.

Table 9.1   Important terminology of breathing.

Term	Definition
Eupnoea	Easy or normal breathing, with a respiration between 12 and 16 breaths per minute
Tachypnoea	Rapid and usually shallow respiration rate, more than 20 breaths per minute
Bradypnoea	Slow respiration rate, less than 10 breaths per minute
Hyperventilation	Increased respiration rate associated with increased ventilation – increased amounts of air entering the alveoli
Hypoventilation	Decreased ventilation – lack of air entering the alveoli
Apnoea	Absence of breathing for more than 15 seconds
Hypopnoea	Shallow breathing with inadequate ventilation
Dyspnoea	Difficult or laboured breathing
Orthopnoea	Difficulty in breathing while lying flat
Cheyne–Stokes breathing	Irregular breathing cycles associated with drug overdose, neurological disturbances and the dying patient

Disorders of the respiratory system

Learning outcomes

On completion of this section the reader will be able to:

- Explain the principles of respiratory failure.
- Describe the pathophysiology of tuberculosis (TB) and pneumonia.
- Discuss the pathophysiology of obstructive and restrictive disorders.
- Describe the physiological changes that occur due to pleural disorders.
- Outline the management of pneumonia, asthma, COPD and pleural disorders.

Respiratory failure

Respiratory failure occurs when respiration is unable to sustain the metabolic needs of the body (Schwartzstein and Parker, 2006). In other words, the lungs are not extracting enough oxygen from the atmosphere. The majority of oxygen (around 98%) is attached to haemoglobin (Hb), which is found in abundance in erythrocytes (red blood cells). A pulse oximiter can gauge what percentage of haemoglobin is carrying oxygen. This reading is called the 'oxygen saturation' (SpO_2). In health, SpO_2 should be between 95% and 99%; however, tremors, anaemia, polycythaemia, cold extremities and nail varnish can all reduce the accuracy of the reading. For this reason, SpO_2 should only be used in conjunction with other observations (Clark et al., 2006). A reduced amount of oxygen in arterial blood is called hypoxaemia. One major symptom of severe hypoxaemia is central cyanosis, a visible bluish hue or tinge visible in the lips and mouth. Hypoxaemia naturally leads to the development of hypoxia, a lack of oxygen in tissue cells. However, hypoxaemia is not the only cause of hypoxia; if you recall, effective transport of oxygen also requires a fully functioning cardiovascular system. Heart failure or haemorrhage, for example, could also result in hypoxia. When a patient is hypoxaemic they are said to be in respiratory failure type 1. Ultimately, the underlying cause should be treated but oxygen may be prescribed to increase SpO_2.

Around 10% of all carbon dioxide is dissolved in plasma and the rest diffuses into the erythrocytes. Once inside the erythrocyte, 20% of the carbon dioxide binds to haemoglobin and the remainder combines with water to form carbonic acid. The carbonic acid then quickly dissociates into bicarbonate ions and hydrogen ions:

$$\underset{\text{Carbon dioxide}}{CO_2} + \underset{\text{Water}}{H_2O} \rightleftarrows \underset{\text{Carbonic acid}}{H_2CO_3} \rightleftarrows \underset{\text{Hydrogen ions}}{H^+} + \underset{\text{Bicarbonate ions}}{HCO_3^-}$$

Naturally the carbon dioxide dissolved in plasma will also generate carbonic acid. However, the reaction that occurs within the erythrocyte is much faster due to the presence of the enzyme carbonic anhydrase. The production of hydrogen and bicarbonate helps to regulate arterial blood pH. A normal arterial blood pH should remain within a very narrow range (7.35–7.45). As levels of hydrogen ion rise and the pH starts to fall below 7.35, more hydrogen ions are combined with bicarbonate to form carbonic acid. As hydrogen ion levels fall and the pH starts to rise, more carbonic acid dissociates. Effective respiration can, therefore, help regulate hydrogen ion concentration (Clancy and McVicar, 2007).

Respiratory disease often leads to respiratory muscle fatigue, which in turn may lead to a shallower and weaker rate and depth of breathing. Any reduction in ventilation will lead to an accumulation of carbon dioxide, a phenomenon known as hypercapnia. Any patient that is hypoxaemic and hypercapnic is said to be in respiratory failure type 2. Because high carbon dioxide levels lead to a reduction in arterial blood pH, respiratory failure type 2 is also referred to as respiratory acidosis. The only way to reduce carbon dioxide is to 'breathe' it away by improving ventilation. Patients with respiratory failure type 2 may be placed on a mechanical ventilator, which can increase their depth of breathing. One common example of mechanical ventilation used in both hospital and community settings is non-invasive positive pressure ventilation (NIPPV). NIPPV is provided by a special portable machine that delivers breaths via a flexible hose and special facial mask (British Thoracic Society, 2002).

Lower respiratory tract infections

Tuberculosis

TB is a lung infection mainly caused by *Mycobacterium tuberculosis*, an airborne slow-growing bacillus.

The signs and symptoms of TB include:

- haemoptysis
- weight loss

- pyrexia
- fatigue
- night sweats.

When the individual is first infected, usually in the upper lobes, lymphocytes and neutrophils congregate at the infection site. The bacilli are then trapped and walled off by fibrous tissue. This phase of TB is referred to as the primary infection and the infected individual is often asymptomatic and unaware. At some point thereafter, re-exposure to TB or another bacterium causes a secondary infection. The bacilli are then reactivated and start to multiply, after which the patient soon becomes symptomatic and infectious. Bacilli are very arduous and can survive trapped in fibrous tissue for long periods. Individuals can remain unaware that they have TB for many years.

The incidence of TB is growing worldwide and its rise is attributed to increased international travel, immigration and poverty. TB, however, can be successfully treated on an outpatient basis with a 6-month course of a combination of antibiotics. Because of the recent increases in drug-resistant strains of TB, the major aspects of care are infection control and the maintenance of compliance (National Institute for Health and Clinical Excellence, 2011a).

Pneumonia

Pneumonia is an infection of the alveoli and small airways. Inflammation and oedema cause the alveoli to fill with debris and exudate. The exudate quickly fills with neutrophils, erythrocytes and fibrin, and a solid mass called consolidation is formed. Consolidation can be patchy and spread throughout both lungs, or concentrated in one mass affecting one or more lobes. Consolidation in the alveoli disturbs external respiration and less oxygen diffuses from the alveoli into the pulmonary circulation; as a result the patient becomes hypoxaemic and breathless.

Aetiology

Pneumonia can develop secondary to aspiration or other airway infections (e.g. influenza); however, in the majority of cases, pneumonia is caught from inhaled pathogens. Up to 12% of all GP prescriptions for lower respiratory tract infections are for pneumonia (British Thoracic Society, 2009).

Pneumonia can either be community or hospital acquired. In one-third of cases of community-acquired pneumonia the cause remains unknown; however, key known pathogens include *Streptococcus pnuemoniae*, *Chlamidya pnuemoniae* and *Legionella* (Legionnaires' disease). Alcoholism, smoking, drug abuse and chronic heart and lung disease all increase the risk of contracting pneumonia. The immunosuppressed are also vulnerable; however, the invading bacteria in such cases are usually either candida (fungus) or *Pneumocystis jiroveci,* formally known as *Pneumocystic carinii.*

As its name suggests, hospital-acquired pneumonia is contracted during a hospital admission. Inpatients are exposed to a wide variety of risks whilst in hospital. Unconscious patients, for example, require intubation and postoperative patients may have a suppressed cough, increasing the risk of aspiration. Furthermore, long-term patients are often immunosuppressed and repeatedly exposed to a multitude of pathogens. Hospital-acquired pneumonia is often caused by bacteria such as *Escherichia*, *Klebsiella* or *Psuedomonas* and, regrettably, occurs in 1–5% of all admissions (Patel *et al.*, 2007).

253

Signs and symptoms

- hypoxaemia
- tachypnoea and dyspnoae
- tachycardia
- pyrexia – in response to bacterial infection
- dehydration – pyrexia causes fluid loss; also the body loses humidified air on expiration
- reduced lung expansion – consolidation makes it hard to expand the lungs and breathing becomes difficult
- pain – inflammation can spread to the pleura, causing pleuritic pain (pleurisy)
- productive cough – the exudate present in the alveoli often produces rust-coloured sputum
- lethargy

Investigations

Table 9.2 summarises the investigations used to establish a diagnosis of pneumonia.

Care and management

Pneumonia can develop into a severe infection and up to 42% of cases will require inpatient care, of which between 5% and 10% of patients will require transfer to intensive care (British Thoracic Society, 2009). The healthcare professional can play an important role in the early detection of deterioration. The main goals of care include:

- Safe administration of prescribed antibiotics.
- Safe administration of prescribed oxygen – to correct hypoxaemia and maintain oxygen saturations above 90%.
- Patient positioning – placing the patient in an upright position will promote diaphragm and intercostal muscle activity and enhance ventilation.
- Establishing and minimising pain levels – to make the patient more comfortable and enhance breathing. An appropriate pain assessment tool should be used (see Chapter 15).

Table 9.2 The main investigations of pneumonia.

Investigation	Rationale
Full blood count	A white blood cell count above 11×10^9/L indicates inflammation, infection or an immune system response
Urea and electrolytes	Raised urea (>7 mmol/L) is an indicator of severe infection
Blood and sputum cultures	To identify the causative agent and appropriate antibiotic treatment
Liver function test	Acute pneumonia can affect liver function
X-ray	To establish the extent of infected lung tissue

Hoare and Lim (2006).

- Temperature management – safe administration of antipyretic agents, such as aspirin, paracetamol or ibuprofen, electric fans, reducing bed clothes.
- Close monitoring of vital signs – respiration rate greater than 30 respirations per minute, new hypotension (systolic less than 90 mmHg or diastolic less than 60 mmHg) and new mental confusion could indicate life-threatening pneumonia (British Thoracic Society, 2009). Vital signs should therefore be recorded hourly until the patient's condition stabilises.
- Fluid balance – as the patient is dehydrated. A minimum of 2.5 L every 24 hours is required. Fluids may be administered intravenously if required (Dunn, 2005).
- Communication – to reduce anxiety and promote comfort.

Case study

255

Ludovic Brozek is a 32-year-old plumber who emigrated from his native Poland 3 years ago. He lives in a one-bedroom flat in a tower block in North London. Three weeks ago he caught a bad cold, which became progressively worse. Today he presented at his local GP surgery with breathlessness on exertion and pleuritic pain. He is also coughing up rust-coloured sputum. Ludovic informs the doctor that he smokes 20 cigarettes a day and drinks alcohol socially.

Take some time to reflect on this case and then consider the following.

1. What do you think is the most likely diagnosis for Ludovic's condition?
2. What health promotion advice would you give to Ludovic?
3. What treatments are likely to be prescribed by the doctor?

Obstructive lung disorders

Obstructive lung disorders involve a degree of obstruction to airflow. In conditions such as asthma and COPD, the obstruction to airflow is associated with narrow airways and increased airflow resistance. If the lumen of an airway is halved, then resistance to airflow will increase 16 times. As resistance increases and more and more gas molecules collide, a noise is generated, accounting for the characteristic wheeze often heard in respiratory patients (Meredith and Massey, 2011). In many patients, airway resistance can be overcome by increasing the work of the respiratory muscles. However, normal passive expiration may not be enough to promote adequate alveoli emptying. Forced expiration generates high intrathoracic pressures that force smaller airways to close, trapping air in the chest.

Investigations

The extent of air trapping can be measured using spirometry, which measures the force and volume of a maximum expiration after a full inspiration. The volume of air that can be forced out is referred to as the forced vital capacity (FVC) and the volume that can be exhaled in the first second of expiration is the forced expiratory volume (FEV_1) (Figure 9.10). By comparing FEV_1 with FVC, the FEV_1 : FVC ratio and the severity of airway obstruction can be ascertained. An individual with an FEV_1 : FVC ratio of less than 80% has obstructed airways (Sheldon, 2005).

Another important measure of airway resistance is peak expiratory flow rate (PEFR) or 'peak flow'. PEFR measures the force of expiration in litres per minute. It measures the patient's

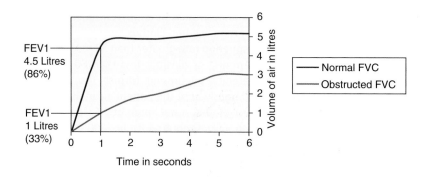

Figure 9.10   Spirometry – a normal forced vital capacity compared to an obstructed forced vital capacity.

maximum expiratory flow rate via their mouth. An inability to meet a predicted value based on age, sex and height could indicate airway obstruction. Peak expiratory flow rates provide a quick and simple assessment of the airways; however, regular peak flow measurements are more reveal-ing than single arbitrary readings and carers should be mindful that peak expiratory flow rates are effort dependent.

Asthma

Asthma is a chronic inflammatory disorder of the lungs. It causes the bronchi and bronchioles to become inflamed and constricted. As a result, airflow becomes obstructed, often resulting in a characteristic wheeze. In the UK, 11% of men and 12% of women have doctor-diagnosed asthma (British Thoracic Society, 2006).

Asthmatics periodically react to triggers. Triggers are substances or situations that would not normally trouble an asthma-free person's airways. Asthma is said to be either extrinsic or intrinsic. In extrinsic asthma, airway inflammation is a consequence of hypersensitive reactions associated with allergy, i.e. pollen, dust mites or foodstuffs, whereas intrinsic asthma is linked to hyperre-sponsive reactions to other forms of stimuli, e.g. infection, sudden exposure to cold, exercise, stress or cigarette smoke. Extrinsic asthma is more common in childhood, with many sufferers 'growing out' of it in adolescence; intrinsic asthma usually develops in adulthood. Many patients, however, have a combination of both types and, irrespective of causative agents, the physiological changes, symptoms and treatments are the same.

Pathophysiology

The pathophysiology of asthma is complicated and intricate. The bronchi and bronchioles contain smooth muscle and are lined with mucous-secreting glands and ciliated cells (Figure 9.11). Close to the airway's blood supply, there are large quantities of mast cells. Once stimulated, mast cells release a number of cytokines (chemical messengers), which cause physiological changes to the lining of the bronchi and bronchioles. Three such cytokines are histamine, kinins and prostaglan-dins, which cause smooth muscle contraction, increased mucus production and increased capillary permeability. The airways soon narrow and become flooded with mucus and fluid leaking from blood vessels (Figure 9.12). As the airways become obstructed, the patient finds it increasingly hard to breathe and to cough up the mucus. If unresolved, fatigue can occur and the patient's

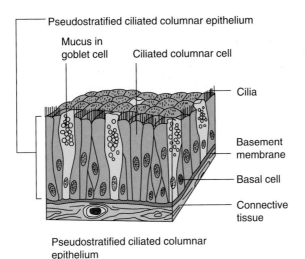

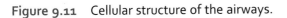

Figure 9.11 Cellular structure of the airways.

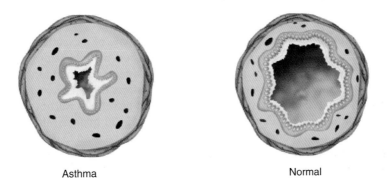

Figure 9.12 Airway pathophysiology, normal compared to status asthmaticus.

respiratory effort becomes weak and inadequate, causing hypoxaemia and in severe cases, hyper-capnia (Sims, 2006).

Care and management

In the UK, around 1500 people a year die from asthma (British Thoracic Society, 2006); therefore, healthcare professionals must be aware of the signs of severe and life-threatening asthma (Table 9.3). Asthma is reversible and care should focus on close monitoring and health promotion. The main care goals are:

- Continuous monitoring of vital signs until the patient is stabilised.
- Safe administration of prescribed oxygen to maintain oxygen saturation above 92%.
- Safe administration of prescribed bronchodilators and steroids – to alleviate dyspnoea (Tables 9.4 and 9.5).

Table 9.3   Features of acute/severe and life-threatening asthma.

Main symptoms of asthma	Features of acute/severe asthma	Features of life-threatening asthma
• Cough, which may become productive with thick sticky mucus • Dyspnoea and chest tightness • Wheeze • Peak flow less than predicted or best	• Peak flow of less than 50% predicted or best • Dyspnoea – unable to complete a sentence in one breath • Tachypnoea – respiration rate greater than 25 breaths per minute • Tachycardia – pulse greater than 110 beats per minute	• Peak flow less than 33% of predicted or best • Oxygen saturation (SpO₂) less than 92% • Silent chest • Weak and feeble respiratory effort • Cyanosis • Bradycardia or hypotension • Confusion, exhaustion or coma

Adapted British Thoracic Society and Scottish Intercollegiate Guidelines Network (2009).

- Communication – as speaking requires a constant flow of air, patients experiencing acute breathlessness are only able to talk only for very short periods before the need to breathe interrupts them. The patient's inability to complete a sentence, therefore, provides a sensitive measure of the extent of a patient's respiratory distress (Higginson and Jones, 2009).
- Regular PEFR measurement – singular or infrequent peak flows will not accurately reflect the patient's status. PEFR should be measured every 15–30 minutes after commencement of treatment and until conditions stabilise. PEFR can also be used to measure the effectiveness of bronchodilator therapy; therefore, PEFR should be measured pre- and post-inhaled or nebulised beta-2 agonists at least four times a day throughout a patient's stay in hospital.
- Comfort and reassurance – dyspnoea can be a traumatic experience and fear and anxiety also promote hyperventilation. The patient's anxieties should be listened to and continuous explanations provided for the multidisciplinary team's actions.
- Sputum collection – yellow or green sputum can indicate infection.
- Health promotion – avoidance of triggers, compliance with prescribed pharmacological therapies, smoking cessation and weight reduction in obese patients may reduce the frequency of asthma attacks.

Chronic obstructive pulmonary disease

Approximately 600 000 people in the UK have COPD and it accounts for 5.4% of all male deaths and 4.2% of all female deaths. COPD has been defined as airflow obstruction that is progressive, not fully reversible and does not change markedly over several months. It has one major cause – smoking. COPD is a term now used to describe the traditional diagnosis of chronic bronchitis or emphysema. Chronic asthma sufferers are also at risk of developing fixed airway obstruction as airways become re-modelled over time. Their symptoms may be indistinguishable from COPD and many COPD patients may also have asthma. Accurate diagnosis therefore is often problematic (Devereux, 2006; National Institute for Health and Clinical Excellence, 2010).

Table 9.4   Summary of bronchodilator therapies given in asthma and chronic obstructive pulmonary disease.

Type	Actions	Examples	Routes	Care considerations
Beta-2 agonists	Mimics the actions of epinephrine. Beta-2 agonists stimulate beta-2 receptor sites in the airways, promoting rapid bronchodilation within 15 minutes, with a duration of 4–8 hours – depending on dose	Salbutamol Terbutaline Fenoterol Salmeterol	Inhaler Nebuliser Oral Subcutaneous	Patient will need to be advised of the potential for tachycardia and hand tremor
Anticholergenics	Blocks the action of acetylcholine, a neurotransmitter released by the parasympathetic nervous system. Acetylcholine promotes bronchoconstriction and bronchial secretion. Peak bronchodilator effects occur within 1 hour, with a duration similar to beta-2 agonists	Ipratropium bromide	Inhaler Nebuliser	Patient may need frequent mouthwashes as may cause dry mouth and a bitter taste
Methylxanthines	Increases concentration of intracellular cyclic adenosine monophosphate (cAMP). Increased cAMP concentration causes bronchodilation	Theophylline	Oral Intravenous (as aminophylline)	Optimal effects occur when plasma theophylline levels are between 10 and 20 mg/L. Regular blood tests are required

Adapted from Barnes (2008) and Joint Formulary Committee (2011).

Table 9.5   Summary of main corticosteroids used in the treatment of respiratory disease.

Indication	Corticosteroids*	Route	Care considerations
Prophylaxis and reduction of frequency of exacerbations	Beclametasone Budesonide Fluticasone	Inhaler	Inhaled corticosteroids can cause hoarseness, loss of voice and candidiasis. Advise patients to rinse their mouths after taking these inhalers
Exacerbation	Prednisolone Hydrocortisone	Oral Intravenous	Patients taking prednisolone and hydrocortisone will need careful monitoring as can cause the following side effects: • osteoporosis • diabetes • weight gain • increased body hair • altered mood

*Corticosteroids are potent anti-inflammatory agents. They are used to reduce bronchial hyperactivity in patients with asthma, chronic obstructive pulmonary disease and other respiratory diseases where reversibility is present. Adapted Barnes (2008) and Joint Formulary Committee (2011).

Signs and symptoms

- reduced FEV_1 which is less than the predicted value
- dyspnoea – due to airway obstruction and air trapping
- productive cough
- reduced exercise tolerance
- respiratory failure types 1 and 2
- cor pulmonale – chronic hypoxia causes hypertension within pulmonary circulation. Eventually, the right ventricle becomes enlarged and fails, ultimately leading to peripheral oedema

Emphysema

Emphysema is defined as the permanent enlargement of airspaces beyond the terminal bronchiole and the destruction of the alveolar wall. The mechanisms behind this degeneration of tissue are thought to relate to the actions of destructive enzymes called proteases, which are released from neutrophils and macrophages in response to infection. In health, lung tissue produces a substance called alpha antitrypsin, which counteracts the destructive action of protease. Smoking, however, is thought to reduce the effect of alpha antitrypsin and increase protease activity, allowing alveolar destruction to continue unabated (Hogg and Senior, 2002). Proteases destroy the elastic fibres essential for elastic recoil, which is much needed during exhalation. As a result, the alveoli become overinflated as air becomes trapped within the lung (Figure 9.13). The increased volume of air within the thorax pushes the diaphragm downwards, disturbing its natural concave shape and making breathing difficult. Frequent infections can also develop as it becomes increasingly difficult to cough up secretions. The destruction of the alveolar wall and adjacent capillaries

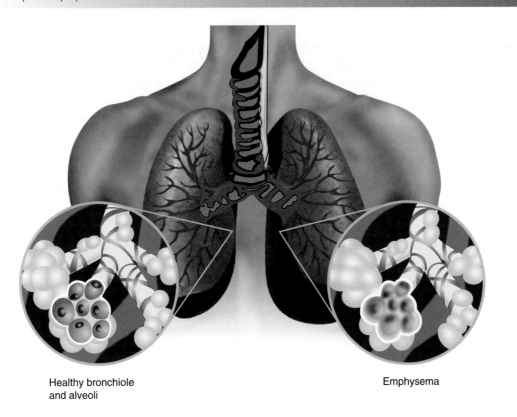

Healthy bronchiole
and alveoli

Emphysema

Figure 9.13   Comparison of a normal bronchiole and alveoli to those in an emphysema sufferer.

will mean that there is less lung tissue available for external respiration and the patient will be at risk of developing hypoxaemia and hypoxia (Gould, 2006).

Chronic bronchitis

Chronic bronchitis is defined as the presence of a productive cough lasting for 3 months in each of 2 consecutive years when other pulmonary and cardiac causes of cough have been ruled out (Braman, 2006). It is characterised by an increase in mucus production and damaged cilia in the bronchi (Figure 9.14). As a result, the bronchi become clogged with mucus, which continues to stimulate the airway's irritant receptors, producing a cough. This chronic irritation causes inflammation and the bronchial wall thickens, causing airway obstruction. The lack of functioning cilia makes mucus clearance difficult and as a result, mucus collects and blocks the smaller airways. Secondary infections then occur, causing yet more irritation and inflammation. As more and more airways become blocked, external respiration is reduced and less oxygen is transferred into the bloodstream. The pathophysiological processes behind increased mucus production and cilia dysfunction are thought to involve an inflammatory response to the constant bombardment of cigarette smoke (MacNee, 2006).

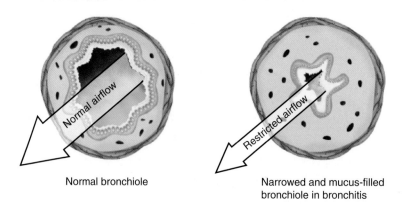

Normal bronchiole   Narrowed and mucus-filled
                                     bronchiole in bronchitis

Figure 9.14   Comparison of a normal bronchiole to that in a chronic bronchitis sufferer.

Table 9.6 FEV_1 as an assessment of airway obstruction.

FEV_1	Severity of airway obstruction
50–80% predicted	Mild
30–49% predicted	Moderate
Less than 30%	Severe

National Institute of Health and Clinical Excellence (2010).

Care and management of chronic obstructive pulmonary disease

The severity of COPD is determined by the FEV_1 (Table 9.6). However, wherever possible the patient should be managed by the multidisciplinary team in their own home. Factors that may lead to acute exacerbation and necessitate hospital admission for COPD include:

- inability to cope at home
- poor social circumstances
- cyanosis
- rapid onset
- impaired level of consciousness
- long-term oxygen therapy
- confusion or disorientation
- SpO_2 less than 90%
- respiratory failure type 2
- chest X-ray changes
- significant co-morbidity, i.e. diabetes, heart disease (National Institute for Health and Clinical Excellence, 2010).

COPD is a diverse and varied condition and its management requires a holistic approach centred upon self-management and symptom control. The main management goals are:

- smoking cessation advice
- education on prescribed oxygen and bronchodilator therapies – to maximise relief of breathlessness
- immunisation – to minimise the frequency of exacerbations
- dietary advice – severe weight loss is a feature of both emphysema and chronic bronchitis
- pulmonary rehabilitation
- promotion of self-management techniques – COPD is associated with high levels of anxiety and depression.

Case study

Alison is a 40-year-old single mother of two. She has been admitted to accident and emergency with severe shortness of breath. She finds answering the nurse's questions very difficult and she cannot complete a sentence without pausing for breath. Her respiration rate is 30 respirations per minute, her pulse is 120 beats per minute, her blood pressure is 126/88 mmHg and her oxygen saturation is 93%. She feels too breathless to blow a peak flow. Alison rarely drinks alcohol but has smoked 20 cigarettes a day since she was 16 years old. She is currently unemployed and lives in a small council flat on the outskirts of town.

Take some time to reflect on this case and then consider the following.

1. Which of Alison's physiological observations do you think are a cause for concern and why?
2. What pharmacological therapies could be used to alleviate Alison's breathlessness?
3. What risk factors may have contributed to Alison's current condition?

Bronchiectasis

Bronchiectasis describes an irreversible lung condition caused by recurrent infection and inflammation. The condition is associated with abnormal dilation of the bronchi together with a loss of functioning cilia. Destruction of alveolar walls and fibrosis also occur. It is characterised by a chronic productive cough, in which the patient produces large amounts of purulent sputum. Other symptoms include dyspnoea, pleuritic pain and wheeze. Treatments include chest physiotherapy and antibiotics.

Bronchiectasis is a chronic lung disorder that usually develops secondary to a problem during childhood. Inflammation as a result of severe pneumonia, measles or whooping cough during childhood damages and weakens the bronchial walls. Diseases that cause bronchial obstruction, such as tumours and TB, can also lead to bronchiectasis when infections occur beyond the obstruction. Less common are congenital causes such as cystic fibrosis, in which the overproduction of viscous mucus causes recurrent lung infections, and immunoglobulin deficiencies, which cause recurrent infections (Goeminne and Dupont, 2010).

Restrictive disorders

Patients with restrictive disorders have difficulty in expanding their thorax. Spirometry shows a reduced FVC and FEV_1 but unlike obstructive disorders, the FEV_1:FVC ratio is normal. This is because the airways are not obstructed, but rather chest expansion is restricted. There are two main reasons why chest expansion could be impeded are:

- A condition that directly affects the chest wall, such as kyphosis or scoliosis.
- A disease that affects lung compliance. Poliomyelitis, amyotrophic lateral sclerosis, and botulism, for example, can cause respiratory muscle paralysis, whereas muscular dystrophy causes muscle weakness.

Disorders that restrict lung tissue are in the main chronic conditions caused by the inhalation of industrial or commercial pollutants. The upper respiratory tract is often unable to handle the vast quantities of airborne particles generated by various work practices, e.g. coal dust. Small particles that become lodged within the lungs cause chronic inflammation. Over time connective tissue within the lungs is eroded and the lungs become less compliant, making chest expansion difficult. This group of respiratory diseases is called pneumoconioses and the individual diseases are often named after the job or pastime that generated them, e.g. coal worker's lung (Gould, 2006). Chest expansion can also be restricted by acute problems such as adult respiratory distress syndrome, which occurs after lung trauma or pulmonary oedema.

Lung cancer

Lung cancer has the highest mortality rate of all known cancers in the Western world. In the UK alone, it accounts for around 36 000 deaths a year (British Thoracic Society, 2006). The most significant risk factor is smoking. Ex-smokers remain at risk although the likelihood reduces over time. Also susceptible are those exposed to passive smoking, albeit at a much lower probability. Smoking or other irritants (i.e. occupational pollutants) damage the pseudostratified epithelium of lung tissue, rendering it more susceptible to inflammation. Certain chemicals present within cigarette smoke are carcinogenic, and promote the development of tumours within the lung tissue. The vast majority of lung cancers (95%) are bronchial carcinomas of which there are two major types – non-small cell and small cell. Non-small cell carcinomas account for 70% of all lung cancers and can be subdivided again into squamous cell carcinomas, which tend to develop within the larger bronchi, and adencarcinomas and large cell carcinomas, which are found in the smaller airways, making them much harder to detect. Small cell carcinomas tend to grow near a large bronchi and are the most aggressive bronchial carcinomas. There are no specific signs of lung cancer but a diagnosis is usually made in smokers who present with the following symptoms:

- cough
- haemoptysis
- dyspnoea
- chest pain
- wheezing
- in some cases, finger clubbing (National Institute for Clinical Excellence, 2011b).

Pleural disorders

Only a minute amount of fluid occupies the pleural space (the space between the parietal and visceral pleura). Any condition that causes air or fluid to collect in the pleural space can cause the lung to partially or fully collapse (Figure 9.15). The collapse of a lung results in areas that are

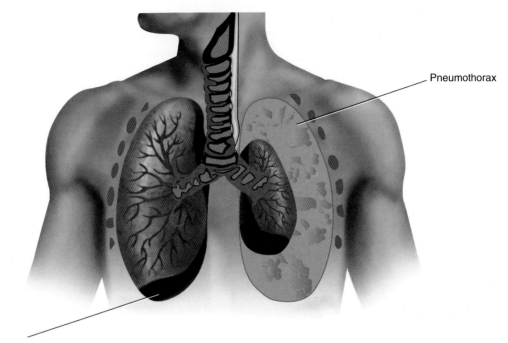

Pneumothorax

Pleural effusuon

Figure 9.15 Pleural effusion and a pneumothorax.

underventilated, a phenomenon known as atelectasis. The surface area for external respiration is dramatically reduced and the patient may develop hypoxaemia (West, 2007). The main investigation for pleural disorders is a chest X-ray; the critically ill patient, however, may require a computed tomography (CT) scan.

One fluid that can leak in the pleural space is blood. Trauma, cancer and surgery can all cause bleeding into the pleural space, a phenomenon referred to as haemothorax. Exudate and transudate pleural effusions can cause other kinds of fluid to collect in the pleural space. Exudate pleural effusions occur when there is a problem within lung tissue. The fluid that collects in the pleural space is rich in protein and white blood cells because it is generated as a result of inflammation secondary to a tumour or an infection, such as pneumonia or TB. Inflammation increases capillary permeability, allowing fluid to leak out of blood vessels and into the pleural space. Transudate pleural effusions occur as a result of a problem outside of the lungs. A prime example is left ventricular failure, which causes an increase in capillary hydrostatic pressure that forces fluid out of the bloodstream and into the pleural space. A decrease in blood osmotic pressure will also force fluid from blood vessels into the pleural space; causes of reduced blood osmotic pressure include hypoproteinaemia. Some patients may develop an empyema, the formation of pus in the pleural effusion (Dobbin and Howard, 2009). Table 9.7 summarises the signs and symptoms of pleural effusions.

The presence of air in the pleural cavity is called a pneumothorax. A pneumothorax can occur as a result of chest trauma, e.g. a stabbing or a broken rib. Patients with chronic respiratory disease

Table 9.7   Signs and symptoms of pleural disorders.

Pleural effusion	Pneumothorax
Dyspnoea	Tachypnoea
Pleuritic pain	Use of accessory muscles
Dry cough	Asymmetrical chest expansion
Cyanosis	Cyanosis
Tachycardia	Tachycardia
	Hypertension or hypotension
	Pulsus paradoxus
	Sweating
	Dry cough
	Restlessness or confusion

are also at risk of developing a pneumothorax. Some individuals have a congenital defect or bleb within the alveolar wall which can rupture spontaneously. Tall young men are at particular risk of this kind of pneumothorax (Ryan, 2005). In certain circumstances, a flap of tissue creates a one-way valve effect and airflow into the pleural space is promoted with each inspiration. As the pneumothorax grows, pressure is exerted on the inferior vena cava, impeding the blood flowing back to the heart (venous return). As a result, the patient becomes hypoxic and breathless. This medical emergency is called a tension pneumothorax (Table 9.7).

Care and management

Chest drains are often used to assist the re-inflation of the affected lung. The monitoring of both the patient and the drain is the responsibility of the healthcare professional and attention should be paid to the following:

- Patient positioning – placing the patient in an upright position will encourage drainage and aid expansion of the thorax.
- Position of the chest drain – the drainage bottle must be kept below the patient's chest level to prevent fluid re-entering the pleural space. Coiled and looped tubing should also be avoided as it can impede drainage flow and lead to a tension pneumothorax or surgical emphysema.
- Continuous monitoring of vital signs until the patient's condition stabilises.
- Close monitoring of the chest drain:
  - Swinging – the level of the fluid in the underwater seal of the drain should fluctuate between 5 and 10 cm when the patient breathes. Absence of swinging could indicate a kink or blockage in the tubing.

- Bubbling – bubbles often occur in the water seal bottle without suction when the patient exhales or coughs. Continuous bubbling indicates a problem with the drain or insertion site.
- Administration of prescribed analgesics for pleuritic pain.
- Accurate recording of drainage – the quantity, colour and consistency of the fluid being drained should be noted.
- Infection control – the insertion site should be checked daily for signs of infection, i.e. redness, swelling, heat, pain and discharge (Sullivan, 2008).

Conclusion

This chapter has examined how respiratory disorders can interfere with respiration. Respiration involves four distinct physiological processes: pulmonary ventilation, external respiration, transport of gases and internal respiration. Respiration ensures that the body receives enough oxygen whilst disposing of excess carbon dioxide. In doing so, respiration plays a vital role in the maintenance of homeostasis. Any disease that interferes with pulmonary ventilation or external respiration will disturb homeostasis by reducing oxygen levels and possibly increasing carbon dioxide. The respiratory system has a complex anatomical structure and therefore there are a multitude of respiratory diseases. TB and pneumonia, for example, affect the alveoli and neighbouring tissue, whereas COPD and asthma obstruct the airways. Whatever the primary cause of the respiratory disorder, pulmonary ventilation and external respiration will almost always be affected and hypoxaemia and hypoxia can result. Patients with respiratory disease present with a multitude of symptoms such as dyspnoea, tachypnoea, pleuritic pain, reduced peak expiratory flow rate, low SpO_2, cyanosis and an inability to speak in complete sentences being just a few examples.

Test your knowledge

- Explain what happens in the alveoli during normal breathing.
- Why would someone in respiratory failure type 2 have an arterial blood pH below 7.35?
- Explain why someone with asthma might produce a peak expiratory flow rate (PEFR) less than that predicted for their age, height and sex.
- What are the differences between obstructive and restrictive lung disorders?
- Why might someone with a pleural disorder become hypoxaemic?

Activities

Here are some activities and exercises to help test your learning. For the answers to these exercises, as well as further self-testing activities, visit our website at www.wiley.com/go/fundamentalsofappliedpathophysiology

Fill in the blanks

During inspiration the _____ contracts _____, while the external _____ muscles contract _____ and _____. As the _____ expands, intra-_____ pressure falls below _____ pressure. As a result _____ enters the _____ in bulk flow. Expiration is a _____ process. On expiration the diaphragm and external inter-costal muscles _____ and the _____ empty. When forced expiration is required, the internal intercostal muscles are utilised. In order to maximise _____, muscles such as the _____ and _____ are used. As these muscles are rarely used for pulmonary ventilation, they are referred to as _____ muscles.

Choose from:
Thorax; Diaphragm; Accessory; Lungs; Alveolar; Scalenes; Intercostal; Downwards; Upwards; Sternolcleidomastoids; Passive; Atmospheric; Outwards; Alveoli; Relax; Gaseous exchange; Air; Thoracic

Label the diagram

Using the list of words supplied, label the diagram.

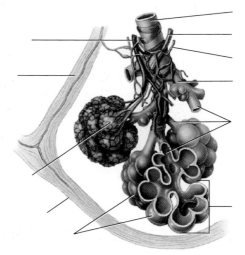

Elastic connective tissue; Terminal bronchiole; Alveolar sac; Visceral pleura; Pulmonary venule; Alveolar ducts; Alveoli; Respiratory bronchiole; Lymphatic vessel; Pulmonary arteriole; Pulmonary (alveolar capillary)

Word search

V	A	S	R	E	C	N	A	C	G	U	N	L	W	B	A
R	E	C	O	X	Y	G	E	N	T	M	D	V	F	R	K
H	H	N	B	W	A	R	B	I	C	S	Y	O	E	O	P
Y	C	C	T	H	L	M	U	T	U	P	S	S	X	N	Z
P	A	L	D	I	W	J	G	I	Y	H	P	E	I	C	S
O	R	Y	N	K	L	B	R	M	F	I	N	W	D	H	I
X	T	A	L	I	P	A	G	E	R	V	O	H	G	I	S
A	Q	M	G	T	A	A	T	A	O	L	E	E	P	E	O
E	P	H	M	S	R	R	T	I	F	J	A	E	N	C	L
M	M	T	R	H	S	I	D	K	O	L	S	Z	E	T	U
I	C	S	P	U	O	S	A	T	R	N	D	E	U	A	C
A	H	A	E	N	R	E	O	F	S	T	F	K	M	S	R
D	I	G	R	T	P	J	E	R	C	E	I	M	O	I	E
D	N	A	V	R	N	A	K	N	U	R	H	H	N	S	B
U	T	S	A	L	B	U	T	A	M	O	L	C	I	A	U
E	S	E	D	I	X	O	I	D	N	O	B	R	A	C	T

Ventilation	Lung cancer	Tuberculosis
Oxygen	Peak flow	Pneumonia
Diaphragm	Chest drain	Asthma
Dyspnoea	Trachea	Salbutamol
Sputum	Respiration rate	Wheeze
Hypoxaemia	Carbon dioxide	Bronchiectasis

Further resources

National Institute for Health and Clinical Excellence (NICE)

http://www.nice.org.uk/
The NICE website provides access to the latest guidance on many respiratory conditions. This guidance is based on the best available research and will inform you on how to keep your practice evidence based and up to date.

British Thoracic Society

www.brit-thoracic.org.uk
The British Thoracic Society website provides a range of information and clinical guidance that is based on best available evidence. Its guidance is essential for all healthcare professionals who wish to provide gold standard care for their respiratory patients. The British Thoracic Society guidance will also ensure that your academic work is up to date.

British Lung Foundation

http://www.lunguk.org
The British Lung Foundation website provides a wealth of information for patients with respiratory disease. By accessing this website, you can gain insight into the support available for people living with lung disease, which may help you in practice and in your academic studies.

Asthma UK

http://www.asthma.org.uk/
The Asthma UK website provides insight into the support and guidance available to people with asthma. This insight can help you to enhance your care.

MacMillan Cancer Support

http://www.macmillan.org.uk
This website has an excellent section on managing breathlessness, which you may find useful when caring for respiratory patients.

Respiratory Education UK

http://www.respiratoryeduk.com/
This website provides access to a range of courses and information that you may wish to utilise for your studies. There are also quizzes and exercises, which you can use to test your understanding.

Glossary of terms

Amyotrophic lateral sclerosis:	a serious neurological disease in which motor neurons gradually deteriorate.
Anaemia:	blood lacking in iron. Often used to mean a deficiency in red blood cells (erythrocytes).
Antipyretic agent:	a drug that can reduce high temperatures (e.g. paracetamol, aspirin, ibuprofen).
Aorta:	the first major blood vessel of arterial circulation. Emerges from the left ventricle of the heart.

Atelectasis:	a partial or complete collapse of lung tissue due to a blocked airway.
Bacillus:	a form of bacteria. Bacilli are rod-shaped, Gram-positive and usually have motility.
Botulism:	a rare but serious bacterial infection which causes muscle weakness and paralysis.
Carcinogen:	something capable of causing cancer.
Carotid artery:	the major artery supplying the brain; stems from the aorta.
Cartilage:	a type of connective tissue that contains collagen and elastic fibres. This strong tough material on the bone ends helps to distribute the load within the joint; the slippery surface allows smooth movement between the bones. Cartilage can withstand both tension and compression.
Cerebrospinal fluid (CSF):	the fluid found within the brain and spinal cord.
Chemoreceptor:	a sensory receptor that detects the presence of a specific chemical.
Central cyanosis:	a bluish hue or tinge visible on the lips and mouth that occurs when arterial oxygen levels are abnormally low.
Cilia:	hair-like extensions on the outer surface of some cells; used to propel liquids.
Cor pulmonale:	right-sided heart failure caused by hypoxia.
Diffusion:	the passive movement of molecules or ions from a region of high concentration to one of low concentration until a state of equilibrium is achieved.
Elastic cartilage:	cartilage that contains more elastin fibres, providing strength and stretchability.
Enzyme:	a protein that speeds up chemical reactions.
Erythrocyte:	another name for a red blood cell.
Expectorate:	to cough up and spit out mucus or sputum.
External intercostal muscle:	a muscle that spans the spaces between the ribs. As opposed to the internal intercostal muscles, the external intercostal muscles sit closer to the outside of the thorax.
External respiration:	the transfer of oxygen from the alveoli in the lungs to the bloodstream and the transfer of carbon dioxide from the bloodstream into alveoli in the lungs.

Extrinsic asthma:	asthma caused by hypersensitive reactions to an allergy.
Exudate:	escaping fluid that spills from a space; contains cellular debris and pus.
Fibrin:	a protein essential for clotting.
Fibrosis:	growth of fibrous connective tissue (scar tissue).
Fibrous:	containing regenerated or scar tissue.
Finger clubbing:	alteration in the angle of finger and toe bases caused by chronic tissue hypoxia.
Goblet cell:	a mucus-secreting cell found in epithelial tissue.
Haemoglobin (Hb):	a protein consisting of globin and four haem groups that is found within erythrocytes (red blood cells). Responsible for the transport of oxygen.
Haemoptysis:	coughing up of blood.
Hydrostatic pressure:	the pressure exerted by a fluid.
Hypercapnia:	elevated levels of arterial carbon dioxide.
Hypertension:	raised blood pressure.
Hypoproteinaemia:	a reduced level of plasma proteins.
Hypotension:	low blood pressure.
Hypoxaemia:	reduced level of oxygen within arterial blood.
Hypoxia:	reduced level of oxygen within the tissues.
Intercostal nerve:	a nerve that links the respiratory centres in the brainstem with the intercostal muscles.
Internal intercostal muscle:	a muscles that spans the spaces between the ribs. As opposed to the external intercostal muscles, the internal intercostal muscles sit closer to the inside of the thorax.
Internal respiration:	the transfer of oxygen from the bloodstream into body cells and the transfer of carbon dioxide from body cells to the bloodstream. This is known as aerobic respiration. Anaerobic respiration does not require oxygen, but does require a substance such as nitrate or iron to do the same job as oxygen (accept electrons during the chemical reaction). Only human cells with mitochondria can undertake aerobic respiration.
Intrinsic asthma:	asthma caused by hyperresponsive reactions to non-allergic stimuli.

Intubation:	the insertion of a special tube into the pharynx and down into the trachea, in order to maintain a patent airway in an unconscious person.
Kyphosis:	curvature of the thoracic spine.
Lymph node:	part of the lymphatic system, it contains many white cells to destroy bacteria that are trapped within the lymph node.
Lymphocyte:	a specialist white blood cell involved in immune responses.
Lymph vessel:	a vessel that carries lymphatic fluid. Part of the lymphatic system which forms part of the immune system.
Macrophage:	a phagocyte produced from monocytes that engulfs and digests cellular debris, microbes and foreign matter.
Mast cell:	a cell found in connective tissue that releases histamine during inflammation.
Medulla oblongata:	lowest region of the brainstem; concerned with the control of the internal organs.
Muscular dystrophy:	a group of diseases characterised by the progressive loss of muscle fibres. Almost all these diseases are hereditary.
Neutrophil:	a type of white blood cell.
Non-invasive positive pressure ventilation (NIPPV):	respiratory support technique that enhances the person's rate and depth of breathing.
Oedema:	the abnormal accumulation of fluid in the interstitial spaces. It may be localised (following an injury = swelling) or it may be generalised (as in heart failure).
Osmotic pressure:	the pressure that must be exerted on a solution to prevent the passage of water into it across a semipermeable membrane from a region of higher concentration of solute to a region of lower concentration of solute.
Peak expiratory flow rate:	the velocity at which a person can expire their total lung volume.
Phrenic nerve:	the nerve that links the diaphragm to the respiratory centre in the brainstem.
Poliomyelitis:	an acute viral disease which affects the central nervous system.
Polycythaemia:	a condition in which there is an abnormally high number of erythrocytes (red blood cells).

273

Pons:	upper region of the brainstem. Connects the midbrain to the medulla oblongata.
Pseudostratified ciliated columnar epithelium:	covering or lining of the internal body surface that contains cilia and mucus-secreting goblet cells.
Pulmonary ventilation:	breathing. The inspiration and expiration of air into and out of the lungs.
Pulse oximetry:	non-invasive measurement of the oxygen saturation of the blood (SpO_2).
Pulsus paradoxus:	a phenomenon in which the pulse is weaker during inspiration than during expiration.
Pyrexia:	elevated temperature associated with fever.
Respiratory acidosis:	a blood pH of less than 7.35 caused by a rise in arterial carbon dioxide.
Scoliosis:	a sideways curvature of the thoracic spine.
Spirometry:	diagnostic tool which measures a person's forced vital capacity (FVC) and forced expiratory volume within the first second of expiration (FEV_1).
Surgical emphysema:	air trapped in the tissues, usually as a result of a surgical or invasive procedure.
Systemic circulation:	the flow of blood from the left ventricle to all parts of the body .
Tachycardia:	a fast heart beat (usually defined as above 100 beats per minute).
Thorax:	the body trunk above the diaphragm and below the neck.
Tracheostomy:	a procedure in which an incision is made in the trachea to facilitate breathing.
Transport of gases:	the movement of oxygen and carbon dioxide between the lungs and body cells.

274

References

Barnes, P.J. (2008). Drugs for airway disease. *Medicine*. 36(4): 181–190.

Braman, S.S. (2006). Chronic cough due to bronchitis: ACCP evidence-based clinical practice. *Chest*. 129: 104S–115S.

British Thoracic Society (2002). BTS guideline non-invasive ventilation in acute respiratory failure. *Thorax*. 57: 192–211.

British Thoracic Society (2006). *The Burden of Lung Disease*. London: BTS.

British Thoracic Society (2009). Guidelines for the management of community acquired pneumonia in adults: update 2009. *Thorax*. 64 (Suppl III): iii1–iii55.

British Thoracic Society and Scottish Intercollegiate Guidelines Network (2009). *British Guideline on the Management of Asthma: A National Clinical Guideline*. London: BTS.

Clancy, J. and McVicar, A. (2007). Immediate and long term regulation of acid-base homeostasis. *British Journal of Nursing.* 16(17): 1076–1079.

Clark, A.P., Giuliano, K. and Chen, H. (2006). Pulse oximetry revisited 'but his O_2 sat was normal!'. *Clinical Nurse Specialist.* 20(6): 268–272.

Devereux, G. (2006). ABC of chronic obstructive disease definition, epidemiology and risk factors. *British Medical Journal.* 332: 1142–1144.

Dobbin, K.R. and Howard, V.M. (2009). Understanding empyema. *Nursing.* June: 56cc1–56cc5.

Dunn, L. (2005). Pneumonia: Classification, diagnosis and nursing management. *Nursing Standard.* 19: 50–54.

Goeminne, P. and Dupont, L. (2010). Non-cystic fibrosis bronchiectasis: diagnosis and management in the 21st century. *Postgraduate Medical Journal.* 86: 493–501.

Gould, B.E. (2006). *Pathophysiology for the Health Professions*, 3rd edn. Philadelphia: Elsevier.

Higginson, R. and Jones, B. (2009). Respiratory assessment in critically ill patients: airway and breathing. *British Journal of Nursing.* 18(8): 456–461.

Hoare, Z. and Lim, W.S. (2006). Pneumonia: Update on diagnosis and management. *British Medical Journal.* 332: 1077–1079.

Hogg, J.C. and Senior, R.M. (2002). Chronic obstructive pulmonary disease 2: Pathology and biochemistry of emphysema. *Thorax.* 57: 830–834.

Joint Formulary Committee. (2011). *British National Formulary*, 61st edn. London: Pharmaceutical Press.

MacNee, W. (2006). ABC of chronic obstructive pulmonary disease pathology, pathogenesis and pathophysiology. *British Medical Journal.* 332: 1202–1204.

Martini, F.H. and Nath, J.L. (2009). *Fundamentals of Anatomy and Physiology*, 8th edn. San Francisco: Pearson Benjamin Cummings.

Meredith, T, and Massey, D. (2011). Respiratory assessment 2: more key skills to improve care. *British Journal of Cardiac Nursing.* 6(2): 63–68.

National Institute for Health and Clinical Excellence (2010). *Clinical Guideline 101. Chronic Obstructive Pulmonary Disease. Management of Chronic Obstructive Pulmonary Disease in Primary and Secondary Care*. London: NICE.

National Institute for Health and Clinical Excellence (2011a). *Clinical Guideline 117. Tuberculosis. Clinical Diagnosis and Management of Tuberculosis, and Measures for its Prevention and Control*. London: NICE.

National Institute for Health and Clinical Excellence (2011b). *Clinical Guideline 121. Lung Cancer: Diagnosis and Treatment of Lung Cancer*. London: NICE.

Ochs, M., Nyengaard, A.J., Knudsen, L., Voigt, M., Wahlers, T., Richter, J. and Gundersen, H.J.G. (2004). The number of alveoli in the human lung. *American Journal of Respiratory and Critical Care Medicine.* 169: 120–124.

Patel, H., Gwilt, C., McGowan, P. (2007). *Crash Course Respiratory System*, 3rd edn. London: Mosby.

Paul, P. (2010). Tracheostomy care and management in general wards and community settings: literature review. *Nursing In Critical Care.* 15(2): 76–85.

Ryan, B. (2005). Pneumothorax assessment and diagnostic testing. *Journal of Cardiovascular Nursing.* 20(4): 251–253.

Schwartzstein, R.M. and Parker, M.J. (2006). *Respiratory Physiology: A Clinical Approach*. Philadelphia: Lippincott Williams & Wilkins.

Sheldon, R.L. (2005). Pulmonary function testing. In: Wilkins, R.L., Sheldon, R.L. and Krider, S.J. (eds). *Clinical Assessment in Respiratory Care*, 5th edn. St. Louis: Elsevier Mosby.

Sims, J.M. (2006). An overview of asthma. *Dimensions of Critical Care Nursing.* 25(6): 264–268.

Sullivan, B. (2008). Nursing management of patients with a chest drain. *British Journal of Nursing.* 17(6): 388–393

West, J.B. (2007). *Pulmonary Pathophysiology: The Essentials*, 8th edn. Philadelphia: Lippincott Williams & Wilkins.

Wheeldon, A. (2011). The respiratory system. In: Peate, I. and Nair, M. (eds). *Fundamental Anatomy and Physiology for Student Nurses*. Chichester: Wiley-Blackwell.

275

10

The nervous system and associated disorders

Janet G. Migliozzi

Senior Lecturer, Department of Adult Nursing and Primary Care, University of Hertfordshire, Hatfield, Hertfordshire, UK

Contents

Fundamentals of Applied Pathophysiology: An Essential Guide for Nursing and Healthcare Students, Second Edition. Edited by Muralitharan Nair and Ian Peate.
© 2013 John Wiley & Sons, Ltd. Published 2013 by John Wiley & Sons, Ltd.

Key words

- Autonomic nervous system
- Brainstem
- Central nervous system
- Cerebrovascular accident
- Epilepsy
- Glasgow Coma Scale
- Limbic system
- Meninges
- Multiple sclerosis
- Parkinson's disease
- Peripheral nervous System
- Spinal cord

Test your prior knowledge

- List the structures of the central nervous system (CNS) and peripheral nervous system (PNS).
- What are the functions of the four areas of the brain?
- What are the major functions of the spinal cord?
- List the lobes of the cerebral hemispheres.
- Explain the term blood–brain barrier.

Learning outcomes

On completion of this section the reader will be able to:

- Outline the structure and function of the central and peripheral nervous systems.
- Describe the function of the autonomic nervous system and understand the function of its divisions.
- Discuss the functions of the 12 cranial nerves.
- Understand the care of the patient with a common disorder of the nervous system.

Don't forget to visit to the companion website for this book (www.wiley.com/go/ fundamentalsofappliedpathophysiology) where you can find self-assessment tests to check your progress, as well as lots of activities to practise your learning.

Introduction

The nervous system is the body's 'computer' as it is responsible for and controls all aspects of voluntary and involuntary action, and plays a major role in the co-ordination of the body's organ system to maintain homeostasis.

This chapter will discuss the structure and function of the central and peripheral nervous systems. Common disorders of the nervous system – multiple sclerosis, stroke, Parkinson's disease, Alzheimer's disease, epilepsy and traumatic head injury will also be explored and their management outlined.

Structure of the nervous system

The nervous system is divided into two major sections – the central nervous system (CNS) and the peripheral nervous system (PNS). The CNS consists of the brain and spinal cord. The PNS lies outside of the CNS and consists of the nerves that carry impulses to and from the spinal cord; it includes the cranial nerves from the brain and the spinal nerves from the spinal cord. The PNS can also be divided into the somatic and autonomic nervous system, which is divided further into the parasympathetic and sympathetic divisions (Figure 10.1).

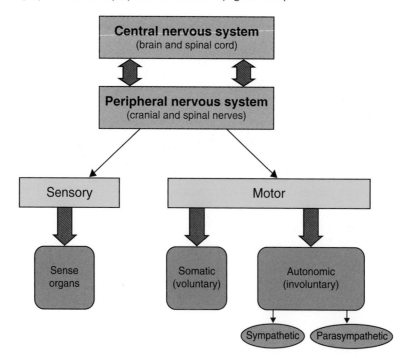

Figure 10.1   Divisions of the human nervous system.

Central nervous system

Brain

The brain or encephalon, which is encased in the cranium (or skull), is the body's control system and can be divided into four main parts (Figure 10.2):

- cerebrum
- cerebellum
- diencephalon
- brainstem.

Cerebrum

The cerebrum (or cerebral cortex) makes up the largest part of the brain and lies uppermost in the skull. The cerebrum consists of two frontal lobes, two parietal lobes, two temporal lobes and two occipital lobes, and is divided into the right and left cerebral hemispheres by fissures or sulci. The cerebral hemispheres are connected at their lower midpoint by the corpus callosum. The

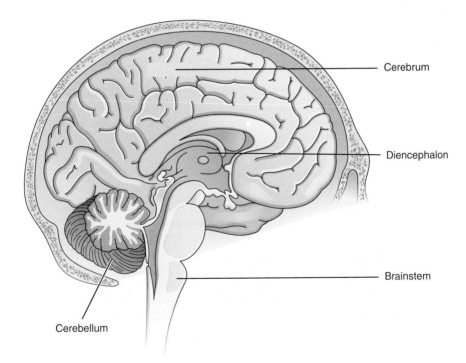

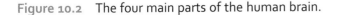

Figure 10.2   The four main parts of the human brain.

hemispheres' surface appears wrinkled due to the numerous convolutions or gyri – raised areas that fold in on each other to increase the brain's surface area. The surface of the cerebrum is known as the cerebral cortex and is composed of a thin layer of grey matter. The inner layer of the cerebrum consists mainly of white matter, but does contain some grey matter in the form of basal ganglia, which play an important role in producing automatic movements and the body's posture.

The cerebrum is divided into four lobes, each of which has a specific function (Table 10.1).

Table 10.1   The lobes of the cerebral hemispheres.

Lobe	Function
Frontal lobe	Conscious thought, abstract thinking, affective reactions, memory, judgement and initiation of motor activity.
Parietal lobe	Sensory functioning and sensory perception association
Temporal lobe	Processing of auditory information and auditory association (Wernicke's area)
Occipital lobe	Visual processing and association

Cerebellum

The cerebellum, which is separated from the brainstem by the fourth ventricle, lies under the occipital lobe of the cerebrum and is the second largest part of the human brain. It consists of an inner layer of white matter and an outer layer of grey matter, and plays a major role in balance, posture, fine movement and co-ordination.

Diencephalon

The diencephalon or interbrain lies between the brainstem and the cerebrum, where it encircles the third ventricle. It consists of the thalamus and hypothalamus. The pineal gland, which is responsible for the secretion of the hormone melatonin, is also located in the diencephalon.

The thalamus consists of grey matter and is a dumbbell-shaped structure that encloses the third ventricle of the brain. It acts as a relay centre that receives information from the body via the spinal cord and forwards this on to the appropriate areas of the brain. The thalamus plays a crucial role in the conscious awareness of pain and the limbic system of the brain, which controls instinctual and emotional drives, e.g. hunger, fear, sexual drive and short-term memory.

The hypothalamus is located just below the thalamus (as its name suggests) and is the major link between the body's endocrine and nervous system, where it has many roles to play in the regulation of homeostasis (Stanfield and Germann, 2008). The hypothalamus also forms part of the limbic system of the brain.

Brainstem

The brainstem connects the spinal cord to the remainder of the brain and is responsible for many essential functions, including the entry to and exit from the brain of 10 of the 12 cranial nerves (Table 10.2).

The brainstem contains the midbrain, the pons, the medulla oblongata and the reticular formation.

The midbrain or mesencephalon is a short section of the brainstem between the diencephalon and the pons, and is the centre for auditory and visual reflexes (Shier *et al.*, 2012). The midbrain consists of bundles of nerve fibres that join the lower parts of the brainstem and the spinal cord with the higher parts of the brain, and also plays a role in the control of the wakefulness of the brain.

The pons is Latin for 'bridge' and it connects the midbrain to the medulla and cerebrum. The pons plays an important role in the control of the rate and length of respiration.

The medulla oblongata, which consists of grey and white matter, is approximately 3 cm long and is, arguably, an extension of the spinal cord as it lies just inside the cranial cavity above the large hole in the occipital bone called the foramen magnum. Within it are contained a number of

Table 10.2   Cranial nerves.

Nerve	Brain location	Transmits nerve impulses to and from
I Olfactory	Olfactory bulb	Olfactory receptors for sense of smell
II Optic	Thalamus	Retina (sight)
III Oculomotor	Midbrain	Eye muscles (including eyelids, lens, pupil)
IV Trochlear	Midbrain	Eye muscles
V Trigeminal	Pons	Teeth, eyes, skin, tongue
VI Abducens	Pons	Jaw muscles (chewing) Eye muscles
VII Facial	Pons	Taste buds Facial muscles, tear and salivary glands
VIII Vestibulocochlear	Pons	Inner ear (hearing and balance)
IX Glossopharyngeal	Medulla oblongata	Pharyngeal muscles (swallowing)
X Vagus	Medulla oblongata	Internal organs
XI Spinal accessory	Medulla oblongata	Neck and back muscles
XII Hypoglossal	Medulla oblongata	Tongue muscles

reflex centres for control of blood vessel diameter, heart rate, breathing, coughing, swallowing, vomiting and sneezing. On either side of the medulla oblongata is a round oval protrusion called the olive, which plays a part in controlling balance, co-ordination and the intonation of sound impulses from the middle ear.

The reticular formation (RF) is a dense network of neurons that evolves from the medulla and midbrain and extends through the brainstem, and is important in the control of consciousness, arousal and the sleep–wake cycle (Stanfield and Germann, 2008).

Blood supply to the brain

The brain receives approximately 15% of the body's total circulating volume of blood, which is equivalent to 750 mL of blood per minute (Hickey, 2009), and this is supplied by the vertebral and internal carotid arteries. These two sets of arteries interconnect at the base of the brain to form the cerebral arterial circle or circle of Willis (Figure 10.3), which provides a collateral supply of blood to the whole of the brain in the event that one of the carotid arteries becomes compromised.

Blood–brain barrier

The brain (unlike other organs) is unable to withstand changes in levels of circulating nutrients, hormones and ions. Therefore, maintenance of a constant environment is crucial to the brain's

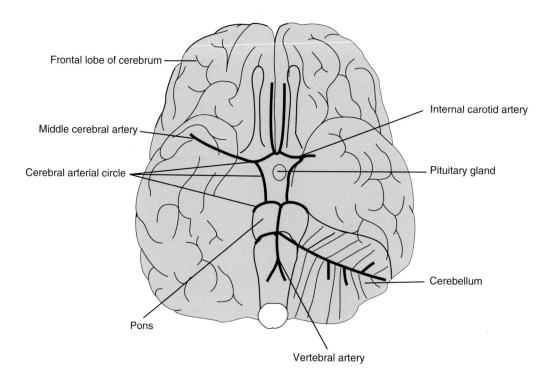

Figure 10.3   The circle of Willis.

ability to function, and the blood–brain barrier, which is an impermeable network of brain capillaries, acts as a 'filter' between the brain tissue and blood-borne substances to provide the brain with some protection against harmful toxins and metabolites. However, the blood–brain barrier provides little protection against fat-soluble molecules and respiratory gases (Marieb, 2011); consequently, some substances, e.g. nicotine, anaesthetic gases and alcohol, can cross the barrier and affect the brain.

Ventricles of the brain

The brain contains four interconnecting ventricles or cavities which produce, circulate and absorb cerebrospinal fluid (CSF) and also provide a protective barrier between the CSF and the brain. CSF, which protects and nourishes the brain, consists of water, glucose, protein and electrolytes, and is continually secreted by specialized epithelial cells called the choroid plexus.

283

Meninges

The dura mater, arachnoid mater and pia mater or meninges are the three layers of connective tissue that protect and cover the brain and spinal cord.

Spinal cord

The spinal cord is located in the vertebral column and provides the communication route between the brain and parts of the body not supplied by cranial nerves. There are 31 pairs of spinal nerves, which are grouped as either the cervical, thoracic or lumber spinal nerves according to their location along the vertebral column (Figure 10.4).

Peripheral nervous system

The peripheral nervous system consists of the nerves connecting the brain and spinal cord to other parts of the body, and includes the cranial and spinal nerves (Figure 10.4) that connect the brain and spinal cord to the peripheral structures, e.g. the skin and skeletal muscles. The PNS is divided into the somatic and autonomic nervous systems of which the autonomic nervous system has two divisions – the parasympathetic and sympathetic divisions.

Somatic nervous system

The somatic nervous system consists of motor neurons that connect the CNS to the skin and skeletal muscles, and plays a major role in the regulation of skeletal muscle contractions and conscious activities.

Autonomic nervous system

The autonomic nervous system (ANS) plays a major role in the maintenance of homeostasis by regulating the body's automatic, involuntary functions. In common with the rest of the nervous system, it consists of neurons, neuroglia and other connective tissue. However, its structure is unique in that it is divided in two – the sympathetic division and the parasympathetic division.

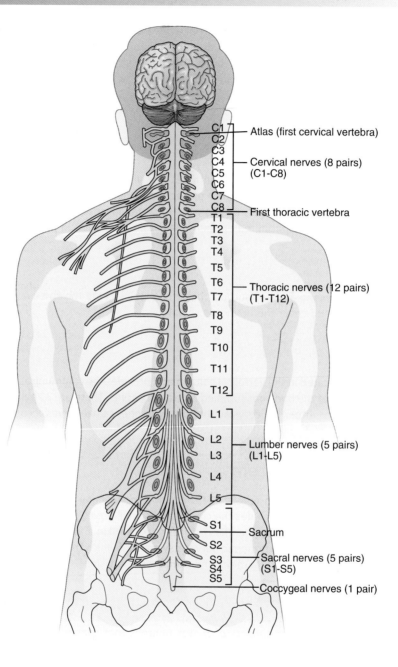

C1 — Atlas (first cervical vertebra)
C2
C3
C4 — Cervical nerves (8 pairs)
C5   (C1-C8)
C6
C7
C8 — First thoracic vertebra
T1
T2
T3
T4
T5
T6 — Thoracic nerves (12 pairs)
T7   (T1-T12)
T8
T9
T10
T11
T12
L1
L2 — Lumber nerves (5 pairs)
L3   (L1-L5)
L4
L5
S1 — Sacrum
S2
S3 — Sacral nerves (5 pairs)
S4   (S1-S5)
S5
Coccygeal nerves (1 pair)

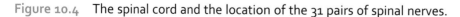

Figure 10.4   The spinal cord and the location of the 31 pairs of spinal nerves.

The sympathetic division controls many internal organs when a stressful situation occurs. This can take the form of physical stress, e.g. if undertaking strenuous exercise, or emotional stress, e.g. at times of anger or anxiety. In emergency situations, the sympathetic nervous system releases norepinephrine which assists in the 'fight or flight' response.

The parasympathetic division utilises acetylcholine to control all the internal responses associated with a state of relaxation and therefore has the opposite effect on the body to the sympathetic nervous system.

Table 10.3 provides a summary of the physiological effects of the sympathetic and parasympathetic divisions of the nervous system.

Table 10.3   Physiological effects of the sympathetic and parasympathetic nervous systems.

Organ/system	Sympathetic effects	Parasympathetic effects
Cell metabolism	Increases metabolic rate, stimulates fat breakdown and increases blood sugar levels	No effect
Blood vessels	Constricts blood vessels in viscera and skin Dilates blood vessels in the heart and skeletal muscle	No effect
Eye	Dilates pupils	Constricts pupils
Heart	Increases rate and force of contraction	Decreases rate
Lungs	Dilates bronchioles	Constricts bronchioles
Kidneys	Decreases urine output	No effect
Liver	Causes the release of glucose	No effect
Digestive system	Decreases peristalsis and constricts digestive system sphincters	Increases peristalsis and dilates digestive system sphincters
Adrenal medulla	Stimulates cells to secrete epinephrine and norepinephrine	No effect
Lacrimal glands	Inhibits the production of tears	Increases the production of tears
Salivary glands	Inhibits the production of saliva	Increases the production of saliva
Sweat glands	Stimulates to produce perspiration	No effect

Disorders of the nervous system

Learning outcomes

At the end of this section the reader will be able to:

- List some of the common diseases associated with disorders of the central nervous system.

- Describe the pathophysiological processes related to some specific central nervous system disorders.

- Outline the management and interventions related to the disorders described.

- Discuss some of the non-pharmacological interventions used in the treatment of the disorders.

Raised intracranial pressure

Intracranial pressure (ICP) is the recordable pressure within the skull caused by three intracranial components – brain tissue, cerebrospinal fluid (CSF) and blood. As the skull is a rigid structure, any increase in volume in any of the three components will lead to an increase in ICP. Several conditions can lead to an increase in ICP, including bleeding in the brain due to a head injury, a space-occupying lesion, e.g. a brain tumour, or infection, e.g. a brain abscess. Left untreated, raised ICP can lead to poor perfusion of the brain as the cerebral arteries and veins become compressed and the brain herniates or shifts as it becomes compressed within the skull. Common signs and symptoms of increased ICP in the early stages are:

- decreasing levels of consciousness
- headache
- sluggish pupil reaction
- visual disturbances
- abnormal breathing patterns
- impaired motor responses.

In the later stages the individual may experience:

- further deterioration in level of consciousness
- a rise in systolic blood pressure
- a fall in diastolic blood pressure
- irregular shallow, slow breathing
- slow pulse
- a high temperature.

Care and management of the patient at risk of increased intracranial pressure

Patients at risk of neurological deterioration require frequent, accurate neurological assessment in order to detect problems early. Therefore, healthcare professionals need to be able to perform a basic neurological assessment and also understand the significance of the findings (Waterhouse, 2005).

A neurological assessment should include:

- conscious level
- pupil size and reactivity
- vital signs, e.g. temperature, heart rate, respiratory rate, blood pressure and blood oxygen saturation
- limb movements (National Institute for Health and Clinical Excellence, 2007b).

Glasgow Coma Scale

The National Institute for Health and Clinical Excellence (2007a) advocates the use of the Glasgow Coma Scale (GCS) for assessment and classification of all head-injured patients.

The GCS was specifically designed as a tool for detecting and monitoring changes in the patient's neurological status by evaluating three categories of behaviour – eye opening, verbal response and motor response (Table 10.4). Within each category, each level of response is allocated a

Table 10.4   The Glasgow Coma Scale.

Feature	Response	Score
Best eye response	Open spontaneously	4
	Open to verbal command	3
	Open to pain	2
	No eye opening	1
Best verbal response	Orientated	5
	Confused	4
	Inappropriate words	3
	Incomprehensible sounds	2
	No verbal response	1
Best motor response	Obeys commands	6
	Localising pain	5
	Withdrawal from pain	4
	Flexion to pain	3
	Extension to pain	2
	No motor response	1

Adapted from National Institute of Health and Clinical Excellence (2007a).

numerical value (Waterhouse, 2005) and the lower the patient scores on the scale, the more serious the neurological condition, e.g. a score of 15 indicates a fully conscious, alert, responsive patient, whereas a score of 3 means that the patient is deeply unconscious.

Vital signs recording

The National Institute for Health and Clinical Excellence (2007a) recommends that the head-injured patient with a GCS of less than 15 should have their vital signs monitored half-hourly until a GCS of 15 is achieved. After the initial assessment (usually in the emergency department), the frequency of observations of patients with a GCS equal to 15 should be:

- half-hourly for 2 hours
- then 1-hourly for 4 hours
- then 2-hourly thereafter.

If the patient with a GCS of 15 deteriorates at any time after the initial 2-hour period, observations should revert back to half-hourly and follow the schedule as outlined above. Additionally, the patient should undergo an urgent reappraisal by medical staff if they experience any of the following (National Institute for Health and Clinical Excellence, 2007a):

- development of agitation or abnormal behaviour
- development of severe or increasing headache or persistent vomiting
- a sustained (at least 30 minutes) drop of one point in the GCS (a drop of one point in the motor response score requires more urgent attention)
- a drop of three or more points in the eye-opening or verbal response scores of the GCS or two or more points in the motor response score
- new or evolving neurological signs or symptoms, e.g. pupil inequality or loss of movement/strength to one side of the body or face.

Case study

Mrs Ankora, a 60-year-old woman, presented to the accident and emergency department complaining of a frontal headache one weeks duration. On the day of admission she experienced an increase in intensity of the headache, it being more global in nature. Mrs Ankora also complained of being weak all over and feeling unsteady on her feet. She denied any change in hearing or vision.

Mrs Ankora has a history of high blood pressure but stopped taking her antihypertensive medication a year ago because of the side effects. She gave up smoking 20 years ago and only occasionally drinks alcohol. She is not currently taking any medications and has no known allergies. On admission to the department, Mrs Ankora's vital signs recordings are:

- temperature 36.7°C
- heart rate 55 beats per minute
- respirations 20 breaths per minute
- blood pressure 260/120 mmHg
- oxygen saturation level 98%.

On examination Mrs Ankora was sleepy, but when aroused she was alert and orientated. Her GCS was 14 and her pupils were equal and reactive. Mrs Ankora was then sent for a head CT scan which revealed a left frontal and parietal intracerebral haemorrhage. Upon return from the CT scan, Mrs Ankora was noted to have expereinced a decrease in her level of consciousness and her GCS was now 9.

Take some time to reflect on this case and then consider the following.

1. What type of stroke has Mrs Ankora experienced?
2. Discuss the signs and symptoms that Mrs Ankora is experiencing.
3. Discuss the role of antihypertensive medication in managing Mrs Ankora's condition.
4. Outline the immediate care that Mrs Ankora will require.

Stroke (cerebrovascular accident)

A cerebrovascular accident (CVA) or 'stroke' occurs as a direct result of impaired blood flow to the brain either because of vessel occlusion or haemorrhaging due to a ruptured vessel. The nature and extent of neurological impairment that the patient may suffer is dependent on the amount and location of oxygen starvation that the brain tissue has experienced and/or the severity of cerebral bleeding that has occurred.

Stroke is the third most common cause of death (approximately 66 000 deaths each year) and a leading cause of adult disability in the UK (Turner and Jowett, 2006). Whilst stroke is primarily a disease experienced by older people and is more likely to be experienced by men (although women who experience a stroke are more likely to die), other factors exist that make certain groups more at risk of having a stroke (The Stroke Association, 2004):

- smoking
- obesity
- history of heart disease or high blood pressure (hypertension)
- high cholesterol (hyperlipidaemia)
- diabetes
- Afro-Caribbean or South Asian descent
- a family history of stroke at a young age (less than 50 years of age).

Pathophysiology

The brain is unable to store nutrients or glucose for use and is therefore dependent on a steady supply of these from the circulation of blood via the internal carotid and vertebral arteries. Any interruption of blood supply to the brain tissue will result in ischaemia and if prolonged, results in death of brain cells. There are two main types of stroke – ischaemic stroke and haemorrhagic stroke.

Ischaemic stroke, which accounts for 85% of all strokes (Hickey, 2009), occurs when a blood clot blocks an artery to the brain, causing an interruption of blood flow to the brain cells. A high cholesterol level causing a 'furring' of the arteries is a common cause of this type of stroke

Table 10.5   Signs and symptoms of stroke according to side of brain affected.

Damage to left side of brain	Damage to right side of brain
Loss of motor function to the right side of the body	Loss of motor function to the left side of the body
Language impairment – either an inability to express self – expressive aphasia, or difficulty in understanding or using speech appropriately although able to speak fluently – receptive aphasia	Language centres not affected
Right visual field deficit	Left visual field deficit
Frustration and depression over loss of independence	Apparent unconcern over loss of independence
Intellectual impairment	Poor judgement and impulsive behaviour

Haemorrhagic stroke occurs when a blood vessel in or around the brain bursts, causing bleeding and increased pressure in the skull, resulting in compression and eventual ischaemia to brain tissue. Untreated high blood pressure (hypertension) is a common cause of this type of stroke.

Following a stroke it is possible to determine the area of the brain that has been damaged by observing the signs and symptoms the patient may experience (Table 10.5).

Transient ischaemic attack

A transient ischaemic attack (TIA) or 'mini' stroke is a temporary interruption in blood flow to the brain which can result in numbness, temporary paralysis and impaired speech. Whilst the symptoms experienced are not permanent and by definition resolve within 24 hours (Monahan et al., 2007), a TIA is often a warning of an impending, more serious cerebrovascular accident.

Pharmacological management

The pharmacological treatment of stroke aims to prevent the reoccurrence of stroke or TIA whilst also taking into consideration the cause of the stroke.

- In the first 3 hours of an ischaemic stroke occurring, the use of thrombolytic therapy, e.g. alteplase, is advocated (National Institute of Health and Clinical Excellence, 2007b).
- Aspirin or dipyridamole (Persantin) may be prescribed to reduce platelet aggregation in the case of TIA or ischaemic stroke.
- Antihypertensives may be prescribed for patients who have high blood pressure.
- Cholesterol-reducing drugs such as simvastatin should be prescribed to prevent recurrent ischaemic stroke or TIA (Turner and Jowett, 2006).

Non-pharmacological management

- Carotid endarterectomy (removal of fatty plaques from the wall of the carotid artery) may be performed in patients with stenosis (narrowing) of the carotid arteries that supply blood to the brain.

- The patient should be educated as to the importance of a varied diet that is low in fat in order to keep their blood cholesterol within safe limits. Patients who are overweight or obese need support to lose weight and be encouraged to take regular exercise.
- Patients should be offered support to stop smoking and reduce alcohol intake.
- Regular monitoring of blood pressure is important to ensure that it is kept within safe limits and patients should be encouraged to reduce their salt intake.

Care and management

Management of a patient who has suffered a stroke varies according to the area of the brain affected and the neurological and functional deficits that the individual experiences. However, the care of the patient during the acute phase of stroke will differ from the care required once the patient has stabilised and is in the rehabilitative phase.

291

Key considerations during the acute phase focus on early detection and prevention of neurological deterioration and life-threatening complications:

- Frequent monitoring of the patient's vital signs and neurological function during the acute phase using an appropriate assessment tool, e.g. the Glasgow Coma Scale, to detect any deterioration in the patient's level of consciousness.
- Keeping the patient nil by mouth until an assessment of the swallowing reflex can be carried out.
- Undertaking a nutritional status assessment within the first 48 hours of admission.
- Protecting the patient from injury due to possible seizures, motor and visual deficits.
- Preventing pressure sore formation as immobility and incontinence place the patient at increased risk.
- Providing explanations to the patient and their family concerning treatment and care interventions in order to alleviate anxiety and fear.

During the rehabilitative phase of stroke, care is geared towards maximising the patient's independence and key considerations include:

- Collaborating with other healthcare professionals to teach the patient adaptive measures to enable them to carry out their activities of daily living, e.g. bathing, eating, dressing and toileting, as independently as possible.
- Minimising the risk of injury and complications associated with impaired mobility.
- Involving a speech therapist to ensure that the patient who has impaired communication is able to express themselves effectively.
- Providing information and support for the patient and their carers/family.
- Liaising with other healthcare professionals and social services prior to the patient's discharge from hospital to ensure that the patient's home environment is suitably adapted to deal with any residual disabilities that the patient may have.

Parkinson's disease (paralysis agitans)

Parkinson's disease (PD) is a disease of the brain that mainly affects older people (but not exclusively) and progresses over time (National Institute of Health and Clinical Excellence, 2006b). This is caused by the loss of cells that produce a messenger called dopamine, which is involved in controlling muscles.

The disease is estimated to affect between 100 and 180 per 100 000 of the UK population and has an incidence of 4–20 per 100 000 (National Institute of Health and Clinical Excellence, 2006b). Whilst the causes of PD are unknown, there is an increased risk of PD with age and also men are more likely to be affected.

Pathophysiology

The symptoms of PD are directly attributable to the loss of the neurotransmitter dopamine from the basal nuclei nerve cells in the substantia nigra of the basal ganglia within the cerebrum.

Levels of dopamine are closely linked with the levels of other chemicals in the brain, including acetylcholine, and low levels of dopamine, together with changes in other chemicals, lead to the symptoms of PD (Monahan *et al.*, 2007):

- slow movements (bradykinesia)
- tremors (initially in the hand but also seen in the limbs, head, face and jaw)
- muscle stiffness and rigidity
- tendency to walk forward on the toes with small, shuffling steps
- changes in balance
- stooped posture
- confusion
- depression
- difficulty with fine motor functions, e.g. writing and eating
- 'mask'-like face
- general weakness and muscle fatigue.

At present, it is not known what causes the loss of the cells that produce dopamine; however, both inherited and sporadic forms of PD have been identified and in both cases degenerative changes have been found within the affected brain tissue (Hickey, 2009).

Pharmacological management

Treatment for PD aims primarily to replace dopamine in the brain and minimise the effects of the disease. Drugs commonly used include:

- L-dopa or levodopa, which is the precursor to dopamine, is the mainstay of treatment for PD. However, as the drug does not cross the blood–brain barrier effectively, it has to be combined with either carbidopa (Sinemet) or benserazide (Madopar) to increase its uptake by the brain.
- Selegiline (Eldepryl) is commonly prescribed for patients who are newly diagnosed with PD as it delays the progression of the disease by blocking the metabolism of dopamine and delaying the need for L-dopa (Monahan *et al.*, 2007).
- Amantadine (Symmetrel) – an antiviral agent that is also used in the early stages of PD as it acts by allowing more dopamine to accumulate at and enter the nerve synapse, which delays the need for L-dopa.
- Anticholenergic drugs, such as trihexyphenidyl (Artane) and benztropine mesylate (Cogentin), are often used in addition to L-dopa (or in patients who cannot tolerate it) to treat tremor and rigidity.

Non-pharmacological management

- Surgery to create lesions on one side of the thalamus (thalamotomy) or destroy part of the basal ganglia (pallidotomy) to control rigidity and tremor was the treatment for PD prior to L-dopa becoming available. It has become popular once again due to the complication associated with the long-term use of, or intolerance to, L-dopa (Hickey, 2009).
- More recent therapy has involved the use of deep-brain stimulation to send impulses deep into the brain and block the signals that cause parkinsonian movements (Mader, 2011).
- The use of stem cells from the umbilical cords of the newborn or the creation of the patient's genetically identical cells using donor eggs are experimental treatments currently being explored (Hickey, 2009).

Care and management

Whilst the majority of patients with PD are managed in the community, as the disease progresses to the later stages, the patient may require residential/nursing home care. Key considerations include:

- Reducing the threat of injury from falls; due to physical immobility, weakness, rigidity and slow movement the patient with PD is at greater risk. This may also require undertaking a risk assessment of the patient's home environment to ensure that any potential hazards are removed.
- Ensuring that the patient is able to express themselves effectively; due to vocal changes and difficulty with writing, the patient's ability to communicate may be affected. Therefore, it might be necessary to involve a speech therapist and other support measures to ensure that the patient will be able to communicate effectively.
- Monitoring the patient's body weight and the provision of adequate nutrition that the patient is able to tolerate; due to possible difficulties with swallowing (dysphagia), there is a risk of malnutrition and weight loss.
- Assisting the patient with meeting their hygiene needs as necessary.

Alzheimer's disease

There are approximately 750 000 people in the UK with dementia. The condition mainly affects those over the age of 65 years and the likelihood increases with age. However, there are 16 000 people in the UK under the age of 65 years who have dementia.

The term 'dementia' describes a set of symptoms that include loss of memory, mood changes, and problems with communication and reasoning. These symptoms occur when the brain is damaged by certain diseases, including Alzheimer's disease (AD), or by a series of small strokes.

Pathophysiology

Although the cause of AD remains unclear, the disease does cause structural changes in the brain, predominately plaques and tangles. Additionally, the disease has also been associated with a shortage of acetylcholine, loss of nerve cells and structural changes in the memory and cognition areas of the brain. Therefore, the sufferer exhibits memory loss, poor judgement, disorientation, confusion, changes in personality that can lead to mood swings, and sometimes violent outbursts.

Table 10.6   Stages of Alzheimer's disease.

Stage of disease	Common signs and symptoms
1 (2–4 years)	Loss of interest in people, environment and present affairs Hesitant in using own initiative, becomes uncertain about making decisions/actions and is forgetful
2 (2–12 years)	Memory loss becomes more apparent, has difficulty in undertaking simple tasks or carrying out simple instructions Loses documents, forgets to pay bills or undertake household chores Unable to meet own needs, loses inhibitions, has periods of irritability, paranoia and anxiety Prone to wandering particularly at night, becomes lost in familiar surroundings and may forget way home
3 (Final stage)	Loses the ability to communicate verbally or in writing Becomes bedridden and incontinent of urine and faeces Does not recognise loved ones Becomes emaciated due to lack of eating

Inability to maintain self-care, wandering and hallucinations are common in the later stages. Table 10.6 outlines the stages of the disease.

Pharmacological management

Whilst there is no cure for AD, there are a number of drugs that can alleviate or slow down the symptoms of the disease:

- Donepezil (Aricept), rivastigmine tartrate (Exelon) and galantamine (Reminyl) work by maintaining existing levels of acetylcholine in patients with mild to moderate dementia.
- Memantine (Ebixa) can be used in patients with middle to late stage dementia; it prevents excess entry of calcium ions into brain cells. Excess calcium is known to damage brain cells and prevent them from receiving messages from other brain cells.

In addition, drug therapy can be used to manage behavioural changes associated with the disease. These include:

- antidepressant medication to treat depressive symptoms
- neuroleptic drugs to treat psychosis and delusional behaviour
- sedatives to treat agitation.

Non-pharmacological management

Patients with mild to moderate disease should be offered the opportunity to participate in a structured group cognitive stimulation programme (National Institute of Health and Clinical Excellence, 2006a).

Care and management

The progressive nature of AD, which results in the patient's loss of independence, personality and cognitive function, presents the healthcare professional and the patient's family with many challenges. Key considerations include:

- Maintenance of a safe environment; due to loss of judgement, cognitive decline and poor memory, the patient is at increased risk of injury.
- Maintenance of hygiene and nutritional needs; due to loss of independence and the inability to make decisions, the patient is unable to meet or plan for their own needs.
- Promotion of restful sleep as the patient is likely to be awake at night and prone to wandering.

Case study

Joe Devlin, a 32-year-old graphic artist, has been admitted to the neurology ward for further investigations. Mr Devlin has a history of fatigue and numbness to his left lower leg and foot, and has recently experienced falls because of this. He is now also complaining of numbness to his hands. He is very anxious because his maternal grandmother also experienced similar symptoms and was found to be suffering from multiple sclerosis.

On neurological examination, he has absent abdominal reflexes with brisk tendon jerks and bilateral extensor plantar responses. Blood investigations are normal, including haemoglobin and white cell count. A lumbar puncture is carried out. The cerebrospinal fluid (CSF) investigation results show oligoclonal IgG bands that are not found in normal CSF, but are found in 90% of patients with multiple sclerosis; in the absence of clinical signs of infection, this test is almost diagnostic of multiple sclerosis.

Take some time to reflect on this case and then consider the following.

1. Discuss the signs and symptoms that Mr Devlin is experiencing.
2. Discuss the role of pharmacological interventions in managing Mr Devlin's condition.
3. Outline the immediate care that Mr Devlin will require.
4. Discuss the health promotion advice Mr Devlin may require to remain safe?

Multiple sclerosis

Multiple sclerosis (MS) is a chronic degenerative disease in which demyelination of the brain and spinal cord damages the nerve pathways, with loss of function in the affected area. The disease is progressive; however, the patient may experience periods of remission before relapsing again.

Whilst the cause of MS is unclear, it is thought to be linked to an impaired immune system following a viral infection that initiates an autoimmune response.

Pathophysiology

MS affects primarily the white matter of the brain and spinal cord by causing areas of demyelination and a breakdown of the myelin sheath that surrounds the nerve fibres and axons (Figure 10.5), preventing conduction of normal nerve impulses.

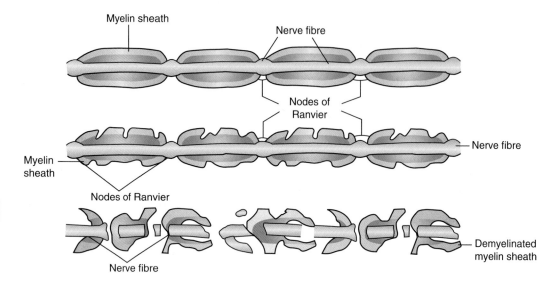

Figure 10.5   The process of demyelination.

Signs and symptoms

The signs and symptoms of MS vary greatly from patient to patient and may vary over time in the same patient (Hickey, 2009). Common signs and symptoms are:

- muscular weakness/feeling of heaviness to the legs
- numbness to face or extremities
- loss of short-term memory
- visual field defects
- bladder and bowel dysfunction
- sexual dysfunction
- fatigue
- depression.

Pharmacological management

Whilst MS is an incurable, extremely debilitating disease, it is rarely fatal (Monahan *et al.*, 2007) and drug therapy can help with the management of the condition. Drug therapy falls into two broad categories:

- Treatment to slow or arrest the disease process – includes the use of interferon and steroids, e.g. prednisolone, to treat acute relapses and aid recovery.
- Treatment to manage the symptoms of MS:
  - baclofen to treat muscle spasticity
  - stool softeners and laxatives to manage constipation
  - oxybutynen (Ditropan) to manage bladder function
  - fluoxetine, (Prozac), amitriptyline (Elavil) or imipramine (Tofranil) to treat depression.

Care and management

Due to the unpredictable nature of its progression, MS presents the healthcare professional, the patient and their family with many challenges. Therefore, the care of the patient with MS will require a multidisciplinary approach to ensure that all aspects of care are met. The healthcare professional plays a key role in this process and key considerations include:

- Minimising risk of injury due to weakness, impaired co-ordination and sensory deficits.
- Preventing complications related to immobility and physical weakness.
- Ensuring that the patient's activities of daily living are met.
- Providing the patient with education and psychological support to understand and adapt to the unpredictable nature of their illness.
- Educating the patient as to how to avoid relapses where possible, e.g. keeping stress to a minimum, reducing the risk of infection.

Epilepsy

There are approximately 600,000 people with epilepsy in the UK, i.e. one in every 103 people has epilepsy (Joint Epilepsy Council, 2011). The disease affects all age groups and 32,000 new cases are treated each year.

Pathophysiology

A seizure or 'fit' is caused by an abnormal electrical discharge in the brain in either the sensory system, motor system or autonomic nervous system, and in the majority of cases the cause is unknown (Martini and Nath, 2011). However, seizures of all kinds are accompanied by a marked change in the pattern of electrical activity in the brain. The change starts in one part of the brain and may spread to nearby areas or continue across the whole of the cerebral cortex. Consequently a seizure may take many different forms, depending on the area and amount of the brain involved. The International League against Epilepsy has developed a widely used system of classifying seizures (Table 10.7).

Status epilepticus

Status epilepticus is an episode of seizure activity lasting at least 30 minutes or repeated seizures without a full recovery period in between (Monahan et al., 2007). Prolonged seizures can be life threatening as they lead to cellular destruction and death if not stopped, and should be treated as a medical emergency.

Care and management of the patient with seizures

Healthcare professionals need to act quickly when a patient has a seizure. Key considerations include:

- Easing the patient to the floor if seated when the seizure occurs.
- Protecting the patient from injury by moving nearby furniture or objects out of the way and putting a pillow under the head.
- Not restraining the patient or forcing anything into the patient's mouth.

Table 10.7   Classification of seizures.

Type of seizure	Effect on consciousness	Signs and symptoms	Postictal state
Partial seizures			
Simple partial seizure	Not impaired	Twitching or tingling and numbness of a body area Loss of speech Sensory disturbance or 'aura', e.g. seeing lights, strange smells, feeling of déjà vu Feeling of fear or doom	No
Complex partial seizure	Impaired	Begins as a partial seizure but progresses to a tonic clonic. Automatic behaviour or automatism experienced, e.g. chewing, lip smacking or picking at clothes	Yes
Generalized seizures			
Tonic-clonic (in any combination) Absence – Typical Atypical Absence with special features Myclonic absence Eyelid myoclonia			
Focal seizures			
Unknown Epileptic spasms			
NB Seizure that cannot be clearly diagnosed into one of the preceding categories should be considered unclassified until further information allows their accurate diagnosis. This is not considered a classification category, however.			

(Berg *et al.*, 2010).

- When the seizure has stopped, ensuring that the airway is clear and administering oxygen if necessary.
- Documenting the duration and type of seizure as well as how long it takes for the patient to become fully responsive to their surrounding (post-ichtal phase).
- Staying with the patient throughout the seizure and orientating/informing the patient about the event once they are awake.

Care and management of the patient with status epilepticus

As status epilepticus is a medical emergency, key considerations include:

- Maintenance of the patient's airway to ensure adequate ventilation – this may include suction of the airway to prevent obstruction.
- Providing oxygen therapy via nasal cannulae as prescribed.
- Protecting the patient from injury.
- Administering prescribed medication, usually diazepam or lorazepam, until the seizures stop.

Pharmacological management

Up to 70% of people with epilepsy have the condition controlled with anti-epileptic (also known as anticonvulsant) drugs and many people become seizure-free on the first drug that is used (Bingham, 2004). Commonly drugs used include:

- carbamazepine (Tegretol)
- sodium valporate (Epilim)
- phenytoin (Dilantin).

Non-pharmacological management

- Surgical intervention, such as removal of the temporal lobe (temporal lobectomy), and vagal nerve stimulation may be performed for patients who do not respond to medication.
- As treatment for epilepsy is usually long-term or life-long, the patient needs to be educated as to the importance of compliance with drug therapy.
- The patient needs to be educated as to lifestyle changes that may be required as a result of having epilepsy, e.g. occupation, driving, etc.

Conclusion

Due to the complex nature of the nervous system, impairment to any part of it means that the symptoms that the patient experiences are dependent on the areas of the nervous system affected and the extent of damage incurred. Therefore, caring for the patient with a neurological disorder presents healthcare professionals with many challenges and the overall aim of this chapter was to provide the reader with insight into some of the more common related problems of the nervous system and their management.

Test your knowledge

- Compare and contrast the differing function of the parasympathetic and sympathetic divisions of the autonomic nervous system.

- What are the three structural types of neurons?

- Discuss the reason why calcium is needed for the release of neurotransmitter at the synapse.

- Describe the structure and function of the four areas of the brain.

- Devise a care plan for a patient who has sustained a traumatic head injury.

- Outline the common signs and symptoms that an individual is likely to experience at each stage of Alzheimer's disease.

- List the pharmaceutical agents commonly used to treat Parkinson's disease and describe their mode of action.

Activities

Here are some activities and exercises to help test your learning. For the answers to these exercises, as well as further self-testing activities, visit our website at www.wiley.com/go/fundamentalsofappliedpathophysiology

Fill in the blanks

The _____ nervous system (PNS) is a collective term for the nervous system structures that do not lie within the _____. The PNS is divided into the _____ and _____ nervous systems. The somatic part consists of the nerves that _____ the skin, joints, and muscles. The autonomic nervous system consists of two parts: the _____ and the _____. The PNS collects _____ from numerous sources both _____ and _____ the body and _____ it to and from the central nervous system to various _____ of the _____.

Choose from:
Information; Somatic; Innervate; Inside; Body; CNS; Peripheral; Autonomic; Relays; Parts; Parasympathetic nervous system; Outside; Sympathetic nervous system

Label the diagram

Using the list of words supplied, label the diagram.

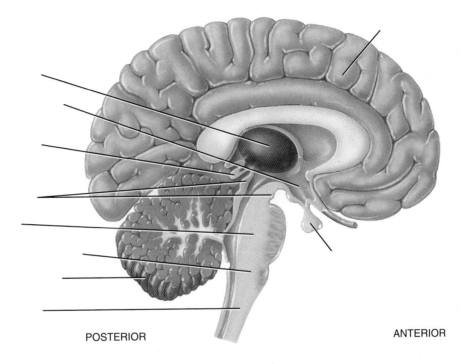

POSTERIOR   ANTERIOR

Cerebellum; Thalamus; Hypothalamus; Pituitary gland; Pineal gland; Pons; Cerebrum; Epthalmus; Brainstem; Medula oblongata; Spinal cord

Word search

Q	G	G	O	R	X	A	F	W	E	W	G	F	E	B
D	N	Y	T	O	U	C	I	Y	N	Q	Z	Y	Y	J
E	C	E	F	Z	I	E	A	J	I	F	A	K	Y	N
M	E	L	M	S	I	T	S	F	M	P	A	G	M	O
E	R	C	J	Z	I	Y	R	O	A	I	P	W	R	I
N	N	I	B	K	J	L	E	Y	P	W	M	J	K	T
T	E	R	G	L	E	C	M	S	O	O	Y	W	A	A
I	R	T	K	K	K	H	I	P	D	Q	U	Q	T	N
A	U	N	T	U	O	O	E	E	Y	Z	X	L	J	I
J	Z	E	R	V	R	L	H	L	P	P	M	Y	N	L
W	I	V	A	S	T	I	Z	I	O	C	T	Z	U	E
L	E	T	C	Z	S	N	L	P	X	F	P	C	A	Y
W	S	L	N	O	K	E	A	E	P	D	O	M	S	M
J	R	P	S	N	O	S	N	I	K	R	A	P	O	E
A	I	S	E	N	I	K	Y	D	A	R	B	F	T	D

Acetylcholine	Ventricle	Stroke
Dementia	Epilepsy	Bradykinesia
Demyelination	Seizure	Parkinsons
Dopamine	Alzheimers	

Further resources

Alzheimer's Association

http://www.alz.org

This is a comprehensive website that students may find useful for understanding all aspects of Alzheimer's disease. The Alzheimer's Association works on a global, national and local level to enhance care and support for all those affected by Alzheimer's and related dementias.

NHS Clinical Knowledge Summaries

http://www.cks.nhs.uk/head_injury

The NHS Clinical Knowledge Summaries are a reliable source of evidence-based information and practical 'know how' about a range of common conditions. This is a useful website for students wishing to understand more about the treatment and management of head injury.

Department of Health

http://www.dh.gov.uk/en/Publicationsandstatistics/Publications/PublicationsPolicyAnd Guidance/DH_4010537

This government website contains useful information on an array of health topics. This link provides access to an action plan for improving services for people with epilepsy in response to the National Clinical Audit of Epilepsy-Related Death.

NICE Pathways

http://www.nice.org.uk/stroke

The National Institute for Clinical Excellence has recently developed 'NICE Pathways', an online tool for health and social care professionals. It brings together all related NICE guidance and associated products in a set of interactive topic-based diagrams, and provides an easier and more intuitive way to find, access and use NICE guidance. NICE Pathways is a useful tool for students wishing to find out about particular health topics and includes a pathway for stroke.

Multiple Sclerosis

http://guidance.nice.org.uk/CG8/NICEGuidance/pdf/English

This is a useful resource for students wishing to understand more about current NICE guidance on multiple sclerosis.

Parkinson's Organisation

http://www.parkinsons.org.uk/pdf/B126_Professionalsguide.pdf

This is a useful website providing information on Parkinson's disease. This link provides details of a multidisciplinary project to create the professional's guide to Parkinson's disease.

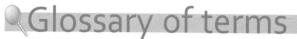 Glossary of terms

Acetylcholine:	a neurotransmitter found widely in the central and peripheral nervous system.
Choroid plexus:	the tissue in the ventricles of the brain which produces cerebrospinal fluid.
Dementia:	the loss of mental ability.
Demyelination:	the loss of the myelin sheath from around the axon of the nerve cell.
Dopamine:	a neurotransmitter found in the central nervous system.
Foramen magnum:	a large hole in the occipital bone through which the vertebral column and spinal cord pass.
Norepinepherine (noradrenaline):	a neurotransmitter in the central and peripheral nervous system.
Schwann cell:	a cell that forms myelin around the axon of a nerve cell
Substantia nigra:	the part of the midbrain that connects to the basal ganglia.
Ventricle:	a cavity filled with cerebrospinal fluid.

References

Berg, A.T., Berkovic, S.F., Marin, J.B., Buchhalter, J., Cross, J.H., van Emde Boas, W., Engel, J., French, J., Glauser, T.A., Mathern, G.W., Moshe, S.L., Nordli, D., Plouin, P. and Scheffer, I.E. (2010). Revised terminology and concepts for organization of seizures and epilepsies: Report of the ILAE Commission on Classification and Terminology, 2005-2009. *Epilepsia.* 51(4): 676–685.

Bingham, E. (2004). Diagnosis and support for people with epilepsy. *Practice Nursing.* 15(2): 64–70.

Hickey, J. (2009). *The Clinical Practice of Neurological and Neurosurgical Nursing*, 6th edn. Philadelphia: Lippincott Williams and Wilkins.

Longenbaker, S.N. (2011). *Maders Understanding Human Anatomy and Physiology*. London: McGraw Hill.

Marieb, E.N. (2011). *Essentials of Human Anatomy and Physiology*, 9th edn. London: Pearson Education.

Martini, F.H., Nath, J.L. and Bartholomew, E.F. (2011). *Fundamental of Anatomy & Physiology*, 9th edn. Boston: Pearson Education Ltd.

Monahan, F.D., Neighbors, M., Sands, J.K. and Marek, J.F. (2007). *Phipps' Medical and Surgical Nursing – Health and Illness Perspectives*, 8th edn. St Louis: Mosby.

National Institute for Health and Clinical Excellence (2006a). *Dementia: Supporting People with Dementia and Their Carers in Health and Social Care*. Clinical Guideline 42. London: NICE.

National Institute for Health and Clinical Excellence (2006b): *Parkinson's Disease: Diagnosis and Management in Primary Care*. Clinical Guideline 3. London: NICE.

National Institute for Health and Clinical Excellence (2007a). *Head Injury: Triage, Assessment, Investigation and Early Management of Head Injury in Infants, Children and Adults*. Clinical Guideline 56 (a partial update of clinical guideline 4). London: NICE.

National Institute for Health and Clinical Excellence (2007b). *Alteplase for the Treatment of Acute Ischaemic Stroke*. NICE technology appraisal guidance 122. London: NICE.

Shiere, D., Butler, J. and Lewis, R. (2012). *Hole's Human Anatomy and Physiology*, 13th edn. London: McGraw Hill Companies.

Stanfield, C.L. and Germann, W.J. (2008). *Principles of Human Physiology*, 3rd edn. San Francisco: Pearson.

The Stroke Association (2004). http://www.stroke.org.uk [accessed 11 September 2012]

Turner, A.M. and Jowett, N.I. (2006). The role of statin therapy in preventing recurrent stroke. *Nursing Times.* 102(38) 25–26.

Walsh, M. (2007). *Watson's Clinical Nursing and Related Sciences*, 7th edn. London: Bailliere Tindall.

Waterhouse, C. (2005). The Glasgow Coma Scale and other neurological observations. *Nursing Standard.* 19(33): 56–64.

11

The gastrointestinal system and associated disorders

Louise McErlean

Senior Lecturer, Department of Adult Nursing and Primary Care, School of Health and Social Work, University of Hertfordshire, Hatfield, Hertfordshire, UK

Contents

Fundamentals of Applied Pathophysiology: An Essential Guide for Nursing and Healthcare Students, Second Edition. Edited by Muralitharan Nair and Ian Peate.
© 2013 John Wiley & Sons, Ltd. Published 2013 by John Wiley & Sons, Ltd.

Key words

- Oral cavity
- Duodenum
- Large intestine
- Peristalsis
- Oesophagus
- Jejunum
- Digestion
- Peritoneum
- Stomach
- Small intestine
- Chyme

Test your prior knowledge

- What are the main functions of saliva?
- List five functions of the stomach.
- Differentiate between chemical and mechanical digestion.
- Name the accessory organs of digestion.

Learning outcomes

On completion of this section the reader will be able to:

- Describe the organs of digestion.
- List the accessory organs of digestion.
- List the main functions of the digestive system.
- Explain the differences between chemical and mechanical digestion.

Don't forget to visit to the companion website for this book (www.wiley.com/go/ fundamentsofappliedpathophysiology) where you can find self-assessment tests to check your progress, as well as lots of activities to practise your learning.

Introduction

The gastrointestinal system is also known as the digestive system or alimentary canal or tract. The principle structures of digestion are the mouth, pharynx, oesophagus, stomach and intestines. These structures are supported by the accessory organs of digestion – the salivary glands, liver, pancreas and gallbladder (Figure 11.1).

   The main function of the gastrointestinal system is to break down nutrients from the diet into the raw materials required by the cells of the body so that they can carry out their specific

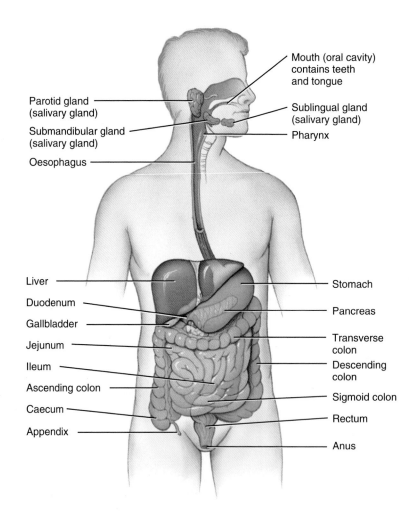

Figure 11.1   The gastrointestinal tract.

functions. The gastrointestinal system does this by digesting the dietary intake, absorbing the nutrients obtained from the process of digestion and eliminating any unwanted material.

The gastrointestinal system is a continuous tract. From the start, at the mouth, to the end at the anus, the gastrointestinal tract measures approximately 10 m. This chapter discusses the structure and functions of this system, the accessory organs of digestion and some common disorders and their related care and management.

Digestion

Food from the diet is broken down throughout the length of the gastrointestinal tract by two types of digestion:

- Chemical digestion is the chemical breakdown of food. It occurs as a result of enzymes being added to the foods as they pass down the length of the gastrointestinal system. Secretion of the enzymes is dependent upon the action of many hormones. The enzymes denature the food, helping to break it down into smaller nutrient molecules.
- Mechanical digestion is the mechanical breakdown of food. It occurs as a result of the food being chewed, moved and mixed as it passes through the digestive system. This activity begins in the oral cavity with chewing and grinding, and continues down the length of the digestive tract as a result of smooth muscle contractions of the muscularis layer that runs throughout the length of the digestive system. This mixing and grinding denatures the food, breaking it down into smaller molecules that can be acted upon by the chemicals of digestion. Smooth muscle contraction occurs as a result of parasympathetic nervous system activity.

Structure of the gastrointestinal system

Oral cavity

The mouth, also known as the oral cavity, is the start of the gastrointestinal tract. It receives food and begins the mechanical breakdown of food by the action of chewing and grinding the food. The chemical digestion of food also begins in the oral cavity. Food mixes with salivary amylase found in saliva and this starts the breakdown of dietary carbohydrate into smaller sugar molecules (Shier *et al.*, 2009). Mixing the food with saliva adds moisture, which is important in order to taste food and helps form the food into a bolus; the latter allows food to move onwards from the oral cavity into the oesophagus.

The activity of breaking down foodstuff by chewing is called mastication. The lips, gums, teeth, cheeks, tongue and palate all assist in the process of mechanical digestion within the oral cavity. The space between the tongue and the palate is the cavity of the mouth, and the space between the lips, gums and the teeth is the vestibule (Figure 11.2).

Lips

The lips form the opening into the mouth. They are fleshy folds, which contain skeletal muscles and sensory receptors (Shier *et al.*, 2009). These structures have a role in assessing the temperature and texture of foods, and direct food into the oral cavity. The lips have a rich blood supply, hence their usual ruby red colouring. The junction between the upper and the lower lips forms

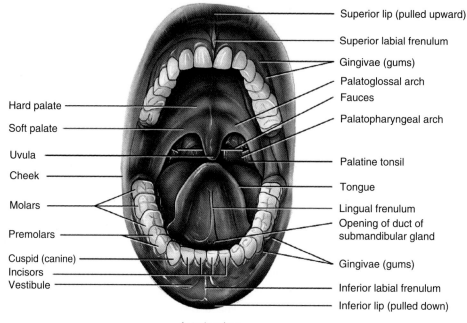

Superior lip (pulled upward)
Superior labial frenulum
Gingivae (gums)
Palatoglossal arch
Fauces
Palatopharyngeal arch

Hard palate
Soft palate
Uvula
Cheek
Molars
Premolars
Cuspid (canine)
Incisors
Vestibule

Palatine tonsil
Tongue
Lingual frenulum
Opening of duct of
submandibular gland
Gingivae (gums)
Inferior labial frenulum
Inferior lip (pulled down)

Anterior view

Figure 11.2   The oral cavity.

the angle of the mouth. These angles can become sore and dry during periods of ill health and this condition is known as angular cheilitis.

Cheeks

The cheeks form the fleshy sides of the face and they run from the corner of the mouth to the side of the nose. Subcutaneous fat, muscles and mucous membranes line the cheeks. The cheeks assist in the chewing of food.

Palate

The palate is divided into the hard and the soft palates (Figure 11.2); both form the roof of the mouth, whereas the tongue lies at the bottom of the oral cavity and forms the floor of the mouth. The hard and the soft palates are covered by mucous membranes and participate in the mechanical breakdown of food.

Tongue

The tongue is a thick muscular organ composed of skeletal muscles and mucous membranes. It contains approximately 10 000 taste buds (Silverthorn, 2009). It tells the person about the taste of food, e.g. whether the food is sweet or sour. Marieb and Hoehn (2010) state that the tongue detects four basic tastes: sweet, salt, bitter and sour. Silverthorn (2009) identified a fifth taste called umami. This word is derived from the Japanese word meaning 'deliciousness', and the taste is associated with glutamate and some nucleotides. Hence, in some Asian countries, monosodium glutamate (MSG) is sometimes used to enhance flavour when cooking.

The tongue is an accessory organ; it helps to blend food when chewing and to push food particles to the back of the mouth when swallowing. Tongue movement can alter the volume of the oral cavity and, in addition to taste, also has an important role in speech, chewing and swallowing.

Teeth

Humans develop two sets of teeth – milk teeth and permanent teeth. There are approximately 20 milk teeth (Figure 11.3), which usually begin to develop from the age of 6 months. Often one pair of milk teeth grows per month and they usually fall out between the ages of 6 and 12 years. Once the milk teeth fall out, they are replaced by permanent teeth. Usually, there are 32 permanent teeth (Figure 11.4), which have the potential to last a lifetime. The first permanent molars appear at the age of 6 years, the second at the age of 12 years and the third may develop after the age of 13 years. The functions of the teeth include cutting, tearing and chewing food.

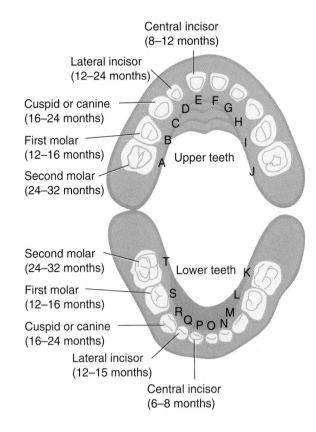

Central incisor
(8–12 months)

Lateral incisor
(12–24 months)

Cuspid or canine
(16–24 months)

First molar
(12–16 months)

Second molar
(24–32 months)

D E F G
C H
B I
A Upper teeth J

Second molar
(24–32 months)

First molar
(12–16 months)

Cuspid or canine
(16–24 months)

Lateral incisor
(12–15 months)

T
S Lower teeth K
R L
Q P O N M

Central incisor
(6–8 months)

Figure 11.3   The milk teeth.

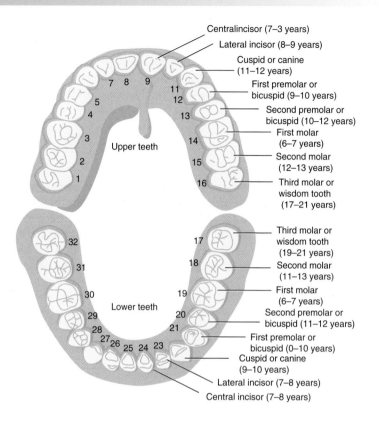

Centralincisor (7–3 years)
Lateral incisor (8–9 years)
Cuspid or canine (11–12 years)
First premolar or bicuspid (9–10 years)
Second premolar or bicuspid (10–12 years)
First molar (6–7 years)
Second molar (12–13 years)
Third molar or wisdom tooth (17–21 years)

Third molar or wisdom tooth (19–21 years)
Second molar (11–13 years)
First molar (6–7 years)
Second premolar or bicuspid (11–12 years)
First premolar or bicuspid (0–10 years)
Cuspid or canine (9–10 years)
Lateral incisor (7–8 years)
Central incisor (7–8 years)

Figure 11.4   The permanent teeth.

Salivary glands

There are three main pairs of salivary glands (Figure 11.5):

- parotid
- submandibular
- sublingual.

The salivary glands are covered by a fibrous capsule and contain secretory cells. The saliva from these secretory cells drains into larger ducts which lead into the mouth. The salivary glands secrete approximately 1 L of saliva per day (Marieb and Hoehn, 2010).

Composition of saliva

Saliva consists of:

- water
- salts

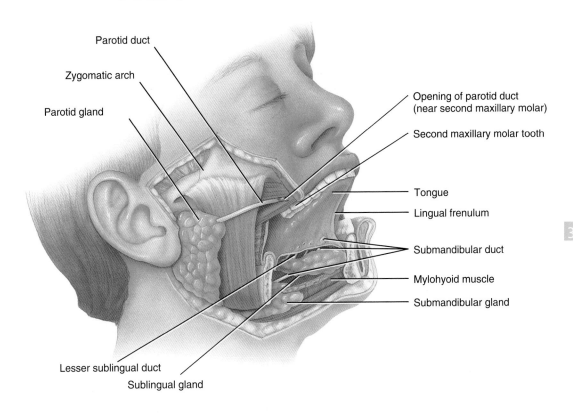

Figure 11.5   The salivary glands.

- salivary amylase
- mucin (a protein that help form mucus)
- lysozyme (a bacteriolytic enzyme).

Functions of saliva

The oral cavity is permanently moist due to a continuous coating of saliva. Saliva makes swallowing easier. The secretion of saliva is under autonomic nervous system control and is not influenced by the action of hormones. The action of salivary amylase begins the chemical digestion of carbohydrate. The bactericidal activity of lysozyme present in saliva helps to prevent bacteria that may be present in food from reaching the lower digestive tract. The pH of saliva ranges from 5.8 to 7.4 (Waugh and Grant, 2010).

Pharynx

The pharynx lies behind the nose and mouth. It is approximately 12 cm in length and is divided into three sections – the nasopharynx, oral pharynx and laryngeal pharynx. The pharynx connects with the mouth superiorly and the oesophagus and larynx inferiorly (Mader, 2011). It also connects with the two small nasal cavities and two eustachian tubes. When food is swallowed, the

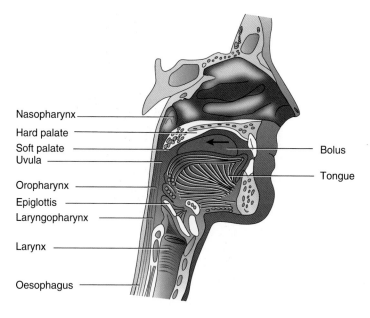

Nasopharynx

Hard palate

Soft palate

Uvula

Bolus

Tongue

Oropharynx

Epiglottis

Laryngopharynx

Larynx

Oesophagus

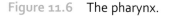

Position of structures before swallowing

Figure 11.6   The pharynx.

soft palate closes the nasal passages and the epiglottis moves over the glottis to close the larynx and the trachea (Figure 11.6). This allows the foodstuff to move down the oesophagus rather than into the respiratory tract (Figure 11.7).

Oesophagus

This is a muscular tube that is approximately 25 cm long, running from the pharynx to the stomach. It lies at the back of the trachea and in front of the spinal column (backbone). The oesophagus is sometimes known as the food pipe (gullet) (Mader, 2011). It is a collapsible muscular tube that channels food into the stomach. The movement of food down the oesophagus occurs as a result of waves of smooth muscle contractions known as peristalsis. It is not possible for a person to swallow and breathe at the same time; this part of swallowing is a reflex action.

Stomach

The stomach is a 'J'-shaped muscular organ situated below the diaphragm, made up of four regions – an upper portion called the cardiac region, an elevated part called the fundus, a middle section called the body and a pyloric region (Figure 11.8). The layers of the stomach include an outer layer called the visceral peritoneum (also known as the serosa), a muscularis layer, a sub-mucosal layer and a mucosal layer (Figure 11.9).

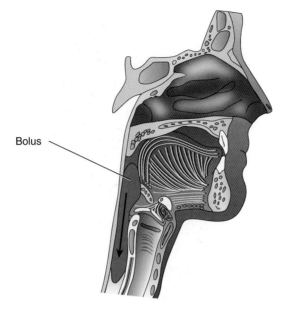

During the pharyngeal state of swallowing

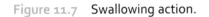

Figure 11.7   Swallowing action.

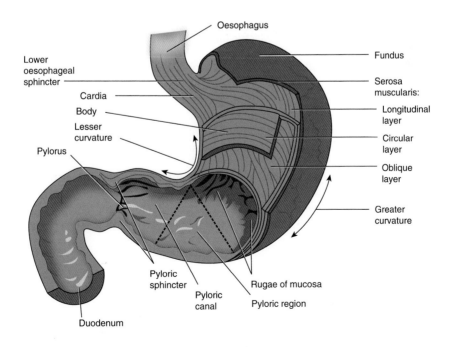

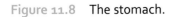

Figure 11.8   The stomach.

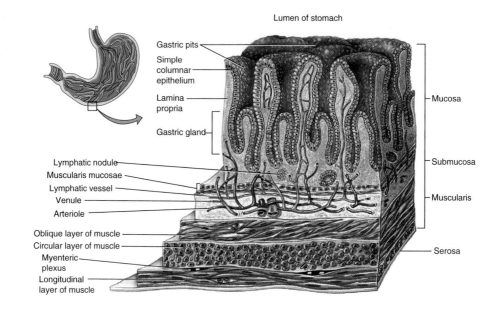

Lumen of stomach

Gastric pits

Simple columnar epithelium

Lamina propria

Gastric gland

Mucosa

Lymphatic nodule
Muscularis mucosae
Lymphatic vessel
Venule
Arteriole

Submucosa

Muscularis

Oblique layer of muscle
Circular layer of muscle
Myenteric plexus
Longitudinal layer of muscle

Serosa

Figure 11.9   Layers of the stomach.

Secretions

The cells of the stomach mucosa secrete numerous enzymes and other substances. These are collectively known as gastric juice. Gastric juice contains:

- Mucus – lubricates food and also lines the stomach, protecting it from digestive enzymes and hydrochloric acid.
- Hydrochloric acid – destroys bacteria that may be ingested in food; an acid environment is essential for the digestion of proteins.
- Intrinsic factor – helps in the absorption of vitamin B_{12} in the small intestine.
- Pepsinogen – required for the chemical digestion of proteins.

Production of gastric juice is dependent upon the hormone gastrin. Gastrin is secreted when food enters the stomach and secretion stops when the stomach pH drops below 1.5.

The secretions and the ingested food are mixed together into a thick, pasty, semisolid and acidic substance called chyme. Chyme leaves the stomach by way of the pyloric sphincter (Figure 11.8) and enters the duodenum.

Functions

The stomach performs numerous functions:

- It is a temporary reservoir for food until it is ready to be passed into the duodenum.
- Nutrients are liquefied, broken down and mixed with hydrochloric acid to form a semisolid substance called chyme.

- Chemical digestion of proteins begins. Proteins are converted into smaller polypeptides by pepsins.
- Mechanical digestion of food occurs as the three smooth muscle layers of the stomach, the muscularis (Figure 11.8), contract and relax, effectively mixing and churning the stomach contents.
- Milk is curdled and casein is released from the milk.
- Digestion of fats begins in the stomach.
- Production of intrinsic factor is essential for the absorption of vitamin B_{12}.

Small intestine

The small intestine extends from the pylorus of the stomach to the ileocaecal valve and is divided into three sections – duodenum, jejunum and ileum (Figure 11.10).

The small intestine is approximately 6 m in length and 3 cm in diameter, and is situated in the abdominal cavity. The small intestine is supported by mesenteries (Figure 11.11). The mesenteries convey blood vessels, lymphatic vessels and nerves to the small intestine.

Duodenum

The duodenum is the 'C'-shaped section of the small intestine (Figure 11.10). This is the shortest section and it is approximately 25 cm in length. The duodenum commences at the pyloric sphincter and ends at the beginning of the jejunum. This section is involved with further digestion of nutrients from the stomach. The cells of the intestine produce intestinal juice which contains some digestive enzymes required for chemical digestion. Pancreatic juice and bile are delivered to the duodenum from the pancreas and gallbladder respectively. As a result of the many enzymes in

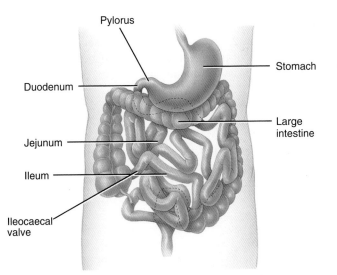

Figure 11.10   The small intestine.

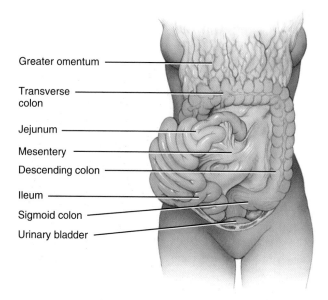

Greater omentum

Transverse colon

Jejunum

Mesentery

Descending colon

Ileum

Sigmoid colon

Urinary bladder

Figure 11.11   The mesentery of the small intestine.

intestinal and pancreatic juice, further chemical digestion of food occurs here. Pancreatic juice is alkaline and it helps to neutralize the acidic chyme as it enters the small intestine.

Jejunum

The jejunum is approximately 2.5 m in length and it commences at the end of the duodenum and terminates at the beginning of the ileum. The main function of the jejunum is to further break down the nutrients coming from the duodenum.

Ileum

The ileum commences at the end of the jejunum and terminates at the ileocaecal valve. It is approximately 3.5 m in length. Absorption mainly takes place in the ileum. The absorption is carried out by small structures called villi (singular – villus) (Figure 11.12).

Large intestine

The large intestine, also known as the colon, commences at the ileocaecal valve and terminates at the rectum. The large intestine is approximately 2 m in length and 6 cm in diameter. The large intestine consists of the caecum; the ascending, transverse, descending and sigmoid colons; and the rectum and anus (Figure 11.13).

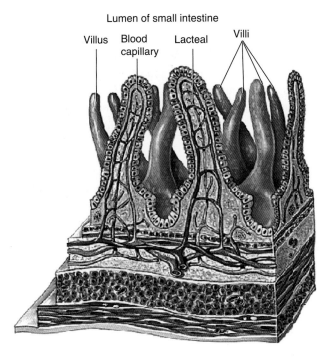

Figure 11.12   Section of the small intestine showing the villi.

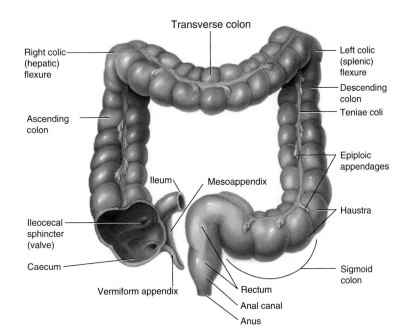

Figure 11.13   The large intestine.

Functions

The functions of the large intestine include:

- absorption of water, electrolytes and vitamins
- secretion of mucus for the lubrication of faeces
- storage of indigestible foodstuff such as cellulose and vegetable fibre
- production of vitamin K and some B complexes (B_1, B_2 and folic acid)
- defecation.

Accessory organs of digestion

Liver

The liver is the largest organ in the body and weighs approximately 1.5 kg. The liver is reddish in colour, wedge-shaped and covered by connective tissue, and is divided into the right and left lobes (Figure 11.14). It is situated in the upper right quadrant of the abdominal cavity beneath the

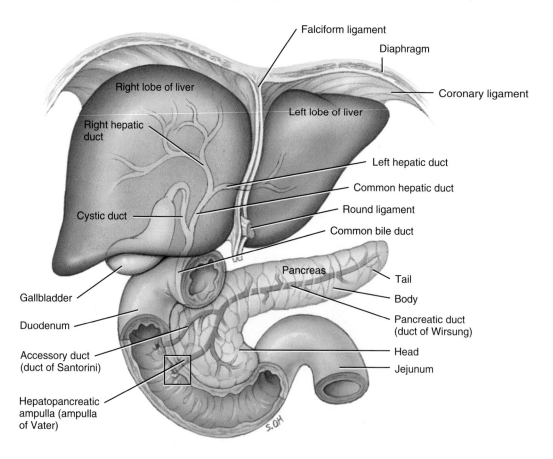

Figure 11.14   The liver.

diaphragm. It is partially protected by the ribs. The right and the left lobes are separated by the falciform ligament and the liver is covered by a serous membrane called peritoneum.

Blood vessels of the liver

The main blood vessels of the liver include the:

- hepatic artery – this is a branch of the celiac artery and it supplies oxygenated blood to the liver
- The hepatic portal vein – drains venous blood from the gastrointestinal tract, which contains nutrients absorbed from the small intestine, into the liver.
- The hepatic vein – drains venous blood from the liver to the inferior vena cava.

Functions

321

The liver has numerous functions:

- carbohydrate, protein and fat metabolism
- modifies waste products and toxic substances, i.e. drugs such as paracetamol, aspirin and alcohol
- produces and stores glycogen
- maintains blood glucose levels
- converts ammonia into urea, which is a waste product
- forms red blood cells in fetal life
- plays a part in the destruction of red blood cells
- stores minerals such as iron and copper
- stores the fat-soluble vitamins A, D, E and K, and water-soluble vitamin B_{12}
- manufactures plasma proteins such as prothrombin
- produces clotting factors
- produces heat
- produces bile, which emulsifies fats in the diet for absorption.

Gallbladder

The gallbladder is a pear-shaped muscular sac, which lies beneath the right lobe of the liver (Figure 11.14). It is divided into the fundus, the body and the neck. The gallbladder is approximately 7–9 cm in length and its main function is to store and concentrate bile, which is produced in the liver (Figure 11.15). Bile is released from the gallbladder in the presence of a hormone called cholecystokinin (CCK). The presence of chyme in the duodenum stimulates the production of CCK by the entero-endocrine cells of the duodenum. This hormone is transported in the bloodstream to the gallbladder where it stimulates the smooth muscles of the gallbladder to contract, thus ejecting bile.

Pancreas

The pancreas is a triangular-shaped organ. It is approximately 12–15 cm in length and 2.5 cm thick. It is divided into three sections – head, body and tail. The head of the pancreas lies in the loop of the duodenum (Figure 11.14) and the tail touches the spleen. It has an endocrine function and an exocrine function.

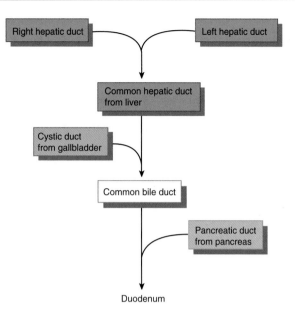

Figure 11.15   Production and storage of bile.

Exocrine function

The pancreas produces pancreatic juice, which is secreted directly from the pancreas into the duodenum via the pancreatic duct (Figure 11.14). The pancreatic juice contains the following enzymes:

- pancreatic amylase completes the digestion of carbohydrates
- trypsin for the digestion of proteins
- lipase for the digestion of fats.

Approximately, 1500 mL of pancreatic juice are produced per day.

Endocrine function

The pancreas also produces hormones that are secreted directly into the bloodstream. The hormones and their functions include:

- glucagon from pancreatic alpha cells – increases blood glucose levels
- insulin from pancreatic beta cells – lowers blood glucose levels
- somatostatin from pancreatic delta cells – regulates both glucagon and insulin levels.

For a more detailed discussion of the endocrine pancreas, see Chapter 13.

Disorders of the digestive system

The digestive system is a large system responsible for processing the diet and the production of a myriad of enzymes and chemicals; as such it has the potential to succumb to disorder along its vast length. The remainder of the chapter will examine some of the disorders associated with the digestive system.

Learning outcomes

On completion of this section the reader will be able to:

- List some of the common disorders of the digestive system.
- Describe the pathophysiology of specific digestive system disorders.
- Discuss the management of digestive system disorders.

Gingivitis

Also known as inflammation of the gums, gingivitis may lead to ulceration and necrosis of the gums.

Aetiology

Gingivitis is largely associated with poor oral hygiene. Bacteria are then able to infect the gums and the toxins produced by the bacteria cause inflammation of the gums. Long-term plaque deposits may also cause gingivitis. Dental plaque, a sticky substance deposited on the exposed portion of the teeth, is made up of bacteria, food particles, mucus and colloid materials found in saliva. Colloid materials can mineralise into hard deposits called tartar and accumulate at the base of the teeth.

Certain drugs, e.g. phenytoin, some birth control pills and ingestion of heavy metals such as lead and bismuth may cause inflammation of the gums. Badly fitting orthodontic appliances, i.e. dentures, bridges and crowns, can irritate the gums and cause inflammation, leading to gingivitis.

Other possible causes of gingivitis are vigorous brushing and flossing of the teeth. Some individuals who have diabetes mellitus are at increased risk of developing gingivitis. Some pregnant women can develop gingivitis associated with the hormonal changes that occur at this time (Kozier *et al.*, 2008).

Signs and symptoms

These include:

- swollen and painful gums; tender when touched
- bleeding from the gums; blood may be visible on the toothbrush even with gentle brushing
- excessive salivation
- bad breath (halitosis)
- gums may appear shinny and or bright red.

Care and management

A dentist should be consulted when signs of gingivitis are suspected. The dentist may use dental instruments to remove the plaque and clean the teeth. Meticulous oral hygiene is essential after visiting the dentist. The dentist or the dental hygienist will demonstrate the correct method of brushing and flossing the teeth. The mouth should be rinsed using copious amounts of water after brushing and flossing.

The healthcare professional should encourage patients who are at risk of contracting gingivitis to brush and floss their teeth after each meal, and emphasise the importance of attending regular dental appointments.

Peptic ulcer

Peptic ulcer is the term used to define the development of an ulcer in the lower part of the oesophagus, the stomach or the duodenum. Duodenal ulcers are more common than gastric ulcers. The ulcer develops as a result of exposure of the gastrointestinal epithelium to the acidic gastric secretions of the stomach. The prevalence of the disease is equal in both sexes. Peptic ulcer usually responds well to drug treatment, but if left untreated, can cause severe complications, such as perforation of the gastrointestinal wall, haemorrhage and even stomach cancer. Figure 11.16 shows the common sites for peptic ulcer.

Aetiology

The causes of peptic ulcers include:

- infection from *Helicobacter pylori* (a Gram-negative bacterium)
- excessive consumption of alcohol and cigarette smoking
- excessive gastric secretions as a result of stress

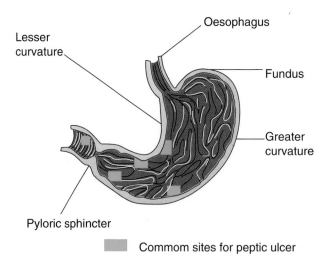

Figure 11.16   Common sites for peptic ulcer. (Adapted from LeMone *et al.*, 2011.)

- excessive use of non-steroidal anti-inflammatory drugs (NSAIDs) and aspirin derivatives
- excessive consumption of caffeine
- familial history of peptic ulcer.

Investigations

As well as taking a full health history, the following investigations may be carried out to confirm diagnosis:

- Gastroscopy and biopsy of stomach lining to detect changes as a result of *H. pylori* infection.
- Barium swallow may be performed to detect ulcer formation. This involves swallowing a drink containing barium, which is radio-opaque. The barium coats the lining of the stomach and the duodenum and, if an ulcer is present, this is detected on the X-ray.
- Full blood analysis.

Signs and symptoms

Some patients with peptic ulcer have no symptoms. However, the following symptoms have been reported in patients with peptic ulcer:

- dyspepsia
- epigastric pain
- heart burn as a result of the regurgitation of gastric secretion
- nausea and vomiting
- blood may be present in vomit if the ulcer bleeds
- loss of weight
- eructation (belching).

Pathophysiology

Mucus lines the digestive tract and acts as a barrier against the acidic gastric secretions. Too little mucus production coupled with too much acid production will leave the digestive tract vulnerable to acid erosion and ulceration. Erosion of the mucosal lining may result in the formation of a fistula. The fistula allows the acidic gastric contents to leak out into the peritoneum, resulting in peritonitis. Stress, caffeine, cigarette smoking and alcohol consumption increase acid production. Medications such as NSAIDs and aspirin inhibit prostaglandins, which protect the mucosal lining (Hogan and Hill, 2004).

H. pylori bacterial infection leads to death of the mucosal epithelial cells of the stomach and duodenum. The bacteria release toxins and enzymes that reduce the efficiency of mucus in protecting the mucosal lining of the gastrointestinal tract. In response to the bacterial infection, the body initiates an inflammatory response, which results in further destruction of the mucosal lining and ulceration.

Care and management

Once peptic ulcer has been diagnosed, the healthcare professional should help the patient identify any lifestyle factors that may be associated with peptic ulcers, such as stress, heavy alcohol consumption, smoking and drinking a lot of coffee. Once identified, the carer and patient can discuss ways of reducing the risks. The patient may be taught relaxation therapy, such as listening to music in order to reduce stress levels. Referral to counselling services, smoking cessation and alcohol awareness may also be of benefit.

Dietary advice should be offered to the patient. Small regular meals are encouraged – approximately five small meals per day to prevent hunger pain. Spicy food should be avoided as it may irritate the mucosal membrane of the stomach, resulting in inflammation and epigastric pain.

Medications such as aspirin and NSAIDs should be avoided as these drugs may inhibit the action of prostaglandins and may lead to gastrointestinal bleeding.

Pharmacological interventions

The patient with peptic ulcer may be prescribed the following medications:

- antibiotics to treat the *H. pylori* infection
- H_2 antagonists such as ranitidine (Zantac) or cimetidine (Tagamet)
- proton pump inhibitor such as omeprazole.

Case study

Amit Hussain has been working at the London stock exchange for several years. Four years ago he was promoted to a very high powered job. Part of his role involves wining and dining important clients and he eats out 5 days per week. He smokes 20 cigarettes a day.

He recently celebrated his 30th birthday by taking some friends to Ibiza for a week of partying. Work has been very stressful of late and Mr Hussain thought he would benefit from the break. However, on his return, he has had to visit his GP, complaining of severe abdominal pain. He tells his GP he has recently started to suffer from heart burn at night in bed, which is only resolved by taking over-the-counter heart burn remedies and by lying on his left side when in bed to prevent acid reflux. He has also noted a lot more belching of late. The doctor suspects that Mr. Hussain has a peptic ulcer.

Take some time to reflect on this case and then consider the following.

1. What medication might Mr Hussain's GP prescribe to treat the acid reflux?
2. Using your knowledge of the anatomy and physiology of the digestive system, explain why lying down can increase the symptoms of gastric reflux.
3. What lifestyle advice would you offer to Mr Hussain to prevent recurrence of this condition?

Ulcerative colitis

Ulcerative colitis is one of a group of chronic inflammatory bowel diseases that includes irritable bowel disease and Crohn's disease. Ulcerative colitis is the chronic inflammation of the mucous membrane of the colon and the rectum. The lining becomes inflamed and ulcerated. Some possible causes of ulcerative colitis include factors such as poor nutrition, stress, bowel infections, genetic factors and autoimmune dysfunction.

Investigations

The following investigations may be performed to confirm diagnosis:

- Sigmoidoscopy or colonoscopy to examine the mucous membrane of the colon and the rectum. The procedure involves passing a flexible scope via the rectum to examine the lining of the colon.
- A barium enema to identify bowel strictures or ulcerations.
- Stool cultures to rule out any infection.
- Full blood count to exclude anaemia and other complications from ulcerative colitis – a raised white blood cell count indicates infection.
- Plain abdominal X-ray.
- Ultrasound to identify ulcerations.

Signs and symptoms

The following symptoms have been reported:

- severe diarrhoea
- blood, pus or mucus in the diarrhoea
- weight loss
- poor appetite
- abdominal pain
- nausea and vomiting.

Pathophysiology

The inflammatory process occurs in the mucosa and the submucosa of the rectum (proctitis) and spreads along the colon. The inflammation may involve the entire colon up to the junction of the ileocaecal valve. The inflammation and mucosal destruction lead to swelling, oedema and bleeding, and as the disease progresses, ulceration develops. Mucosal destruction also leads to an increase in the urge to defaecate with patients having to go to the toilet over 10 times per day. Some patients will have iron deficiency anaemia. The ulceration spreads through the submucosa, causing necrosis and sloughing of the mucous membrane (LeMone *et al.*, 2011). In the later stages of the disease, the walls of the colon thicken and become fibrous. This leads to a narrowing of the lumen of the large intestine, which can lead to intestinal obstruction. Loss of normal large intestine function can lead to complications such as dehydration and electrolyte imbalance. Abdominal cramping and pain are associated with these attacks.

Long-term complications of ulcerative colitis include an increased risk of developing bowel cancer.

Care and management

The patient with ulcerative colitis may need psychological support and counselling. Depression may be a result of the debilitating disease and the person may feel isolated. As a result of diarrhoea and bowel habits, the patient may be reluctant to engage in social activity and feel a burden to their family. The patient should be allowed to express their anxieties and worries about the disease.

Fluid intake and output must be monitored to ensure that the patient is not dehydrated. Dehydration is a possibility as a result of the diarrhoea. Electrolyte balance needs to be monitored daily as a result of the loss of electrolytes such as sodium and potassium in the vomit and diarrhoea.

Dietary intake should be monitored. A low-residue diet should be advised to prevent irritation of the mucosal lining of the colon from the bulk formation. During the early stage of the disease, the patient may be unable to eat and therefore may need parenteral nutrition (Miller *et al.*, 2006) when diarrhoea is severe. There may be a need for vitamin and mineral supplements in the diet. Healthy eating should be advised once the diarrhoea has settled.

Blood transfusion may be necessary if the patient is anaemic as a result of the bleeding. The healthcare professional must ensure the safe administration of blood and be able to recognise incompatible blood transfusion reactions, such as pyrexia, tachycardia and rashes.

Bowel movements should be monitored and findings recorded, such as frequency, consistency and volume. The stool should be tested for blood and the findings recorded on a stool chart. Diarrhoea is an indication of the severity of the disease and it can indicate the amount of fluid and electrolytes lost.

The patient should be assisted with personal cleansing and dressing. Signs of inflammation or any bleeding should be observed around the perianal area from frequent wiping after the diarrhoea. The patient should lie in a warm bath for a soothing effect and if necessary apply soothing barrier cream to the perianal region.

Pharmacological intervention

The following medications may be prescribed in the treatment of ulcerative colitis:

- analgesia for pain
- anti-inflammatory drugs (steroid therapy)
- aminosalicylates
- antibiotics.

Surgical intervention

In individuals in whom there are few periods of remission, a lack of response to therapy, limited lifestyle, risk of perforation or obstruction, or precancerous changes, then surgical intervention may be required. The surgery will involve the removal of the large intestine and rectum, and the formation of an ileostomy or ileo-anal pouch.

Case study

Mrs Fiona Brown is a 30-year-old computer analyst. She works part time. She has been married to her husband Ed for 3 years. They have no children but would like to have a family some day. They live close to both sets of parents and siblings.

Mrs Brown was diagnosed with ulcerative colitis when she was 19 years old and has had symptoms and treatment on and off since then. She has been admitted to the surgical ward as her ulcerative colitis has been unremitting for several months now.

Her symptoms include:

- weight loss of 10 kg in the past 4 months
- tiredness and lethargy – Mrs Brown has been unable to go to work
- dry skin and mouth
- frequent diarrhoea (up to 12 visits to the toilet per day)
- bloody stools
- nausea and vomiting
- concentrated urine
- crampy abdominal pain
- abdominal distension.

Following a recent biopsy, the doctors have noted some worrying changes in the histology of the tissue. They are also concerned that Mrs Brown's condition is not improving with treatment. They have therefore decided that Mrs Brown would benefit from a total colectomy. The doctors are confident that with Mrs Brown's previous optimistic approach and concordance with prescribed therapy and lifestyle advice, she is a good candidate for the formation if an ileo-anal pouch procedure. This may have to be completed in stages. They have discussed this with Mrs Brown and she has consented to the surgery.

Take some time to reflect on this case and then consider the following.

1. Discuss how the pathophysiology of ulcerative colitis leads to the signs and symptoms Mrs Brown is experiencing.
2. List the postoperative complications Mrs Brown is at risk of developing.
3. Mrs Brown would like to start a family but is worried about the effect of the pregnancy on the pouch. Investigate the possibility of pregnancy and discuss the advice you would offer to Mrs Brown.

Peritonitis

Peritonitis is the inflammation of the peritoneum, which is the lining that covers the abdominal viscera. It may be caused by bacteria or contamination of the acidic contents of the stomach as a result of perforation or rupture of any of the abdominal organs, such as the appendix or urinary bladder. The condition can also occur postoperatively as a result of leakage from an intestinal anastomosis.

Signs and symptoms

The following signs and symptoms may be present in a patient with peritonitis:

- abdominal pain with rebound tenderness
- nausea and vomiting
- board-like rigidity of the abdomen
- paralytic ileus
- dehydration
- shallow respiration

- tachycardia
- hypotension.

Pathophysiology

The peritoneum is a serous membrane that lines the organs of the peritoneum and the peritoneal cavity. When the peritoneum is infected, an inflammatory response is initiated. The surrounding tissues become oedematous with accumulation of fluid in the peritoneal cavity. The patient may become dehydrated as fluid and electrolytes are lost from the systemic circulation into the peritoneal cavity.

The patient may experience severe abdominal pain as a result of the infection and inflammation of the peritoneum. The patient may develop oliguria, electrolyte imbalance and shock. As the inflammation worsens, septicaemia may develop, resulting in multiorgan failure.

Care and management

In the early stages of the disease, the patient should be on bed rest due to extreme weakness and shock. Vital signs should be monitored hourly until they are stable; any changes in the vital signs should be reported immediately in order to allow prompt action to be taken and to prevent sepsis.

The patient may require the passage of a nasogastric tube as a result of abdominal distension and paralytic ileus. The contents of the stomach should be aspirated 2-hourly and the amount and type of aspirate recorded on a fluid chart.

Intravenous fluid therapy may be prescribed for fluid replacement and to correct electrolyte imbalance. The carer should ensure that the fluid is administered as prescribed and a record of fluid input and output maintained. Urine output is monitored hourly until the patient is stable. Some patients may need parenteral nutrition in the early stages of the disease as they may be unable to take nutrients orally.

If surgery is needed, it is the healthcare professional's duty to prepare the patient for theatre, taking into account local protocol for pre-operative care. All care given pre- and post-operatively should be documented in accordance with local policy and guidance issued by professional bodies such as the Nursing and Midwifery Council (2009).

Assistance should be provided in maintaining personal hygiene and the patient should be informed of the importance of moving their limbs in bed to prevent deep vein thrombosis and to improve circulation. Pressure areas should be observed, e.g. the sacral region, for signs of redness or inflammation as these are early signs of a pressure sore (decubitus ulcer) developing.

Pharmacological interventions

The following medications may be prescribed for the patient with peritonitis:

- analgesia for pain
- antibiotics for bacterial infection
- anti-emetic for nausea and vomiting.

Conclusion

The gastrointestinal tract, also referred to as the digestive system, provides water, nutrients and electrolytes for bodily functions. Nutrients are extracted from food and transported throughout the body for cellular function. Any undigested food, along with water, bacteria and dead cells, is eliminated from the body in the form of faeces. Digestive enzymes help to break down foodstuff into smaller molecules, which are then absorbed along the gastrointestinal tract. This chapter has provided the reader with insight into the normal anatomy and physiology of the gastrointestinal tract and some of the disorders associated with the system. It is not the remit of this chapter to discuss all the related disorders; the reader is advised to read further.

All healthcare professionals work as members of the team in assisting or giving advice to patients with gastrointestinal problems. These problems can affect the patient both physically and psychologically and thus may impinge on the patient's ability to perform activities of daily living.

Test your knowledge

- Name the components of gastric juice.

- List the functions of the liver.

- Describe chemical and mechanical digestion.

- Is the gallbladder essential for the digestive process? Explain your answer.

- List the signs and symptoms of pancreatitis.

Activities

Here are some activities and exercises to help test your learning. For the answers to these exercises, as well as further self-testing activities, visit our website at www.wiley.com/go/fundamentalsofappliedpathophysiology

Fill in the blanks

The _____ is a J-shaped organ. Food is delivered via the _____ above it and it empties into the _____ below. Its _____ layer contains three layers of muscle instead of the two found elsewhere in the gastrointestinal tract. This is useful as it allows the stomach to stretch when it is acting as a _____ for food and when the muscular activity of stomach helps with the mechanical _____ of food. The rumbling and gurgling of the stomach can be embarrassing for the individual but it cannot be controlled as it is under the control of the _____ nervous system, also known as the _____ nervous system. The waves of contraction of the muscle layer are known as _____ and the mixture produced by the stomach is known as _____.

Choose from:
Peristalsis; Reservoir; Muscularis; Stomach; Duodenum; Involuntary; Digestion; Oesophagus; Autonomic; Chyme

Label the diagram

Using the list of words supplied, label the diagram.

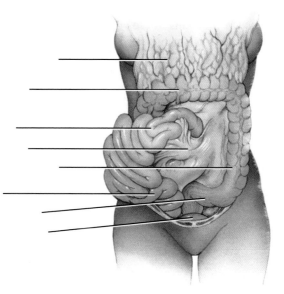

Mesentery; Jejunum; Sigmoid colon; Greater omentum; Ileum; Descending colon; Transverse colon; Urinary bladder

Word search

```
I  S  A  P  F  A  I  L  O  H  C  S  P  S  P  N  S  U  J  I  I
O  S  U  I  E  M  I  N  E  R  A  L  Y  S  O  Z  Y  M  E  E  A
I  R  E  C  L  U  R  M  S  I  R  A  L  U  C  S  U  M  J  M  I
O  S  M  O  V  R  G  A  L  L  B  L  A  D  D  E  R  C  U  R  V
O  S  Y  E  M  Y  Z  N  E  T  O  P  S  C  N  N  A  C  N  S  T
R  I  H  D  I  R  E  O  O  F  H  E  N  O  M  R  O  H  U  E  C
E  T  C  I  S  E  P  I  A  T  Y  R  T  L  D  S  M  D  M  P  I
G  I  N  G  I  V  I  T  I  S  D  I  E  I  A  M  N  M  R  S  M
A  N  A  E  S  I  G  P  S  P  R  S  A  T  E  U  I  O  U  I  L
T  O  O  S  R  L  L  R  R  E  A  T  S  I  F  N  S  M  T  S  R
X  T  N  T  P  S  O  O  P  O  T  A  I  S  P  E  P  S  Y  D  U
N  I  N  I  K  O  T  S  Y  C  E  L  O  H  C  D  E  I  E  P  S
Y  R  D  O  R  E  T  B  S  R  E  S  S  C  S  O  P  E  P  O  V
R  E  Y  N  I  T  I  A  C  U  N  I  O  U  E  U  Q  A  L  P  E
A  P  C  N  E  R  S  N  M  A  C  S  R  P  N  D  L  I  A  I  N
H  A  C  C  A  P  A  A  C  Y  N  O  G  Y  H  A  P  R  S  H  B
P  A  P  O  I  P  P  L  G  I  L  I  V  I  T  A  M  I  N  A  L
O  E  S  A  L  I  V  A  O  Y  S  A  N  E  S  P  G  U  P  S  E
O  T  P  I  I  O  A  E  P  M  M  O  S  E  C  G  P  U  C  D  A
D  K  E  C  B  A  N  S  Y  T  A  I  R  E  C  T  U  M  S  U  E
A  U  M  P  E  T  L  L  I  I  O  E  G  I  I  T  S  I  M  O  S
```

Fundus	Digestion	Enzyme
Hormone	Gastrin	Duodenum
Ulcer	Colitis	Protein
Tongue	Palate	Mucosa
Jejunum	Ileum	Colon
Rectum	Appendix	Peritonitis
Sepsis	Peritoneum	Dyspepsia
Oesophagus	Gingivitis	Plaque
Pharynx	Epiglottis	Mucus
Pepsin	Lipase	Amylase
Bile	Carbohydrate	Incisor
Vitamin	Mineral	Pancreas
Liver	Gallbladder	Saliva
Peristalsis	Absorption	Canine
Cholecystokinin	Fat	Anus
Molar	Lysozyme	Pylorus
Cardia	Chyme	Muscularis

Further resources

The Gastrointestinal Forum

http://www.rcn.org.uk/development/communities/rcn_forum_communities/gastro_and_stoma_care

This forum provides healthcare professionals with up-to-date information and practices in gastrointestinal nursing. It provides a platform to discuss good practice, research areas of concern and share new ideas.

National Association for Colitis and Crohn's Disease (NACC)

http://www.nacc.org.uk/content/home.asp

This link is useful for finding out the latest information about the treatment of sepsis, which can occur alongside peritonitis.

The Surviving Sepsis Campaign

http://www.survivingsepsis.org/Pages/default.aspx

Peritonitis and sepsis can be linked. The Surviving Sepsis Campaign aims to improve diagnosis of sepsis and treatment through education, research and the development of tools, e.g. the sepsis care bundle.

NHS Choices. Your health, your choices

http://www.nhs.uk/Livewell/digestive-health/Pages/digestive-health.aspx

If you want to find out more about maintaining a healthy digestive system so that you are better equipped to advise your patients, this link provides helpful advice on diet, exercise, alcohol and smoking. This is all aimed at improving digestive health.

The British Dental Foundation

http://www.dentalhealth.org/

The website of this charitable organisation contains useful advice about the prevention of gum disease. You can learn more about the recent studies linking gum disease and lack of exercise, and also the links between gum disease and heart disease/stroke.

The Ileostomy and Internal Pouch Support Group

http://www.iasupport.org/pouch_pregnant.aspx

This useful link provides information for people who have had their colon removed. This support group provides a forum for those affected. You can learn more about patient experiences of pregnancy with an ileo-anal pouch.

Glossary of terms

Absorption:	the taking of nutrients from the gastrointestinal tract.
Anastomosis:	surgical joining of two parts.
Angular cheilitis:	soreness and dryness in the corners of the mouth.
Barium meal:	examination of the gastrointestinal tract using a contrast medium; under X-ray control.
Bile:	an alkaline fluid produced by the liver that aids digestion of lipids.
Chyme:	a semisolid substance of the stomach.
Digestion:	the breakdown of foodstuff.
Duct:	a tube.
Dyspepsia:	the feeling of epigastric discomfort.
Endocrine gland:	a ductless gland that secretes hormones into the bloodstream.
Enzyme:	a protein that speeds up chemical reactions.
Eructation:	the act of bringing up air from the stomach.
Exocrine gland:	a gland that secretes hormones into ducts that carry the secretions to other sites (e.g. the intestine).
Fibrous:	containing regenerated or scar tissue.
Fistula:	an abnormal passage from an internal organ to the surface of the skin or between two organs.
Fundus:	the upper portion of the stomach.
Gastroscopy:	examination of the gastrointestinal tract using a flexible gastroscope.
Glycogen:	a carbohydrate (complex sugar) made from glucose. Excess glucose is stored as glycogen in the liver.
Intestine:	the small and large bowel.
Large intestine:	the colon; large bowel.
Mastication:	chewing, tearing and grinding of food.
Oesophagus:	the gullet; food pipe.
Oliguria:	deficient secretion of urine; less than 30 mL per hour.
Oral cavity:	the mouth.
Palate:	the roof of the mouth.
Paralytic ileus:	the absence of peristaltic movement.

335

Parenteral nutrition:	the administration of nutrients other than via the gastrointestinal tract (e.g. intravenously).
Peristalsis:	the involuntary movement of the gastrointestinal tract. A wave-like contraction.
Peritoneum:	the serous membrane that covers the abdominal cavity.
Peritonitis:	inflammation of the peritoneum.
Pharynx:	the throat.
Proctitis:	inflammation of the rectum.
Prostaglandin:	complex unsaturated fatty acid produced by the mast cells and acting as a messenger substance between cells. Intensify the actions of histamine and kinins. They cause increased vascular permeability, neutrophil chemotaxis, stimulation of smooth muscle (e.g. the uterus) and can induce pain.
Ptyalin:	a digestive enzyme; also known as salivary amylase.
Pyloric region:	funnel-shaped portion of the stomach.
Small intestine:	the small bowel.
Stomach:	the organ that receives food from the oesophagus.

References

Hogan, M.A. and Hill, K. (2004). *Pathophysiology: Reviews and Rationales*. New Jersey: Prentice Hall.

Kozier, B., Erb, G., Berman, A., Snyder, S.J., Lake, R. and Harvey, S. (2008). *Fundamentals of Nursing. Concepts, Processes and Practice*. Harlow: Pearson Education.

LeMone, P., Burke, K. and Bauldoff, G. (2011). *Medical – Surgical Nursing; Critical Thinking in Client Care*, 4th edn. New Jersey: Pearson.

Mader, S.S. (2011). *Understanding Human Anatomy and Physiology*, 4th edn. Boston: McGraw Hill.

Marieb, E.N. and Hoehn, K. (2010). *Human Anatomy and Physiology*, 8th edn. San Francisco: Pearson Benjamin Cummings.

Miller, M., Crawshaw, A., Logan, L. and Paterson, R. (2006). Disorders of the gastrointestinal system, liver and biliary tract. In: Alexander, M.F., Fawcett, J.N. and Runciman, P.J. (eds). *Nursing Practice: Hospital and Home – the Adult*, 3rd edn. Edinburgh: Churchill Livingstone.

Nursing and Midwifery Council (2009). *Record Keeping. Guidance for Nurses and Midwives*. London: Nursing and Midwifery Council.

Silverthorn, D.U. (2009). *Human Physiology: An Integrated Approach*, 5th edn. Edgewood Cliffs, NJ: Prentice Hall.

Shier, D., Butler, J. and Lewis, R. (2009). *Holes Human Anatomy and Physiology*, 12th edn. London: McGraw Hill.

Waugh, A. and Grant, A. (2010). *Ross and Wilson: Anatomy and Physiology in Health and Illness*, 11th edn. Edinburgh: Churchill Livingstone.

337

12

Nutrition and associated disorders

Muralitharan Nair

Senior Lecturer, Department of Adult Nursing and Primary Care, School of Health and Social Work, University of Hertfordshire, Hatfield, Hertfordshire, UK

Contents

Fundamentals of Applied Pathophysiology: An Essential Guide for Nursing and Healthcare Students, Second Edition. Edited by Muralitharan Nair and Ian Peate.

Key words

- Anabolism
- Proteins
- Triglycerides
- Micronutrients
- Catabolism
- Vitamins
- Fatty acids
- Glycogen
- Carbohydrates
- Lipids
- Macronutrients
- Gluconeogenesis

Test your prior knowledge

- List the complications of obesity and undernutrition.
- What are micro- and macro-nutrients?
- What is the body's main energy source?
- List the fat-soluble vitamins.

Learning outcomes

On completion of this section the reader will be able to:

- Discuss the roles of carbohydrates, proteins and fats.
- List the micro- and macro-nutrients.
- Describe the role of micro- and macro-nutrients.
- List some of the nutritional assessment tools.

Don't forget to visit to the companion website for this book (www.wiley.com/go/ fundamentalsofappliedpathophysiology) where you can find self-assessment tests to check your progress, as well as lots of activities to practise your learning.

Introduction

Nutrition is a vital component for human existence. An adequate intake of nutrients is essential for the survival of the body systems. Nutrients such as the proteins, carbohydrates, lipids and vitamins found in foodstuff are used by the body for energy production, growth and repair. The digestive organs (see Chapter 11) play a vital role in ingestion, absorption, transportation and elimination. When individuals do not receive sufficient nutrients, their body systems do not function efficiently. Food substances can be divided into macro- and micro-nutrients.

This chapter discusses the roles of micro- and macro-nutrients, identifies the different types of food sources and nutritional requirements of the body, and outlines government recommendations with regards to nutritional intake and nutritional disorders, such as obesity and undernutrition. Nutritional assessment tools and their importance in clinical practice will be discussed. Healthcare professionals play a vital role in ensuring that the nutritional needs of the patient are met. Thus, in hospital, the key responsibilities of the healthcare professional include nutritional assessment of the patient on admission; managing mealtimes, e.g. providing privacy for the patient, ensuring that they are not disturbed during mealtimes; and maintaining an accurate record of the patient's nutritional intake.

Macronutrients

Macronutrients are organic compounds required in relatively large quantities ('macro' means large) for normal physiological functions of the body. Macronutrients include:

- carbohydrates
- proteins
- lipids
- alcohol.

Carbohydrates

Carbohydrates are organic compounds that contain carbon, hydrogen and oxygen molecules. They make up the body's main source of energy and are required in large quantities. Carbohydrates are mainly found in starchy foods (such as grain and potatoes), fruit, pasta and cereals. Other sources of carbohydrates are vegetables, beans and nuts, but in lesser quantities.

One gram of carbohydrate provides approximately 4 kcal/g of energy (Green and Jackson, 2007). Calories are units of energy found in food and drink. The body burns calories to produce energy and any excess is stored as fat. In nutrition, values are given for the actual amount of kilocalories in food, but are commonly referred to in calories.

$$1000 \text{ calories} = 1 \text{ kcal}$$

Carbohydrates are divided into three groups:

- Monosaccharides – also known as simple carbohydrates found in food sources, e.g. glucose (found in fruit, sweetcorn and honey), fructose (fruit sugar) and galactose (produced from lactose – sugar in milk).
- Disaccharides – obtained from sucrose (glucose and fructose), lactose (glucose and galactose) and maltose (glucose).
- Polysaccharides – also known as complex carbohydrates; found in grains and root vegetables.

Carbohydrates are broken down and converted into glucose by the digestive enzyme amylase found in the saliva and pancreas, which the cells utilise to produce energy. An individual may consume more carbohydrate than the body requires and as a result may have an excess of glucose in the system. The excess glucose is then converted to glycogen or fat (LeMone *et al.*, 2011). Glycogen is stored in the liver and muscle cells, and fat is stored in adipose tissue.

The body's capacity to maintain blood glucose levels is achieved by a variety of hormones; the two key hormones are insulin and glucagon. Both these hormones are produced by the pancreas and secreted into the bloodstream. Insulin secretion is increased after a meal has been eaten and the main function of insulin is to transport glucose into the cells for energy production. In the absence of a carbohydrate meal and when the level of blood glucose is low, glucagon stimulates the liver to convert stored glycogen into glucose (a process called glycogenolysis). Thus, the important role of these hormones is to regulate blood glucose levels. However, glucose can be made available by the liver from non-carbohydrate sources, such as proteins and fats, through a process called gluconeogenesis (Jenkins and Tortora, 2013).

Proteins

Protein was the first nutrient to be identified as an important part of a living cell. Proteins are highly complex molecules composed of amino acids. Amino acids are simple compounds containing carbon, hydrogen, oxygen, nitrogen, some sulphur and other elements such as phosphorus, iron and cobalt (Jenkins *et al.*, 2007). Amino acids link together to form chains called peptides.

Most foods contain at least some protein. Good sources of protein include meat, fish, eggs, nuts and seeds, pulses, soya products (tofu, soya milk and textured soya protein such as soya mince), cereals (wheat, oats and rice), eggs and dairy products (milk, cheese and yoghurt). Approximately 1 g of protein yields 4 kcal/g of energy.

Different foods contain different proteins, each with their own unique amino acid composition. The proportions of essential amino acids in foods may differ from the proportions needed by the body to make proteins. Dietary proteins with all the essential amino acids in the proportions required by the body are said to be high-quality proteins. Therefore, the proportion of each of the essential amino acids in foods containing protein determines the quality of that protein.

Proteins are essential for growth and repair. They play a crucial role in virtually all biological processes in the body. All enzymes and many of the hormones are proteins and are vital for the body's function. Muscle contraction, immune protection and the transmission of nerve impulses are all dependent on proteins. Proteins found in the skin and bone provide structural support. The body uses carbohydrate and fat for energy, but when there is excess dietary protein or inadequate dietary fat and carbohydrate, protein is used to produce energy. Excess protein may also be converted to fat and stored in adipose tissue.

One important difference between proteins, carbohydrates and lipids is that a healthy individual can exclude carbohydrate from the diet without much ill effect, and lipids may be excluded for a short while; however, daily protein intake is vital for bodily function. The lifespans of proteins vary: some last for a few minutes while others last a few months. At the end of their lifespan, the protein is broken down into amino acids and these are stored and reused in protein synthesis.

Lipids

Lipid is a term generally used for fats and oils; they are insoluble in water. The dietary lipids are derived from animal (visible fat on meat, milk and milk products such as cream, butter, cheese) and plant sources (Mann and Skeaff, 2007). Approximately 97% of natural lipids are triglycerides, which consist of fatty acids. The fatty acid is common to most lipids. There are three types of fatty acids – saturated fatty acids, monounsaturated fatty acids and polyunsaturated fatty acids. It is estimated that 1 g of fat yields approximately 9 kcal/g and that fat provides 30% of energy intake. Fats and oils in food are mainly in the form of triglycerides.

Lipids are essential for:

- lubrication of food to facilitate swallowing
- transportation of fat-soluble vitamins, such as vitamins A, D, E and K
- synthesis of steroid hormones, such as testosterone and oestrogen
- transportation of lipid-soluble drugs, such as nicotine and caffeine
- biological membranes, such as cell and organelle membranes
- energy production.

Some digestion of fats into free fatty acids begins in the stomach with the aid of the digestive enzyme gastric lipase. The fat is mixed with other nutrients and is passed into the duodenum. Once the contents of the stomach reaches the duodenum, the hormone cholecytokinin is released, which stimulates the release of bile from the gallbladder and pancreatic lipase (see Chapter 11). Fats are then further broken down and absorbed from the gastrointestinal tract.

The absorbed lipids are transported by units called lipoproteins (Figure 12.1). There are five types of lipoproteins:

- chylomicrons
- very low density lipoproteins
- intermediate density lipoproteins
- low density lipoproteins (50% cholesterol, 25% protein)
- high density lipoproteins (20% cholesterol, 40–45% protein).

Alcohol

Alcohol is a substance that is considered to be both a nutrient and a drug that affects brain function (Truswell, 2007). It contains carbon, hydrogen and oxygen, and yields approximately 7 kcal/g of energy; it has a high calorie content, which when consumed in great volume can result in obesity. Moderate intake of alcohol is associated with increased levels of high density lipoprotein, which is useful in protecting the heart against heart disease. Excessive intake can result in dis-

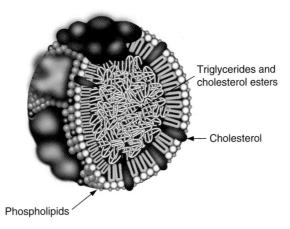

Triglycerides and
cholesterol esters

Cholesterol

Phospholipids

Figure 12.1   A lipoprotein.

eases, e.g. cirrhosis of the liver, stroke, heart disease, cancer of the oesophagus, and other alcohol-related problems such as antisocial behaviour and road traffic accidents (Peate, 2007).

Alcohol is measured in units and each unit of alcohol is equal to 8 g of pure alcohol. It is recommended that men consume no more than 3–4 units of alcohol per day and women no more than 2–3 units per day.

Micronutrients

Micronutrients are organic compounds required in small quantities for the normal physiological functions of the body. They include chemical elements such as hydrogen, nitrogen and carbon, and minerals and vitamins, e.g. vitamins A, B group, C, D, E and K.

Vitamins

Vitamins are organic (carbon-based) substances essential for growth and cellular function. They are required in small quantities and are mainly absorbed from the diet and altered by the body. Some vitamins, such as vitamin D, are synthesised by the body. There are two types of vitamins:

- fat-soluble
- water-soluble.

Vitamins A, D, E and K are fat-soluble vitamins and they circulate in the bloodstream; any excess is stored in adipose tissue and used when the levels are low in the bloodstream. As these vitamins can be stored, it is not essential to take these vitamins daily in the diet. In a healthy individual, fat-soluble vitamin supplements can lead to toxicity. Water-soluble vitamins B group and C circulate freely throughout the body and are not stored (except for vitamins B_{12} and B_6). Excess of these vitamins is excreted in the urine and not stored in the body. Toxicity from these vitamins is less likely and the individual will need a daily intake of these vitamins in the diet. Table 12.1 summarises the vitamins, the food sources containing them and their functions.

Table 12.1   Summary of vitamins and their functions.

	Food sources	Functions
Fat-soluble vitamins		
Vitamin A	In meat as retinol In vegetables as carotenoids	Good vision in dim light Growth and immunity
Vitamin D	Synthesis by ultraviolet rays of the sun Some found in eggs, milk and fish	To maintain calcium level Normal growth, bone and teeth formation
Vitamin E	Green vegetables, eggs, nuts, whole grains and plant oils	Antioxidant Maintains immune system
Vitamin K	Found in leafy vegetables and milk	Important in blood clotting
Water-soluble vitamins		
Vitamin B_1 (thiamine)	Found in a variety of food sources such as liver, pork products, green beans, sunflower seeds and whole grain	Essential for growth and carbohydrate metabolism
Vitamin B_2 (riboflavin)	Milk, milk products, eggs and meat	Involved in citric acid cycle
Vitamin B_3 (niacin)	Tuna, peanuts, mushrooms, chicken and turkey	Involved in glycolysis
Vitamin B_6 (pyridoxine)	Liver, kidneys, meat, poultry and fish	Involved in amino acid metabolism
Biotin	Whole grain, nuts and eggs	Synthesis of nucleic acid and fatty acid
Vitamin B_5 (pantothenic acid)	Meat, milk and vegetables	Involved in glucose production from lipids and amino acids
Folate (folic acid)	Grain products, leafy vegetables and liver	Synthesis of nucleic acid
Vitamin B_{12}	Meat, poultry, seafood and eggs	Production of red blood cells
Vitamin C (ascorbic acid)	Fruit and vegetables	Synthesis of collagen, important component of tendons, blood vessels and bone

Adapted from Seeley *et al.* (2006).

Table 12.2   Minerals and their functions.

Minerals	Functions
Calcium (Ca^2)	For healthy teeth and bone formation, blood clotting, nerve conduction and muscle function
Iron (Fe)	Production of red blood cells and energy production
Magnesium (Mg)	Bone formation, muscle and nerve function
Phosphorus (P)	Teeth and bone formation
Potassium (K)	Muscle and nerve function
Sodium (Na)	Nerve and muscle function; maintains osmotic pressure
Sulphur (S)	Components of hormones, vitamins and proteins
Zinc (Zn)	Essential for enzyme function, carbon dioxide transport and protein metabolism
Selenium (Se)	Antioxidant properties

Adapted from Seeley *et al.* (2006).

Minerals

Minerals form approximately 5% of body weight. Sodium, potassium and calcium form the positive ions (anions) while sulphur and phosphorus form the negative ions (cations).
Minerals are essential for:

- strong bones and teeth
- controlling body fluids between intracellular and extracellular fluid compartments
- turning food into energy.

Table 12.2 summarises the minerals and their functions.
The requirement of minerals varies – an ill person may require more minerals for body function than a healthy individual. A sick patient or a pregnant woman will require more minerals than they would normally need as a result of increased demand for body function.

Nutritional requirements

Nutritional requirements vary according to health status, activity pattern and growth. For example, an elderly person's energy requirement is not the same as that of a baby or a young adult. During a growth spurt, there is more demand for energy. The energy demand also depends on the activity the individual is engaged in. An athlete who is in training will require more energy than a person who is not undertaking any activity, and a patient recovering from surgery or illness will need more energy during the period of recovery.

Nutritional disorders

Learning outcomes

On completion of this section the reader will be able to:

- List some of the common disorders of nutrition.

- Describe the pathophysiological processes related to nutritional disorders.

- List the possible investigations.

- Outline the care and interventions related to the disorders described.

Case study

Mr Martin Fish is a 40-year-old man who lives with his wife Brenda and their two children. Mr Fish is 172 cm tall and Brenda is 160 cm tall. Mr Fish weighs 100 kg and Brenda 88 kg. Mr Fish is a greengrocer and his wife helps him at the stall when the children are at school. Mr Fish tells you, "Brenda and I have struggled with our weight for years. I can see that the children were gaining weight, too. We both work long hours and it is hard to find time to cook. We live mostly on fast food like Chinese and Indian takeaways, kebabs and pizzas".

Mr Fish went to see his GP because lately he noticed that he had frequent headaches, suffered from dizziness and suffered from general tiredness. After several tests, his GP informed him that he is hypertensive and that he should be on antihypertensive tablets. The GP also informed Mr Fish that he is overweight and that he should see the practice nurse to get some advice.

Take some time to reflect on this case and then consider the following.

1. Calculate the body mass index (BMI) for Mr Fish and his wife.
2. Discuss the possible complications of obesity.
3. Outline a plan of care for Mr Fish and his wife with regard to losing weight.
4. What support systems are available in the community for Mr Fish and his family?

Obesity

Obesity is an excessive accumulation of fat cells (adipose tissue) for an individual's height, weight, gender and ethnicity to such an extent that it can lead to health problems (Truswell, 2007). The fat may settle in the abdominal region (apple-shaped), hips or thighs (pear-shaped). One useful tool for calculating obesity is body mass index (BMI). The formula for BMI is:

$$BMI = \frac{\text{weight (kg)}}{\text{height (m)}^2}$$

An individual with a BMI between 19 and 24.9 kg/m^2 is of normal weight, of 25–29.9 kg/m^2 is considered overweight and of over 30 kg/m^2 is considered obese. Obesity can reduce life expectancy and lead to complications:

- heart disease
- diabetes mellitus
- vascular disease
- respiratory disease
- hypertension
- bowel cancer
- deep vein thrombosis
- varicose veins
- cerebrovascular accident.

An increase in weight may be due to an increase in adipose tissue or an increase in muscle mass. For example, a bodybuilder may be very lean and muscular but weigh more than others of the same height. Thus, a bodybuilder may be considered to be overweight as a result of an increased muscle mass but not fat.

Omari and Caterson (2007) report that obesity and overweight are very common and occur in most parts of the world despite health education and numerous interventions. Obesity increases with age, is much more common among the lower socioeconomic groups, and is an escalating problem. In 2007, the government-commissioned Foresight report predicted that if no action is taken, 60% of men, 50% of women and 25% of children in the UK will be obese by 2050. This places a significant burden on the NHS – direct costs caused by obesity are estimated to be £4.2 billion per year and are forecast to more than double by 2050 (Department of Health, 2010).

Aetiology

Both hereditary and environmental factors have been associated with obesity, including physiological, psychological and cultural influences. Some of the causes include:

- endocrine disorders, such as hypothyroidism (under active thyroid) and Cushing's syndrome
- familial history
- depression as a result of, for example, bereavement
- low physical activity and intake of a high calorie diet
- high consumption of alcohol
- stress, which may result in the person overeating
- low self-esteem
- steroid therapy.

Signs and symptoms

Most practitioners use the BMI assessment tool to identify if a person is overweight or obese:

- BMI between 25 and 29.9 kg/m^2 is overweight
- BMI between 30 and 39.9 kg/m^2 is obese
- BMI over 40 kg/m^2 is extremely obese
- visible body fat accumulation on hips, waist and thighs

- increased abdominal girth
- increased weight
- waist–hip ratio.

Screening tools for nutritional assessment

The following tools may be used to determine the level of obesity:

- BMI to identify excess adipose tissue, but this needs to be interpreted with caution as it is not a direct measure of adiposity (National Institute for Health and Clinical Excellence, 2006a).
- Malnutrition universal screening tool (MUST) to determine nutritional status (Malnutrition Advisory Group, 2003).
- Anthropometry measurements to measure skinfold thickness.
- Clinical assessment of the patient.
- Biochemical tests to assess nutrient levels, e.g. protein, nitrogen and lipids.

Care and management

Patients with obesity often suffer from psychological problems, such as depression, low self-esteem, social stigma and reduced mobility. Healthcare professionals will need to be sensitive to the patient's feelings when providing care. The nurse should assist the patient to identify the cause of obesity and offer advice on preventative measures, such as dieting and exercise (Alexander *et al.*, 2007).

Advice on diet and healthy eating (Figure 12.2) should be offered as recommended by the Department of Health (British Nutrition Foundation, 2003). Food sources rich in saturated fat should be avoided, and a diet low in calories and high in fruit and vegetables is advocated. It has been estimated that eating at least five portions of a variety of fruit and vegetables per day could reduce the risk of death from chronic diseases such as heart disease, stroke and cancer by up to 20%. The patient should be encouraged to have their weight checked weekly and to keep a record of this.

The patient should be encouraged to take regular exercise for weight reduction. Unless contraindicated, the British Nutrition Foundation Task Force (2007) recommends 30 minutes exercise, such as walking, cycling or swimming, at least five times per week under the supervision of the practice nurse. The level of activity should be gradually increased to the level the patient can tolerate. The patient should be encouraged to participate in group activities such as Weight Watchers Club, which could help them to lose weight. The aim is to ensure that energy output is greater than energy intake (Figure 12.3) and this may be achieved through exercise and dieting. An individual will put on weight if the energy intake is more than energy expenditure.

Pharmacological interventions

Currently, two medicines have been recommended by National Institute for Health and Clinical Excellence (2006b):

- orlistat – reduces gastrointestinal absorption of fatty acids, cholesterol and fat-soluble vitamins, and increases faecal fat elimination
- sibutramine – blocks the reuptake of serotonin and noradrenaline in the brain.

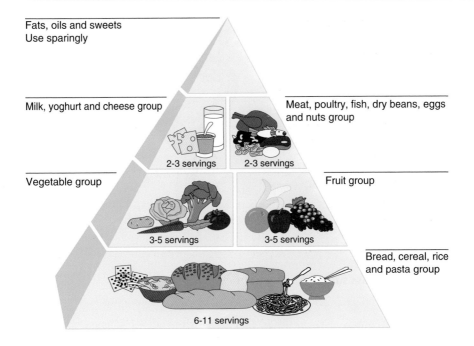

Figure 12.2   Food groups and recommended portions.

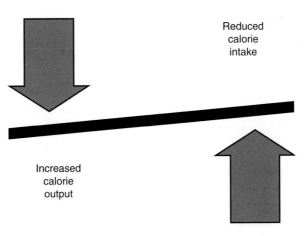

Reduced calorie intake – Increased calorie output = Weight loss

Figure 12.3   Energy balance.

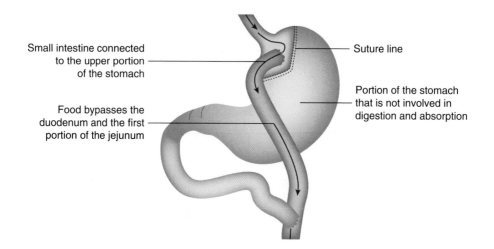

Small intestine connected
to the upper portion
of the stomach

Suture line

Food bypasses the
duodenum and the first
portion of the jejunum

Portion of the stomach
that is not involved in
digestion and absorption

Figure 12.4   Gastric bypass surgery.

These medicines are not recommended for all obese patients, only for patients with a BMI of $30\,kg/m^2$ and above, and should be prescribed in concurrence with advice on diet, physical activity and lifestyle changes.

Surgery

Surgery may be offered to some patients when dieting and exercise have not been successful in reducing their weight (Peate, 2007). Surgical procedures such as gastric bypass (Roux-en-Y connection) may be carried out to limit the quantity of food the individual can eat at any one time (Figure 12.4).

Case study

Miss Fuji Mata is a 29-year-old third-year nursing student. Her friends noticed that Miss Mata does not join them at lunch time for her meals. They also notice that her clothing does not fit her and that she has lost weight. When they invite Miss Mata to join them for lunch, she replies by telling them that she had a big breakfast and that she is not hungry.

A lecturer also noticed that Miss Mata has not been attending her lessons regularly and that she is always late in submitting her course work. Concerned, her lecturer invited her to have a chat. During the conversation Miss Mata broke down in tears and informed the lecturer that she was diagnosed with coeliac disease over 8 years ago and lately it has worsened. She is finding it difficult to concentrate and that she has lost 2 kg over 3 weeks. The lecturer referred Miss Mata to occupational health and advised her to see her GP so that she can get some help.

Take some time to reflect on this case and then consider the following.

1. Discuss the effects of undernutrition on the systems of the body.
2. Explain why Miss Mata is losing weight with coeliac disease.
3. Outline a plan of care for Miss Mata's undernutrition.
4. With the aid of a risk assessment tool, what nutritional advice will you offer Miss Mata?

Malnutrition

Malnutrition is a general term used to define undernutrition as a result of inadequate food intake, dietary imbalance or overnutrition from excess consumption of food. In clinical practice, malnutrition is regarded as undernutrition and overnutrition.

Undernutrition refers to the inability to meet the body's need for nutrition and energy. It can result from low intake of nutrients, high calorie demand of the body or poor absorption of nutrients from the gastrointestinal tract, e.g. as a result of stomach cancer. Undernutrition can be detrimental to health and if untreated, can result in complications:

- tremors
- impaired co-ordination
- cardiovascular problems, e.g. an enlarged heart
- amenorrhoea
- hypotension
- constipation
- muscle wasting
- enlarged liver
- susceptible to infection
- low basal metabolic rate
- severe weight loss.

Multisystem failure and death can from severe weight loss..

Carbohydrates and fats are the main energy source of the body. When dietary intake is not sufficient to meet the energy requirements of the body, stored glycogen, body protein and fats are used to produce energy (LeMone *et al.*, 2011). In a severe state of undernutrition, the body uses fat reserve and converts it into fatty acid and ketones, which provide energy for the brain. As the disease process progresses, body mass is reduced and there is a reduction in energy expenditure. Alexander *et al.* (2007) report that undernutrition is often common in hospitalized patients and identified several possible factors:

- stress as a result of hospital admission
- pain as a result of surgery or chronic disease may reduce appetite
- the presentation and taste of hospital food may not be to the patient's liking
- unfamiliar environment
- hospital meal times may not be suitable for the patient.

Signs and symptoms

- BMI between 17 and 18.5 kg/m^2 – mild undernutrition
- BMI between 16 and 17 kg/m^2 – moderate undernutrition

- BMI less than $16 \, kg/m^2$ – severe malnutrition
- severe muscle wasting
- wrinkled skin in patients with marasmus
- distended abdomen in patients with kwashiorkor
- swollen ankles in patients with kwashiorkor

Aetiology

Causes of undernutrition include:

- elderly and living on their own
- socioeconomic factors, e.g. poverty, isolation
- patients who suffer from osteo and rheumatoid arthritis
- unconscious patients
- chronic disease such as cardiovascular and renal disease
- ill-fitting dentures and periodontal disease
- stomatitis or candida
- loss of appetite, e.g. as a result of chemotherapy or excessive alcohol consumption.

Screening tools

- clinical assessment of the patient
- MUST to determine nutritional status (Malnutrition Advisory Group, 2003)
- body mass index
- anthropometry measurements

Care and management

Prior to planning care, a full assessment of the patient should be undertaken, including a physical assessment, nutritional assessment, past nursing and medical history, and any problems the patient may present with that could result in undernutrition. Assessment may reveal:

- changes in dietary habit
- physiological problems such as swallowing difficulties that may have an effect on nutritional intake
- psychological problems, e.g. depression as a result of bereavement
- socioeconomic factors such as lack of finance that may affect purchasing and cooking of food
- cultural and religious beliefs.

With the patient's consent, the information gathered may be shared between the members of the multidisciplinary team, including the dietitian in order to plan optimum care.

The patient should be encouraged to keep a food diary of the quantity of food and fluids consumed each day. The patient should be weighed daily (at the same time and wearing the same clothing) to ensure that they are gaining weight. The weight should be recorded and documented. Advice should be offered on the type of food to purchase that is nutritious and healthy. When giving advice, the healthcare professional needs to consider the patient's preferences and their cultural and religious beliefs. If necessary, information on oral supplements, e.g. Ensure plus, should be offered; it is the healthcare professional's role to ensure that patients take the supplement as prescribed. For patients who find these drinks unacceptable due to their high milk content, fruit-flavoured supplements such as Enlive or Fortijuice may be preferred. The dietitian will be able to give advice on the appropriate supplement for the patient to take. Advice on supplements should be offered in accordance with the National Institute for Health and Clinical Excellence (2006c) recommendations and guidelines on nutritional support in adults.

The patient should be encouraged to take at least 180 mL of water every hour to prevent dehydration and infection – fluid is essential for effective body function. The patient should be educated about the importance of taking adequate fluid. An input and output chart should be maintained and it should be ensured that all carers are aware of the importance of maintaining an accurate fluid balance chart. Any significant changes in fluid balance should be reported immediately to allow prompt action to be taken, e.g. commencement of an intravenous infusion if the patient is dehydrated. Conversely, excessive fluid overload can result in heart or kidney failure.

When presenting food to the patient, the healthcare professional needs to ensure that it looks appetising. The quantity of food offered each mealtime should be related to the amount the patient can consume. Large portions of food should be avoided as these may be unappetising for the patient. Mealtimes should be planned with the patient's relatives in order to make eating a pleasurable and social activity. It is the role of the healthcare professional to ensure that the nutritional needs of the patient are met as recommended in *Essence of Care* (Department of Health, 2003).

The healthcare professional needs to be aware that elderly patients who are on bed rest as a result of ill health are prone to developing complications, such as decubitus ulcers (pressure ulcers), chest infection or urinary tract infection. Good nutrition is essential for growth and tissue repair. In the undernourished patient, loss of muscle mass and adipose tissue increases the risk of developing pressure ulcers; the most affected areas are the ankle, shoulder blades, sacrum and elbows. Pressure areas should be observed every 2 hours for early signs of pressure ulcer development, e.g. inflammation, and appropriate action taken, such as repositioning the patient (Walter, 2010). The healthcare professional will need to adhere to local policies and guidelines in the prevention of pressure ulcers.

Passive and active movement of limbs in bed should be encouraged to improve circulation and prevent complications such as deep vein thrombosis and infection. Deep breathing exercises should be encouraged to prevent complications such as chest infection.

Enteral nutrition

To facilitate enteral nutrition, a tube is inserted directly into the gastrointestinal tract and the patient is fed a liquid diet through the tube. Enteral feeding is used to supplement oral intake or if the patient is unable to take nutrition orally. Indications include (Alexander *et al.*, 2007):

- major surgery, such as gastrectomy
- oesophageal stricture
- carcinoma of the oesophagus or mouth
- coma following head injury
- gastrointestinal fistula
- dysphagia following cerebrovascular accident
- patients who are confused and reluctant to eat
- severe burns
- inflammatory bowel disease.

Say (2010) reports that there are three types of enteral feeding:

- Nasogastric (NG) tube feeding involves the insertion of a nasogastric tube via the nasopharynx into the stomach. This procedure is normally carried out by a registered nurse or medical staff.
- Nasojejunal (NJ) tube feeding involves the insertion of a tube via the nasopharynx and the stomach into the jejunum. Insertion of the NJ tube is carried out by medical staff using endoscopy and it is confirmed to be in place radiologically.
- Percutaneous endoscopic gastrostomy (PEG) or jejunostomy (PEJ) involves the insertion of a tube into the stomach through the abdominal wall. This procedure is carried out surgically by the medical staff.

Care and management of the patient with enteral feeding

Healthcare professionals should ensure that patients receiving enteral feeding are monitored regularly for complications, e.g. breathlessness and abdominal distension, and their vital signs recorded every 2 hours. They should ensure that the enteral feeding tube is correctly positioned before commencing each feed. Local policies, guidelines and the National Institute for Health and Clinical Excellence (2006c) recommendations in the management and care of the patient with enteral feeding should be adhered to.

Healthcare professionals need to ensure that the patient who is receiving an enteral feed has full care, such as oral and nasal hygiene, washing hands before administering the feed and documenting all the care given as per Nursing and Midwifery Council (2009) guidelines.

Parenteral nutrition

Parenteral nutrition is the direct infusion of a solution into a vein and is used when the patient cannot be nourished with oral or enteral feeding. The solution contains all essential nutritional requirements (macro- and micro-nutrients) for the body, including fluid replacement. It is a specialised method of feeding which requires specialist care from healthcare professionals. The patient receiving parenteral nutrition in the community will need co-ordinated support from the district nurse, specialist nutrition nurse, dietitian, pharmacist and GP (National Institute for Health and Clinical Excellence, 2006c). The patient receiving parenteral nutrition is at risk of developing complications such as infection, fluid overload, heart failure, electrolyte imbalance, and respiratory and renal complications. It is not the remit of this chapter to describe this specialist care. Further in-depth discussion regarding the special care of patients receiving parenteral nutrition can be found elsewhere, e.g. Dougherty and Lister (2011).

Conclusion

Nutrition plays a vital role in body function and maintaining homeostasis. Nutrients are classified as macro- and micro-nutrients. The macronutrients include carbohydrates, proteins and fats, while micronutrients are vitamins and minerals. These nutrients are primarily obtained from the diet and are absorbed from the gastrointestinal tract after digestion. Macronutrients are primarily for energy production whilst micronutrients promote growth and development.

Obesity and undernutrition are two major global and national concerns. In the UK, the estimated cost of obesity and undernutrition is approximately £6.6–£7.4 billion per year. Obesity is both a medical condition and a lifestyle disorder. Undernutrition is becoming increasingly prevalent as the elderly population is increasing. Some elderly people and children are more prone to undernutrition as a result of illness or socioeconomic factors.

The role of the healthcare professional is varied as regards nutritional care. The responsibilities include preventing undernutrition in patients and offering health education and support relating to obesity and undernutrition. It is their responsibility to prevent and highlight nutritional problems and to take prompt action to prevent complications, such as heart failure, renal disease, constipation and even death.

Test your knowledge

- Explain the roles of carbohydrates, protein and fats.

- Explain the terms macro- and micro-nutrients.

- List the fat-soluble vitamins and describe their functions.

- List the possible causes of obesity and undernutrition.

- How are lipids transported in the body?

Activities

Here are some activities and exercises to help test your learning. For the answers to these exercises, as well as further self-testing activities, visit our website at www.wiley.com/go/fundamentalsofappliedpathophysiology

Fill in the blanks

_____ causes a _____ in _____ and body tissue mass, and also results in altered _____ and physiological _____, which has adverse effects on health. Muscle wasting and weakness decrease _____ and _____ and impair functions of the lung and heart. _____ is associated with poor _____ healing, impaired immune responses and delayed recovery from illness, with a higher incidence of postoperative _____. Correcting undernutrition has many benefits, including improved disease recovery with fewer complications, and shorter hospital stays. _____ nutrition can lead to _____ and _____ risk factors, a decreased ability to process _____, hyperlipidaemia and _____.

Choose from:
Wound; Complications; Mobility; Function; Obesity; Glucose; Reduction; Metabolic; Stamina; Malnutrition; Cardiovascular; Muscle; Over; Undernutrition; Hypertension

Label the diagram

From the list of words supplied, label the diagram.

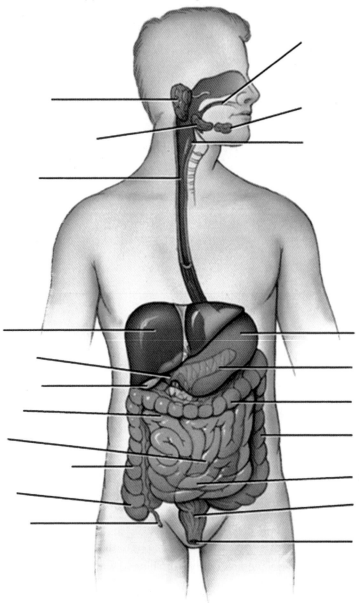

Right lateral view of head and neck and anterior view of trunk

Mouth (oral cavity) contains teeth and tongue; Sublingual gland; Pharynx; Oesophagus, submandib-ular gland; Parotid gland; Stomach; Pancreas; Descending colon; Transverse colon; Sigmoid colon; Anus; Rectum; Appendix; Caecum; Ascending colon; Ileum; Jejunum; Liver; Gallbladder; Duodenum

Word search

S	C	N	T	M	F	P	P	U	E	I	H	I	T	R	N
N	A	P	O	N	R	F	N	R	I	F	B	N	T	E	E
C	O	N	C	T	T	E	O	Y	O	F	R	U	D	F	G
O	V	I	T	A	M	I	N	S	Y	T	H	T	Y	F	O
I	Y	I	T	H	C	R	U	A	M	E	E	R	T	U	C
S	T	N	E	I	R	T	U	N	O	R	C	I	M	B	Y
L	I	P	O	P	R	O	T	E	I	N	S	E	N	M	L
R	S	I	T	L	O	R	P	R	Y	S	O	N	O	O	G
T	E	T	W	O	I	M	U	O	O	S	R	T	C	F	U
Y	B	I	A	O	U	P	T	N	M	T	C	S	O	I	T
A	O	G	Z	F	R	A	I	A	L	E	K	R	E	S	N
R	C	A	R	B	O	H	Y	D	R	A	T	E	N	T	T
O	T	P	A	A	E	T	L	T	S	F	M	R	Z	U	O
R	O	K	R	O	I	H	S	A	W	K	Y	E	Y	L	I
S	U	M	S	A	R	A	M	N	K	U	E	O	M	A	T
I	A	N	C	F	G	Y	D	M	S	E	R	R	E	N	S

Anthropmetry	Coenzyme	Malnutrition
Buffer	Fistula	Kwashiorkor
Carbohydrate	Gastrectomy	Nutrients
Protein	Lipids	Micronutrients
Fats	Marasmus	Glycogen
Vitamins	Obesity	lipoproteins

Further resources

Netdoctor

http://www.netdoctor.co.uk/health_advice/facts/obesity.htm
From this website you can get useful information on obesity for your studies; it also provides reference material which can aid you in health promotion.

Department of Health (DH)

http://www.dh.gov.uk/en/Publichealth/Obesity/index.htm
This link provides information and guidance on obesity, including government targets with regards to reducing obesity in children and adults.

National Institute for Health and Clinical Excellence (NICE) – Obesity

http://guidance.nice.org.uk/CG43/Guidance
There is increasing recognition both in the UK and worldwide that there is an 'obesity epidemic'. The issue has received much attention recently from politicians, professionals, the media and the public. This link gives some insight into a whole range of guidelines from NICE with regards to obesity.

World Health Organization (WHO)

http://www.who.int/topics/nutrition_disorders/en/
Nutritional disorder is not just a UK problem. It is a worldwide issue. Some of the conditions discussed in this chapter, such as obesity and undernutrition, can lead to other physiological problems both in adults and children. WHO provides guidance and recommendations with regards to these health problems. All students should access this website to gain knowledge on these issues.

National Institute for Health and Clinical Excellence (NICE) – Eating disorders

http://guidance.nice.org.uk/CG9/publicinfo/pdf/English
In this NICE guidance you will find information on anorexia nervosa, bulimia nervosa and related eating disorders.

British Medical Journal

http://www.ncbi.nlm.nih.gov/pmc/articles/PMC1118795/
Students may find this link beneficial as there are numerous articles related to eating disorders and the burden these have on finance and resources.

Glossary of terms

Anthropometry:	assessment tool used to measure skinfolds.
Body mass index:	a number calculated from a person's weight and height.
Buffer:	a chemical substance that allows a slight change in pH when acid or base is added to the solution.
Carbohydrate:	an organic compound that is composed of carbon, hydrogen and oxygen. Sugars (including glucose) and starch are carbohydrates. They are very important as an energy store.Coenzyme: a molecule that binds to an enzyme and is essential for its activity, but is not permanently altered by the reaction.
Dysphagia:	difficulty in swallowing.
Enteral:	through the gastrointestinal tract.
Extracellular:	outside the cell.
Fatty acid:	composed of carbon chemically bonded together.
Fistula:	an abnormal passage from an internal organ to the surface of the skin or between two organs.
Gastrectomy:	surgical excision of part or the whole of the stomach.
Glucagon:	a hormone released by the pancreas, which increase blood sugar levels.
Gluconeogenesis:	the production of glucose from non-carbohydrate sources.
Glycogen:	a carbohydrate (complex sugar) made from glucose. Excess glucose is stored as glycogen mainly in the liver.
Glycogenolysis:	the conversion of glycogen into glucose.
Intracellular:	inside the cell.
Ketone:	product of fat metabolism.
Kwashiorkor:	protein-deficiency malnutrition.
Lipid:	an energy-rich organic compound that is soluble in organic substances such as alcohol and benzene.
Lipoprotein:	a transport unit for lipids with proteins.
Macronutrient:	a nutrient that provides energy.
Marasmus:	protein- and carbohydrate-deficiency malnutrition.
Micronutrient:	vitamins or mineral.
Nutrient:	chemical component of foods.

Obesity:	excess of body fat.
Organelle:	a structural and functional part of a cell that acts like a human organ to fulfil all the needs of the cell so that it can grow, reproduce and carry out its functions.
Protein:	an organic nitrogenous compound essential as the building material for growth and repair.
Synthesis:	production.
Triglyceride:	a major form of lipids in the body.
Undernutrition:	failing health as a result of inadequate nutrient.
Vitamin:	an organic compound essential for physiological functions of the body.

References

Alexander, M.F., Fawcett, J.N. and Runciman, P.J. (2007). *Nursing Practice: Hospital and Home – the Adult*, 3rd edn. Edinburgh: Churchill Livingstone.

British Nutrition Foundation (2003). Health eating: A whole diet approach. In: Alexander, M.F., Fawcett, J.N. and Runciman, P.J. (eds) *Nursing Practice: Hospital and Home – the Adult*. Edinburgh: Churchill Livingstone.

British Nutrition Foundation Task Force (2007). Obesity. In: Alexander, M.F., Fawcett, J.N. and Runciman, P.J. (eds) *Nursing Practice: Hospital and Home – the Adult*. Edinburgh: Churchill Livingstone.

Department of Health (2003). *The Essence of Care: Patient-Focused Benchmarks for Clinical Governance*. London: The Stationary Office.

Department of Health (2010) *Healthy Lives, Healthy People: Our Strategy for Public Health in England*. London: The Stationary Office

Dougherty, L. and Lister, S. (2011). *The Royal Marsden Hospital Manual of Clinical Nursing Procedures*, 8th edn. Oxford: Blackwell Science.

Green, S. and Jackson, P. (2007). Nutrition. In: Alexander, M.F., Fawcett, J.N. and Runciman, P.J. (eds) *Nursing Practice: Hospital and Home – the Adult*, 3rd edn. Edinburgh: Churchill Livingstone.

Jenkins, G.W. and Tortora, G.J. (2013). *Anatomy and Physiology*. New Jersey: John Wiley and Sons.

LeMone, P., Burke, K. and Bauldoff, G. (2011). *Medical – Surgical Nursing; Critical Thinking in Client Care*, 4rd edn. New Jersey: Pearson.

Malnutrition Advisory Group (2003). *The MUST Report. Nutritional Screening of Adults: A Multidisciplinary Responsibility*. London: British Association for Parenteral and Enteral Nutrition.

Mann, J. and Skeaff, M. (2007). Lipids. In: Mann, J. and Truswell, A.S. (eds). *Essentials of Human Nutrition*, 3rd edn. Oxford: Oxford University Press.

National Institute for Health and Clinical Excellence (2006a). *Obesity: Guidance on the Prevention, Identification, Assessment and Management of Overweight and Obesity in Adults and Children*. London: NICE.

National Institute for Health and Clinical Excellence (2006b). *Treatment for People Who Are Overweight or Obese*. London: NICE.

National Institute for Health and Clinical Excellence (2006c). *Nutrition Support in Adults – Nutrition Support in Adults: Oral Nutrition Support, Enteral Tube Feeding Parenteral Nutrition*. Clinical Guideline 32. London: NICE.

Nursing and Midwifery Council (2009). *Record Keeping: Guidance for Nurses and Midwives*. London: Nursing and Midwifery Council.

Omari, A. and Caterson, I.D. (2007). Overweight and obesity. In: Mann, J. and Truswell, A.S. (eds). *Essentials of Human Nutrition*, 3rd edn. Oxford: Oxford University Press.

Peate, I. (2007). *Men's Health – the Practice Nurse's Handbook*. Chichester: John Wiley and Sons.

Say, J. (2010). Eating and drinking: Nutrient and fluid replacement for health. In: Peate, I. (ed). *Nursing Care and the Activities of Living*, 2nd edn. London: Wiley-Blackwell.

Seeley, R.R., Stephens, T.D. and Tate, P. (2006). *Anatomy and Physiology*, 7th edn. Boston: McGraw Hill.

Truswell, S. (2007). Alcohol. In: Mann, J. and Truswell, A.S. (eds) *Essentials of Human Nutrition*, 3rd edn. Oxford: Oxford University Press.

Walter, K. (2010). An ergonomic approach to safe manual handling. In: Peate, I. (ed). *Nursing Care and the Activities of Living*, 2nd edn. London: Wiley-Blackwell.

13

The endocrine system and associated disorders

Carl Clare

Senior Lecturer, Department of Adult Nursing and Primary Care, School of Health and Social Work, University of Hertfordshire, Hatfield, Hertfordshire, UK

Contents

Fundamentals of Applied Pathophysiology: An Essential Guide for Nursing and Healthcare Students, Second Edition. Edited by Muralitharan Nair and Ian Peate.
© 2013 John Wiley & Sons, Ltd. Published 2013 by John Wiley & Sons, Ltd.

Key words

- Hormones
- Homeostasis
- Receptors
- Up-regulation
- Down-regulation
- Negative feedback
- Hypothalamus
- Calorigenic effect
- Glucagon
- Corticosteroids
- Hyposecretion
- Hypersecretion

Test your prior knowledge

- Where is the hypothalamus?
- Name one organ of the endocrine system and one hormone it releases.
- What is the treatment for hypothyroidism?
- Name the two major types of diabetes.

Learning outcomes

On completion of this section the reader will be able to:

- Name the major endocrine organs.
- Name the hormones that they secrete.
- Describe the principles of the negative feedback control system that affects most endocrine glands.
- Describe the effects of thyroid hormone on the body.
- Discuss the regulation of blood glucose by the pancreas.

Don't forget to visit to the companion website for this book (www.wiley.com/go/fundamentalsofappliedpathophysiology) where you can find self-assessment tests to check your progress, as well as lots of activities to practise your learning.

Introduction

The endocrine system is the name given to a collection of small organs that are scattered throughout the body, each of which releases hormones (Marieb and Hoehn, 2010). Hormones are chemical substances that are released into the blood by the endocrine system and have physiological control over the function of cells or organs other than those that created them (Guyton and Hall, 2010) (Figure 13.1). The purpose of each hormone varies but their common primary role is to maintain homeostasis (that is keeping a normal physiological balance in the body).

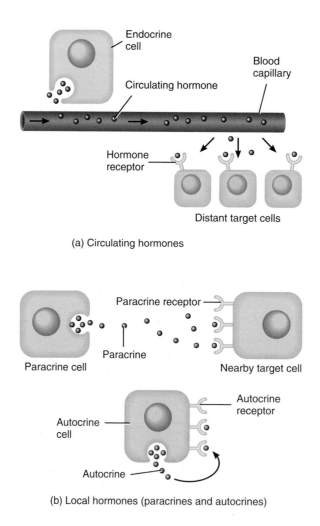

(a) Circulating hormones

(b) Local hormones (paracrines and autocrines)

Figure 13.1   Hormone release and transport.

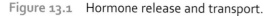

Endocrine-releasing organs can be divided into three main categories:

- Endocrine glands – these are organs whose sole function is the production and release of hormones. The pituitary, thyroid, parathyroid and adrenal glands are all examples of this category.
- Organs that are not pure glands but contain relatively large areas of hormone-producing tissue – examples of these are the pancreas, the hypothalamus and the gonads.
- Other tissues and organs also produce hormones – areas of hormone-producing cells are found in the wall of the small intestine, the stomach, the kidneys and the heart.

The organs and their position in the body are shown in Figure 13.2. Each of these organs will typically have a rich vascular (blood vessel) network and the hormone-producing cells within them are arranged into cords and branching networks around this supply (Marieb and Hoehn, 2010). This arrangement of blood vessels and hormone-producing cells ensures that hormones enter the blood rapidly and are then transported throughout the body.

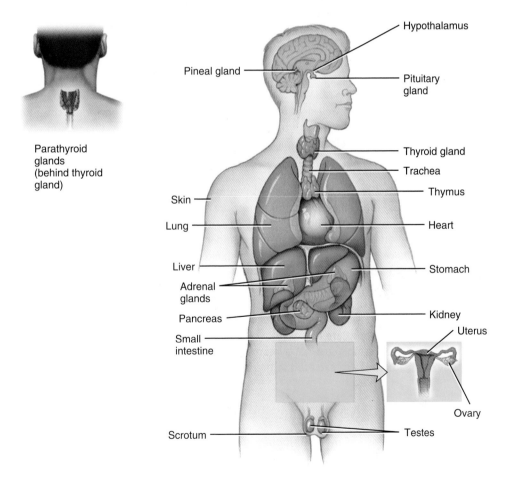

Figure 13.2   Position of the endocrine glands.

Hormones

There are a great number of hormones produced by the endocrine system and each has very different effects and affect different cells and organs in the body. The major bodily processes that hormones influence or regulate are reproduction, growth and development, the body's defence mechanisms against stressors, levels of electrolytes, water and nutrients in the body, and cellular metabolism and energy (Marieb and Hoehn, 2010). Hormones are generally made from either amino acids (most) or cholesterol (the steroid hormones). As hormones are released into the bloodstream they are carried throughout the body, but they do not affect all cells. In order for a hormone to have an effect on a cell, the cell must have receptors for that particular hormone. Cells that have receptors for a particular hormone are known as the target cells for that hormone (Guyton and Hall, 2010). Some hormones are very specific and thus receptors are only found on specific cells (e.g. adrenocorticotropic hormone), whereas thyroid hormone affects nearly every cell in the body.

Receptors for a hormone are proteins that are sited either on the cell wall or inside the cell. The exact location of a receptor depends on the type of hormone that the receptor is for (Tortora and Derrickson, 2011). Amino acid-based hormones cannot cross the cell membrane and therefore their receptors are found on the cell wall; activation of these receptors leads to the activation of secondary messenger systems within the cell. One exception is thyroid hormone, which is very small and can diffuse easily across the cell membrane into the cell. The steroid hormones can cross the cell membrane because they are small and lipid-soluble and thus their receptors are found within the cell itself.

The activation of a target cell depends on the blood levels of the hormone, the number of receptors on the cell and the affinity of the receptor for the hormone. Changes in all three of these factors can happen relatively quickly in response to a change in stimuli. Changes in the number of receptors are known as up-regulation and down-regulation (Guyton and Hall, 2010).

- Up-regulation is the creation of more receptors in response to low circulating levels of a hormone. Thus, the cell becomes more responsive to the presence of the hormone in the blood.
- Down-regulation is the reduction in the number of receptors and is often caused by the exposure of a cell to prolonged periods of high circulating levels of a hormone. Thus, the cell becomes less responsive (desensitised) to a hormone, which protects the cell from over-responding to continued high levels of that hormone.

Hormones can have a very powerful effect even at low concentrations and thus it is essential that the released hormones are disposed of efficiently. Some hormones are rapidly broken down within their target cells; most are inactivated by the liver or the kidneys and then excreted in the urine, but small amounts are excreted in the faeces (Guyton and Hall, 2010).

The control of hormone release

The creation and release of most hormones is commenced by an external or internal stimulus; further creation and release is then regulated by a negative feedback system (Figure 13.3). Thus, the influence of a stimulus, from inside or outside the body, leads to hormone release; following this, some aspect of the target organ function then inhibits further reaction to the stimulus and thus further release of the hormone by the organ.

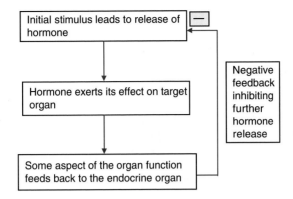

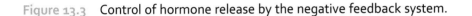

Figure 13.3   Control of hormone release by the negative feedback system.

367

An example of a negative feedback system is the release of insulin by the pancreas. Insulin is released by the pancreas in response to rising levels of glucose, amino acids or fatty acids in the blood. The effect of insulin is to reduce these levels, thus reducing the stimulus for further insulin release.

The initial stimulus for the release of a hormone is usually one of three types, although some organs respond to multiple stimuli (Marieb and Hoehn, 2010):

- Humoral – a response to changing levels of certain ions and nutrients in the blood, e.g. the release of parathyroid hormone is stimulated by falling blood levels of calcium ions.
- Neural – a response to direct nervous stimulation. Only a few endocrine organs are directly stimulated by the nervous system. Increased activity in the sympathetic nervous system directly stimulates the release of catecholamines (epinephrine and norepinephrine) from the adrenal medulla.
- Hormonal – a response to hormones released by other organs. Hormones that are released in response to hormonal stimuli are usually rhythmical in their release (i.e. the levels rise and fall in a specific pattern). Many of the hormones released from the anterior pituitary gland are released in response to releasing and inhibiting hormones from the hypothalamus.

Summary

- Hormones are chemicals that are released into the bloodstream.
- Hormones are released by glands and other organs.
- A hormone's effect on its target cell is through receptors, which are found in the cell wall or contained in the cell itself.
- The stimulus for a hormone's release can be changing levels of ions or nutrients in the blood, direct stimulation by the nervous system or in response to other hormones.
- Further control of hormone release is regulated by a negative feedback system.

The physiology of the endocrine glands

The hypothalamus and pituitary gland

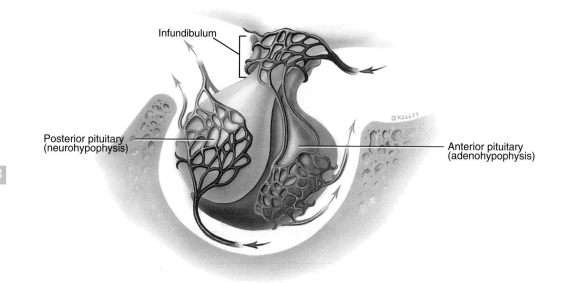

Figure 13.4   The pituitary gland.

The pituitary gland is a pure endocrine gland that is located in the brain just below the hypothalamus. It is about the size and shape of a pea on a stalk. The pituitary stalk (infundibulum) connects the pituitary gland to the hypothalamus and contains both nerve fibres and blood vessels (Figure 13.4). The direct link between the hypothalamus and the pituitary gland is essential as it allows direct hypothalamic control of the release of the pituitary hormones.

Anatomically, the pituitary gland is split into two sections. The posterior lobe (the neurohypophysis) is mostly made up of nerve fibres and nerve endings that have their origin in the hypothalamus; it stores two hormones that are created in the hypothalamus and are then transported down the nerve fibres in the stalk (the hypothalamic–hypophyseal tract) and stored in the nerve endings (Tortora and Derrickson, 2011). The anterior pituitary gland (the adenohypophysis) consists of glandular tissues. Whilst the anterior pituitary gland has no direct neural link from the hypothalamus, it does receive its blood supply directly from the hypothalamus through the pituitary portal system. This blood supply is an essential component in the control of the release of hormones from the anterior pituitary gland as it transports inhibiting and releasing hormones created by the hypothalamus to the anterior pituitary gland (Table 13.1).

Growth hormone (somatotropin) stimulates most body cells to increase in size and divide; however, its major targets are the bones and skeletal muscle. Growth hormone also has several other effects, including increasing the cellular uptake of amino acids to be used in the building of proteins. The secretion of growth hormone is regulated by two hypothalamic hormones – growth hormone-releasing hormone (GHRH) and growth hormone-inhibiting hormone (GHIH). It is usually

Table 13.1   The hormones of the hypothalamus and the anterior pituitary gland.

Hypothalamus	Anterior pituitary gland	Target organ or tissues
Growth hormone releasing factor	Growth hormone	Many
Growth hormone release inhibiting factor	Growth hormone (inhibits release)	Many
Thyroid-releasing hormone	Thyroid-stimulating hormone	Thyroid gland
Corticotropin-releasing hormone	Adrenocorticotropic hormone	Adrenal cortex
Prolactin-releasing hormone	Prolactin	Breasts
Prolactin-inhibiting hormone	Prolactin (inhibits release)	Breasts
Gonadotropin-releasing hormone	Follicle-stimulating hormone	Gonads
	Luteinising hormone	

released in a diurnal cycle (related to the pattern of day and night) and is found at its highest level about an hour after the onset of sleep.

The release of thyroid-stimulating hormone (TSH or thyrotropin) from the anterior pituitary gland in regulated by exposure of the gland to thyrotropin-releasing hormone (TRH) from the hypothalamus and the blood levels of thyroid hormones. The effect of TSH is to stimulate activity in the thyroid gland.

Adrenocorticotropic hormone (ACTH or corticotropin) stimulates the cortex of each adrenal gland to release corticosteroid hormones. The release of ACTH usually follows a diurnal rhythm with the peak being in the morning just after rising (Marieb and Hoehn, 2010). The release of ACTH is stimulated by corticotropin-releasing hormone (CRH) from the hypothalamus; however, other triggers for release include fever, trauma and other stressors (Marieb and Hoehn, 2010).

Gonadotropins is the collective name for follicle-stimulating hormone (FSH) and luteinising hormone (LH) (Marieb and Hoehn, 2010). The release of both hormones is regulated by the secretion of gonadotropin-releasing hormone from the hypothalamus. In the adult, FSH stimulates the production of gametes (sperm or egg) and in females it also regulates ovulation in conjunction with LH. LH promotes the production of gonadal hormones in both males and females (Tortora and Derrickson, 2011).

Prolactin stimulates milk production in the breasts and is controlled by releasing and inhibiting hormones produced by the hypothalamus. Prolactin-inhibiting hormone is produced in high levels in men, whereas in women the production of the releasing and inhibiting hormones varies depending on the amount of oestrogen in the blood.

Two hormones are released from the posterior pituitary gland – oxytocin and antidiuretic hormone (ADH). Oxytocin has an effect on uterine contraction in childbirth and is responsible for the 'let down' response in breastfeeding mothers (the release of milk in response to suckling). In men and non-pregnant women, it plays a role in sexual arousal and orgasm (Marieb and Hoehn, 2010).

The primary role of ADH (vasopressin) is to prevent wide fluctuations in the water balance of the body. Osmoreceptors in the hypothalamus monitor the concentration of dissolved ions in the blood (and therefore water levels). An increase in the concentration of dissolved ions leads to an increase in ADH release from the posterior pituitary gland. The main target of ADH is the renal tubules in the kidneys, causing them to increase the reabsorption of water from the urine and back into the blood (thus decreasing urine output and increasing blood volume). A decrease in blood pressure also stimulates ADH release.

The thyroid gland

The thyroid gland is a butterfly-shaped gland located in the front of the neck on the trachea just below the larynx (Tortora and Derrickson, 2011). It is made up of hollow, spherical follicles which contain thyroglobulin molecules with attached iodine molecules; the thyroid hormone is created from these. One unique factor of the thyroid gland is its ability to create and store large amounts hormone; this can be up to 100 days of hormone supply (Guyton and Hall, 2010). The thyroid gland releases two forms of thyroid hormone – thyroxine (T_4) and tri-iodothyronine (T_3), both of which require iodine for their creation. However, T_4 is the primary hormone released by the thyroid gland; this is then converted into T_3 by the target cells (Marieb and Hoehn, 2010).

Thyroid hormone affects virtually every cell in the body, except the adult brain, spleen, testes, uterus and thyroid gland itself. In the target cells, thyroid hormone stimulates enzymes that are involved with glucose oxidation. This is the calorigenic effect and its overall effects are an increase in basal metabolic rate, oxygen consumption and production of body heat. Thyroid hormone also has an important role in the maintenance of blood pressure as it stimulates an increase in the number of receptors in the walls of blood vessels (Marieb and Hoehn, 2010).

The control of the release of thyroid hormone is mediated by a negative feedback system which involves the hypothalamus and cascades through the pituitary gland (Figure 13.5).

Increased levels of T_4 in the blood inhibit the release of TRH from the hypothalamus, thus reducing the stimulation for the release of TSH from the anterior pituitary gland. The effect of TSH on the thyroid gland is to promote the release of thyroid hormone into the blood; therefore,

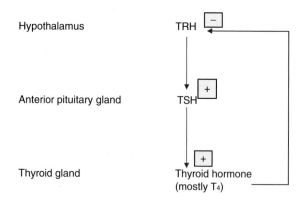

Figure 13.5   The negative feedback control of thyroid hormone production. TSH, thyroid-stimulating hormone; TRH, thyroid-releasing hormone.

a reduction in TSH reduces the release of T_3 and T_4. A reduced level of T_4 in the blood reduces the negative feedback and thus there is an increase in the release of TRH, which leads to an increase in thyroid gland function. Conditions that increase the energy requirements of the body (such as pregnancy or prolonged cold) also stimulate the release of TRH from the hypothalamus and therefore lead to an increase in blood levels of thyroid hormone. In these situations, the stimulating conditions override the normal negative feedback system (Tortora and Derrickson, 2011).

The parathyroid glands

The parathyroid glands are tiny glands normally located on the back (posterior) of the thyroid gland. There are usually two pairs of glands, but the precise number varies and some patients have been reported to have up to four pairs (Marieb and Hoehn, 2010). The parathyroid glands release parathyroid hormone (PTH), which is the single most important hormone for the control of the calcium balance in the body (Tortora and Derrickson, 2011). Physiologically, calcium is important in the transmission of nerve impulses, is involved in muscle contraction and is required for the production of clotting factors in the blood.

The release of PTH by the glands is controlled by the blood levels of calcium; a reduced calcium level stimulates the release of PTH and an increased calcium level inhibits its release. PTH increases blood levels of calcium by its action on three target areas in the body (Marieb and Hoehn, 2010):

- Bones – PTH stimulates the activity of osteoclasts to digest some of the bone and release calcium into the blood.
- Kidneys – PTH increases reabsorption of calcium.
- Intestines – PTH increases the absorption of calcium in the intestines by activating vitamin D (which is required for the absorption of calcium in the gut).

The adrenal glands

The adrenal glands are two pyramid-shaped glands that lie on top of each of the kidneys (Tortora and Derrickson, 2011). Each of the adrenal glands is structurally and functionally two glands in one. The inner core of each of the adrenal glands is called the adrenal medulla; this is surrounded by the much larger adrenal cortex (Figure 13.6). Both the medulla and the cortex secrete different hormones and respond to different stimuli.

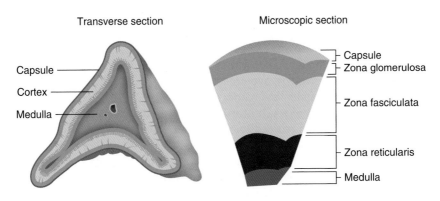

Figure 13.6   Anatomy of an adrenal gland.

The adrenal medulla

The adrenal medulla secretes epinephrine (adrenaline) and (to a lesser extent) norepinephrine (noradrenaline) in response to stimulation by the sympathetic nervous system. Although epinephrine and norepinephrine are essential for normal bodily functioning, the epinephrine and the norepinephrine secreted by the adrenal medulla are not essential and serve only to intensify the effects of sympathetic nervous stimulation (Marieb and Hoehn, 2010).

The adrenal cortex

The adrenal cortex is functionally separated into three different zones (Figure 13.6), each of which produces at least one steroid hormone (hormones made from cholesterol are known collectively as the corticosteroids) (Tortora and Derrickson, 2011):

- zona glomerulosa – produces the mineralocorticoids
- zona fasciculata – produces the glucocorticoids
- zona reticularis – involved in the production of glucocorticoids but also produces small amounts of adrenal sex hormones (the gonadocorticoids).

Mineralocorticoids are hormones whose primary function is the regulation of electrolyte concentrations (especially potassium and sodium) in the blood. Several mineralocorticoid hormones are known; however, aldosterone is the most potent and accounts for 95% of all the mineralocorticoid hormones secreted. The effect of aldosterone on the body is to reduce the excretion of sodium in the urine by regulating the reabsorption of sodium from the urine in the distal portion of the renal tubules. Aldosterone also has an effect on the body levels of water and several other ions (including potassium, bicarbonate and chloride) as their regulation is coupled to the regulation of sodium in the body. The stimulus for the release of aldosterone is primarily related to the blood concentrations of sodium (Na^+) and potassium (K^+), blood pressure (BP) and blood volume. Increased concentrations of potassium, reduced blood concentrations of sodium and a reduction in blood pressure and/or blood volume all stimulate the release of aldosterone, whilst the opposite inhibits release (Figure 13.7).

There are several mechanisms that regulate the release of aldosterone. The primary control mechanism is the production of angiotensin II by the renin–angiotensin system. However, in response to a severe, non-specific stressor, hypothalamic release of CRH stimulates the increased release of ACTH. This increase in ACTH stimulates a slight increase in the release of aldosterone, leading to a slight increase in blood volume and pressure, which will help to ensure the adequate delivery of oxygen and nutrients to the tissues (Marieb and Hoehn, 2010).

The glucocorticoid hormones influence the metabolism of most body cells and are also involved in providing resistance to stressors and promoting the repair of damaged tissues. They also suppress the immune system and inflammatory processes of the body; hence their use in the treatment of inflammatory conditions such as asthma and arthritis. The glucocorticoids include cortisol (hydrocortisone), cortisone and corticosterone; however, only cortisol is secreted in any significant amounts (Marieb and Hoehn, 2010). Cortisol is normally released in a rhythmical pattern, with most being released shortly after the person gets up from sleep and the lowest amount being released just before, and shortly after, sleep commences. Cortisol release is promoted by ACTH from the anterior pituitary gland; increasing levels of cortisol act on both the hypothalamus and the pituitary gland, inhibiting further release of both CRH and ACTH in a negative feedback system.

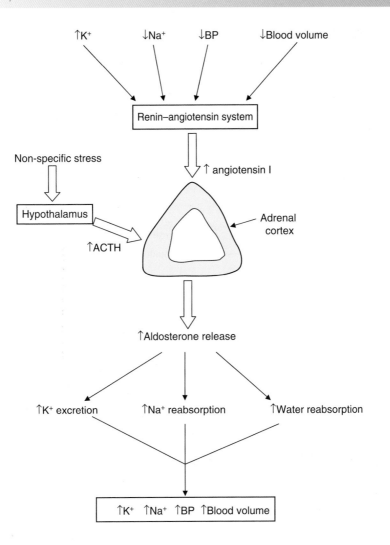

↑K⁺   ↓Na⁺   ↓BP   ↓Blood volume

Renin–angiotensin system

Non-specific stress

↑ angiotensin I

Hypothalamus

↑ACTH

Adrenal cortex

↑Aldosterone release

↑K⁺ excretion   ↑Na⁺ reabsorption   ↑Water reabsorption

↑K⁺ ↑Na⁺ ↑BP ↑Blood volume

Figure 13.7   Mechanisms for the control of aldosterone secretion. BP, blood pressure.

However, this negative feedback system is overridden by acute physiological stress (e.g. trauma, infection or haemorrhage). The increase in sympathetic nervous system activity in response to an acute stress triggers greater CRH release and thus there is a significant increase in subsequent cortisol production (Figure 13.8).

The effect of cortisol on the body is to promote gluconeogenesis (the formation of glucose from fats and proteins), the release of fatty acids into the blood and the breakdown of stored proteins to provide amino acids for tissue repair (Tortora and Derrickson, 2011). Cortisol also enhances the vasoconstrictive effect of epinephrine in the control of vascular tone. Thus, cortisol helps to enable the body to respond to stressors of various types.

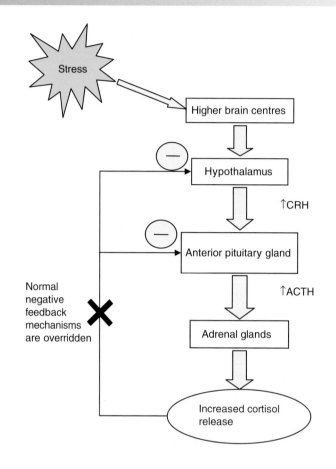

Figure 13.8   Response of the endocrine system to stress.

The pancreas

Located partially behind the stomach, the pancreas is a mixed gland containing both endocrine and exocrine gland cells. The majority of the gland is made up of acinar cells; these cells produce an enzyme-rich fluid that is secreted into the small intestines and aids the digestion of food. Scattered amongst the acinar cells are pancreatic islets, otherwise known as the islets of Langerhans. Each one of these islets is a collection of at least three major endocrine cell types, with each cell type producing a different hormone:

- Alpha cells produce the hormone glucagon.
- Beta cells are the most numerous of the cells and they produce insulin.
- Delta cells release somatostatin, a hormone that inhibits the release of glucagon and insulin.

Both insulin and glucagon are involved in the control of the blood levels of glucose, but they have directly opposite effects. Glucagon promotes the breakdown of glycogen stored in the liver into glucose (glycogenolysis); it also promotes the synthesis of glucose from fatty acids and amino acids (gluconeogenesis) and the release of the newly created glucose from the liver into the bloodstream (Tortora and Derrickson, 2011). Thus, the major effect of glucagon is to raise glucose levels in the blood. The stimuli for the release of glucagon are decreased blood levels of glucose and increased blood levels of amino acids (e.g. after a protein-rich meal).

Insulin reduces the blood glucose levels and plays a role in the breakdown of protein and in the metabolism of fat (Marieb and Hoehn, 2010). The target cells of insulin are virtually every cell in the body, especially the skeletal muscle cells (but not the brain, the liver and the kidneys). The effect of insulin on these cells is to promote the transport of glucose across the cell membrane into the cell body. Insulin also activates and promotes the enzyme systems within the cell to metabolise glucose to produce adenosine triphosphate (ATP), the basic fuel of body cells. Once the energy needs of the cells are met, insulin promotes the conversion of the remaining glucose into glycogen, and in the adipose tissues it promotes the conversion of glucose into fat molecules and the subsequent storage of these fat molecules in the cells (Marieb and Hoehn, 2010). Finally, insulin promotes amino acid uptake by the muscle tissue and the formation of proteins from these amino acids. The release of insulin is stimulated by a rise in glucose levels in the blood, or increased blood levels of amino acids and fatty acids.

As the effect of each of these two hormones leads to the conditions that stimulates the release of the other hormone (e.g. as insulin reduces the blood levels of glucose, so the stimulus for the release of glucagon is increased), insulin and glucagon release is constantly being adjusted. The overall effect is maintenance of homeostasis by preventing large fluctuations in blood glucose.

Disorders of the endocrine system

Learning outcomes

On completion of this section the reader will be able to:

- Describe the potential impact of hypopituitarism on the endocrine system.
- Describe the symptoms of disorders of the thyroid gland.
- Explain the need for close monitoring and observation of the patient suffering from an adrenal crisis.
- Discuss the role of the healthcare worker in the management of diabetes.

General considerations for caring for patients with an endocrine condition

Regardless of the particular endocrine condition, all patients share a need for psychological support and information, as will their relatives (Department of Health, 2006). Patients will require information on the particular disorders that they are suffering from and the signs and symptoms that they can expect the condition to manifest. Providing the patient with a clear understanding will:

- Reduce anxiety as to what the future may hold.
- Allow the patient to attribute signs and symptoms to their condition rather than enduring them.
- Give the patient control of their health and illness.

- Enable the patient to monitor their own disease and report deviations that may be attributed to a worsening condition or poor control.
- Encourage compliance with treatment regimens.

The pituitary gland

Hypopituitarism

Hypopituitarism is the inability of the pituitary gland to produce enough hormones for normal bodily functioning (Schneider *et al.*, 2007). It can be caused by disorders of the pituitary gland itself or the reduction of hypothalamic-releasing hormones due to a disorder of the hypothalamus, thus reducing the stimuli for pituitary gland activity (Figure 13.9).

The most common cause of hypopituitarism is a tumour of either the pituitary gland or the hypothalamus, or a tumour in the same region that is putting pressure on the pituitary gland (Schneider *et al.*, 2007). Other causes include genetic causes and, increasingly, the role of trauma to the brain has been recognised (e.g. stroke, trauma or radiation therapy). If a tumour is identified and surgically removed, then normal pituitary functioning may return; however, if destruction

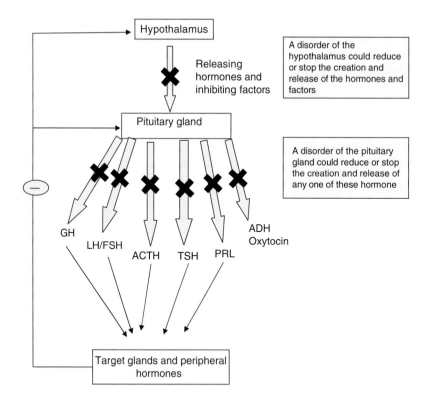

Figure 13.9   Causes of hypopituitarism and its effects on hormone release. GH, growth hormone; LH, luteinising hormone; FSH, follicle-stimulating hormone; ACTH, adrenocorticotropic hormone; TSH, thyroid-stimulating hormone; PRL, prolactin; ADH, antidiuretic hormone.

of pituitary gland tissue has occurred, or the cause is not reversible, the condition is chronic and lifelong.

The signs and symptoms of hypopituitarism are related to the pituitary hormones that are deficient and their effect on target organs and tissues. In patients who have hypopituitarism caused by a tumour, there may be additional signs and symptoms caused by the tumour pressing on other structures in the same area of the brain, e.g. visual disturbances and headaches.

The treatment for the symptoms of hypopituitarism is to replace the hormones that are not being produced. This can either be a direct replacement of pituitary hormones, such as growth hormone, or replacement of the hormones normally produced by a target organ, e.g. thyroxine replacement therapy if TSH production is reduced. The signs and symptoms that patients may exhibit due to a reduction in the relevant target organ activity are dealt with in the associated sections of this chapter.

Diabetes insipidus

Diabetes insipidus is a condition where ADH production and release is reduced (e.g. due to head injury), leading to excessive urine output. A conscious patient can compensate for this increased output by drinking more to replace the fluids passed out as urine. An unconscious patient who may be at risk of diabetes insipidus, e.g. following head injury, requires close monitoring of their urine output. In the event of a reduction in ADH production, the patient will pass large amounts of urine and rapidly dehydrate. The patient should be catheterised and the urine output monitored and recorded at regular intervals. In the event of increased urine output, an unconscious patient cannot replace the excess fluid and will require intravenous fluids, close monitoring of fluid balance and observation for the signs of dehydration.

The thyroid gland

Disorders of the thyroid gland are the most common endocrine disorder encountered in the community setting. These disorders can be classified as either hypersecretion of thyroid hormones (excessive thyroid gland activity – hyperthyroidism) or hyposecretion of thyroid hormones (reduced thyroid gland activity – hypothyroidism). Thyroid disorders can be divided into two categories:

- Primary – due to a disorder of the thyroid gland itself.
- Secondary – alterations in thyroid function due to an increase or decrease in the production of either TRH from the hypothalamus or TSH from the pituitary gland.

The diagnosis of a disorder of the thyroid gland is often delayed as the signs and symptoms are vague and diverse, and in the elderly many signs and symptoms may be attributed to age. The introduction of simple laboratory tests for blood levels of the thyroid hormones has now made the diagnosis much easier, but delays in diagnosis are still common. The most useful tests for thyroid disease are the analysis of blood levels of TSH and free T_4. The expected findings of these tests in clinical thyroid disease are detailed in Table 13.2.

Table 13.2 Common laboratory test findings in the diagnosis of thyroid disease.

	Thyroid stimulating hormone	Free T_4
Hyperthyroidism	Reduced	Normal or elevated
Hypothyroidism	Elevated	Normal or reduced

Case study

Sarah Thompson is an 18-year-old woman who has had a prolonged history of struggling though school. During her time at school she reports she was constantly tired, depressed and "couldn't be bothered". She was constantly in trouble for not paying attention and whenever she had to undertake class work she found it difficult to concentrate. By the age of 17 years she had been to the doctors many times. Nothing wrong was found but she was questioned about her eating habits as she had been gaining weight. Sarah noted that she was constantly cold and even in summer wore a coat to school. Recently her GP had taken a blood test and prescribed her tablets to take (levothyroxine) and since then she has been feeling much better. She says that the GP has asked her to go back for blood tests every 2 months.

Take some time to reflect on this case and then consider the following.

1. What are the likely results of Sarah's blood test (thyroid function test) and why are they like this?
2. What is the most likely cause of Sarah's hypothyroidism?
3. Why does the GP wish Sarah to have such regular blood tests?
4. What advice would you give Sarah about her medication?
5. Sarah is worried that there will be long-term consequences to her health from her condition, including dying prematurely. What would you tell Sarah in answer to her concerns?

Hyperthyroidism

Excessive production of thyroid hormone is commonly due to Graves' disease, an autoimmune disorder where autoimmune antibodies mimic the effect of pituitary TSH, thus stimulating the excessive release of thyroid hormone (Medeiros-Neto *et al.*, 2011). Other causes include thyroid cancer, thyroid nodules (usually non-cancerous), viral thyroiditis, postpartum thyroiditis and iodine-containing drugs (such as amiodarone) (Medeiros-Neto *et al.*, 2011).

The signs and symptoms of hyperthyroidism are related to the increased levels of thyroid hormone:

- nervousness, restlessness, fatigue, insomnia
- tachycardia, palpitations (atrial fibrillation is common in the elderly)
- shortness of breath
- weight loss despite an increased appetite, frequency of passing stools, nausea, vomiting
- muscle weakness, tremors
- warm, moist flushed skin
- fine hair
- staring gaze, exophthalmia
- goitre
- heat intolerance.

The long-term effects of hyperthyroidism can include cardiovascular disease and osteoporosis (Boelaert and Franklyn, 2005). In pregnancy, hyperthyroidism has been linked with higher rates of miscarriage, premature labour, eclampsia and low birth weight of the baby (Girling and Martineau, 2010).

Treatments for hyperthyroidism include:

- Surgery to remove part or all of the thyroid gland (rarely used except for surgical removal of thyroid tumours).
- Radioactive iodine – this treatment relies on the fact that the most active cells in the thyroid gland will take up the most iodine and thus be destroyed. Radioactive iodine is contraindicated in pregnancy.
- Antithyroid drugs (ATDs) – these reduce thyroid hormone production but do not damage the gland. However, in common with all drugs, ATDs have associated side effects and are poorly tolerated in the long-term (Hegedus, 2009).
- Symptomatic relief of tachycardia, palpitations, tremors and nervousness can be achieved with beta-blockers such as atenolol.

Beyond treatment of the overactive thyroid gland, the management of hyperthyroidism also requires the alleviation of signs and symptoms, the provision of education and support, and monitoring of the patient for any deterioration of the condition.

- Anxiety management is essential and the use of beta-blockers should not be ignored. Psychological support and a calm environment are required to prevent exacerbation of nervousness.
- Provision of a well-ventilated cool environment and an electric fan will help the patient to remain comfortable.
- Encouraging regular fluid intake in patients who are perspiring excessively.
- The patient will be fatigued but will find it difficult to rest. The provision of a comfortable environment may aid relaxation and sleep.
- The healthcare worker should be watchful for the potential onset of a thyroid storm (Box 13.1), especially in the newly diagnosed or patients awaiting definitive treatment. Regular monitoring of vital signs and patterns of patient activity/mental state should be carried out.

Box 13.1   Endocrine emergency: thyroid storm.

Thyroid storm is most common in patients with undiagnosed or poorly managed hyperthyroidism; it is due to the effect of high blood levels of thyroid hormone in association with increased sympathetic nervous system activity. There are several known causes of thyroid storm, including emotional or physical trauma and stress (Noble, 2006).

The patient exhibiting thyroid storm will be hyperthermic (temperature over 40 °C), tachycardic (commonly atrial fibrillation is found on ECG monitoring), agitated and confused, and may be vomiting or have diarrhoea.

Patients in thyroid storm require close observation and monitoring in a critical care area. The temperature should be reduced by active cooling; intravenous fluids will be required as the patient will rapidly dehydrate, and the tachycardia may require control with beta-blocking drugs (Gardner, 2007). Control of thyroid function and the reduction of circulating thyroid hormone are also normally required.

379

Hypothyroidism

The causes of hypothyroidism are diverse and include treatment for hyperthyroidism (especially radioactive iodine therapy), radiation therapy of the neck and drugs, such as amiodarone and lithium (Krishnan and Randhir, 2011). However, the most common cause of hypothyroidism is Hashimoto's thyroiditis (an autoimmune disorder).

As with hyperthyroidism, the signs and symptoms of hypothyroidism are varied and it affects virtually every bodily system:

- confusion, lethargy, memory loss, depression
- bradycardia, enlarged heart (cardiomegaly), pericardial effusions
- constipation, weight gain
- muscle cramps, myalgia (generalised muscle aches), stiffness
- dry cool skin
- brittle nails
- coarse hair, hair loss
- oedema of hands and eyelids
- cold intolerance
- vacant expression

However, the development of the symptoms of hypothyroidism is often slow due to the fact that the thyroid gland stores a large amount of thyroid hormone and this is released despite the inability of the gland to produce more.

In pregnancy, hypothyroidism has been linked to recurrent miscarriages and preterm labour; it is also suspected that untreated maternal hypothyroidism has an effect on the development of the fetus, including the pituitary gland, and this is linked to reduced IQ in the child (Rivkees and Mandel, 2011).

The treatment of hypothyroidism is lifelong thyroxine replacement therapy (Okosieme *et al.*, 2011). In the first months of commencing thyroxine therapy, patients will require regular blood tests to ensure that a suitable blood level is achieved and the dose may need to be altered several times during this period (Okosieme *et al.*, 2011). Once a suitable dose has been found, patients will require yearly blood tests to ensure that their needs have not changed; over-replacement of thyroid hormone is one of the leading causes of hyperthyroidism, but can be avoided and is easily rectified. Monitoring of concordance with replacement therapy and the use of strategies to encourage and maintain concordance are essential as many patients are reluctant to take long-term thyroxine therapy (Crilly, 2004). Patients should be counselled as to the possible side effects of thyroid replacement therapy, including temporary hair loss. Patients should be given information regarding what to do in the event of prolonged gastrointestinal disturbance that prevents taking oral medications. Acute illness or trauma may precipitate myxoedemic coma (Box 13.2) and patients must be made aware of the need to seek medical help.

Caution must be exercised in commencing thyroxine therapy in patients with known ischaemic heart disease; these patients are usually commenced on a lower dose and this is then slowly increased, as giving the patient the full replacement dose may worsen the symptoms of angina or even precipitate a myocardial infarction (Boelaert and Franklyn, 2005).

Elderly patients are also usually commenced on a lower dose and their replacement requirements may be lower than those of a younger patient (Feldt-Rasmussen, 2007). Elderly patients in the community may also require regular health checks to ensure concordance with replacement therapy and monitoring of their symptoms (especially as relatives or carers may attribute symptoms to old age rather than thyroid disease).

Box 13.2   Endocrine emergency: myxoedemic coma.

Myxoedemic coma is the end stage of untreated hypothyroidism (Gardner, 2007). This may be due to the previously unrecognised hypothyroidism or the patient stopping replacement therapy; often the crisis is brought on by an underlying illness or trauma. If untreated, it will eventually result in the death of the patient.

The patient in myxoedemic coma will be hypothermic, bradycardic and have a slow, shallow respiratory rate. Blood tests will usually identify low blood levels of sodium and glucose as well as low blood levels of thyroid hormone.

Patients suffering from myxoedemic coma require admission to an intensive care unit for close monitoring, intubation and ventilation, and intravenous replacement of thyroxine, and will require fluid restriction to avoid further diluting the sodium levels in the blood.

The parathyroid glands

Hypoparathyroidism

Prior to the discovery of the parathyroid glands, patients undergoing surgery for removal of the thyroid gland often suffered from hypoparathyroidism as the parathyroid glands were removed along with the thyroid. The patient would subsequently suffer from parasthaesia, tetany and seizures due to the reduced availability of calcium. With the discovery of the parathyroid glands and the reduction of surgery for thyroid disorders, this outcome is now rare. Hypoparathyroidism due to the destruction of the parathyroid gland is now largely due to autoimmune syndromes. These patients require calcium and vitamin D replacement therapy to ensure the availability of calcium for normal muscle functioning.

Hyperparathyroidism

Hyperparathyroidism (excessive production of parathyroid hormone) is most commonly due to an adenoma (a benign tumour) and is more common in women (Fraser, 2009). These patients have raised blood levels of calcium, calcium in the urine and a decreased bone mass; they may also exhibit subtle signs of fatigue and muscle weakness. The current treatment for hyperparathyroidism is the surgical removal of the overactive glands, but many patients remain asymptomatic as the condition progresses slowly (if at all) and monitoring of parathyroid function is all that is required (Fraser, 2009).

The adrenal glands

Cushing's disease

Excessive release of the corticosteroids is rare and normally due to a pituitary tumour increasing the release of ACTH; the most common cause of raised blood levels of the glucocorticoids is their therapeutic use in inflammatory conditions (such as asthma and arthritis). Patients with high levels of glucocorticoids in the blood show the signs and symptoms of Cushing's disease (Nieman *et al.*,

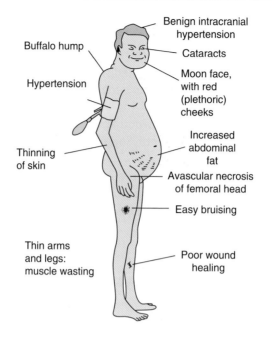

Figure 13.10   Cushing's disease (http://www.bmb.leeds.ac.uk/teaching/icu3/lecture/24/index. htm).

2008). These patients are commonly obese, with the main distribution of fat being around the face (moon facies), neck (buffalo hump), trunk and abdomen (Figure 13.10). Relative to the central obesity, the patient's arms and legs are often thin and spindly and the patient may report muscle weakness. The patient will often have thin, easily bruised skin and may report slow wound healing or frequent fungal infections; the majority of female patients will report increased hair growth on the face. Osteoporosis is common and back pain is the most common presenting symptom (Nieman *et al.*, 2008). The majority of patients with Cushing's disease will exhibit some signs of psychological disturbance, e.g. euphoria, mood swings, irritability, poor memory and difficulty in concentrating; disturbance of sleep patterns is common. The long-term effects of persistently high levels of glucocorticoids in the blood include hypertension, cardiovascular disease, susceptibility to infection and the development of steroid-induced diabetes.

   The treatment of Cushing's disease is to remove or destroy the tumour (Sharma and Nieman, 2011) or reduction of the doses of glucocorticoid treatment where possible.

Adrenal insufficiency

Adrenal insufficiency (the reduced production and release of corticosteroids from the adrenal glands) is divided into two types:

●   Primary adrenal insufficiency (Addison's disease) due to a disorder of the adrenal glands (Figure 13.11a). The leading cause of Addison's disease in the industrialized world is autoimmune adrenalitis (Husebye and Lovas, 2009); other causes include tuberculosis, and fungal

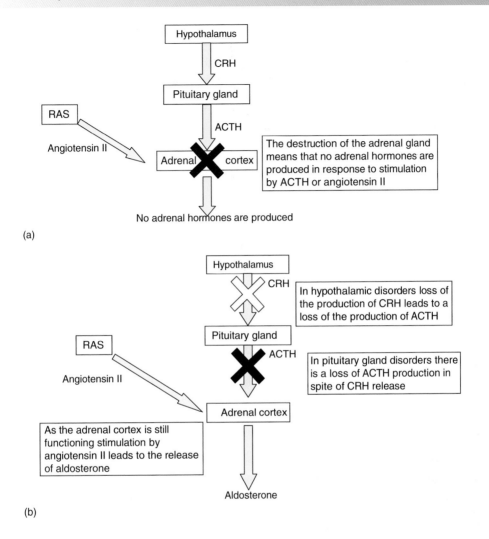

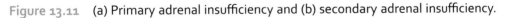

Figure 13.11   (a) Primary adrenal insufficiency and (b) secondary adrenal insufficiency.

infection in immunosuppressed patients (such as HIV/AIDS or therapeutic suppression of the immune system).

- Secondary adrenal insufficiency (Figure 13.11b) is more common and is due to the sudden cessation of glucocorticoid therapy (Hahner and Allolio, 2009); however, tumours of the hypothalamic–pituitary region and their treatment are also a cause of secondary adrenal insufficiency.

The signs and symptoms of primary adrenal insufficiency are related to the lack of both glucocorticoid hormones and mineralocorticoid hormones (in secondary adrenal insufficiency the release of mineralocorticoid hormones is preserved as it is under the control of the renin–angiotensin system and thus symptoms related to a lack of aldosterone are not present). In the event of destruction of the adrenal glands (primary adrenal insufficiency), the loss of the adrenal medulla is not associated with clinically important symptoms as the role of the medullary hormones (epinephrine and norepinephrine) is to magnify the effect of sympathetic nervous system activity, which remains intact.

The signs and symptoms of adrenal insufficiency are vague and thus the majority of patients will exhibit signs and symptoms for up to a year before diagnosis (Husebye and Lovas, 2009):

- fatigue, lack of stamina, loss of energy
- reduced muscle strength
- increased irritability
- nausea
- weight loss
- muscle and joint pain
- abdominal pain
- low blood pressure
- women may report a reduction in or loss of libido due to the lack of adrenal sex hormones.

In addition in primary adrenal insufficiency only:

- Symptoms related to the loss of aldosterone production, including dehydration, hypovolaemia (with possible postural hypotension), low blood levels of sodium and raised blood levels of potassium.
- Hyperpigmentation of the skin due to the stimulation of skin receptors by increased levels of ACTH. This can show as a darkening of the creases of the skin (e.g. in the palms, knuckles and oral mucosa), vitiligo (pale patches of skin) or an overall darkening of the skin (similar to a sun tan).

However, a proportion of patients will present as an acute adrenal crisis, which is often precipitated by trauma or infection (Box 13.3).

Box 13.3   Endocrine emergency: adrenal crisis.

Adrenal (or addisonian) crisis is an acute life-threatening event often precipitated by an acute traumatic event, fever or other serious illness. Patients present with severe hypotension resistant to standard therapies such as inotropes, hypovolaemic shock, acute abdominal pain, vomiting, fever, hypoglycaemia, hyponatraemia and hyperkalaemia (Blanshard, 2011).

Treatment of an adrenal crisis requires close monitoring of a patient, including blood pressure monitoring, cardiac monitoring for potential arrhythmias caused by the high potassium levels in the blood, intravenous hydrocortisone to replace the depleted levels of corticosteroids and intravenous fluids to replace volume. Normal saline is the usual fluid used as it will also replenish the reduced blood levels of sodium. Intravenous glucose may be required and, depending on the levels of potassium in the blood, therapies to reduce these levels may be commenced (e.g. diuretics to promote the excretion of potassium from the kidneys).

Patients who have been taking high-dose glucocorticoid therapy (such as prednisolone) are at risk of developing temporary adrenal gland atrophy (Hahner and Allolio, 2009); if the therapy is stopped suddenly they can present with the signs and symptoms of adrenal insufficiency and even an acute adrenal crisis. Therefore, all patients taking glucocorticoid therapy should never stop their medication suddenly and should carry a 'steroid treatment card' at all times. A reducing dose of glucocorticoids is required to allow for the recovery of the adrenal glands to their full function (British Medical Association/Royal Pharmaceutical Society of Great Britain, 2011).

The treatment of adrenal insufficiency is the replacement of glucocorticoid hormones with oral hydrocortisone in two to three daily doses. In primary adrenal insufficiency, replacement of the mineralocorticoid hormones is also required; this is achieved by the administration of oral fludro-cortisone once a day. However, the quality of life of patients with adrenal insufficiency is often reduced, even with optimum replacement therapy, and patients report fatigue, a lack of energy, depression and anxiety (Erichsen *et al.*, 2009).

Patients with permanent adrenal insufficiency (primary or secondary) will require education on the management of their replacement therapy (Hahner *et al.*, 2009). Adrenal crises are often the result of a patient not increasing their replacement therapy in response to physical stressors (such as strenuous exercise, trauma, infection or fever). Patients admitted to hospital for a surgical procedure will require either intravenous or intramuscular hydrocortisone prior to surgery to prevent the onset of a crisis. In the event of persistent diarrhoea and vomiting that prevent the patient from taking their normal oral medications, hydrocortisone may be administered by intra-muscular injection, and increasingly patients are doing this themselves or with the help of their relatives. Patients are often supplied with an emergency injection kit (hydrocortisone for intra-muscular injection, needles and syringes) for the immediate management of an acute traumatic event or illness, and both the patient and their relatives should be trained in its use and their training and knowledge regularly refreshed (Hahner *et al.*, 2009). It is strongly recommended that all patients with adrenal insufficiency wear a medical alert talisman (typically a bracelet or necklace).

The pancreas

Hypersecretion of insulin is very rare, and the cause of increased blood levels of insulin in the vast majority of patients is over-administration of insulin in the management of diabetes mellitus (Marieb and Hoehn, 2010).

Diabetes mellitus (diabetes) is a group of disorders characterised by raised blood levels of glucose (World Health Organization, 2006). There are two main types of diabetes – type 1 and type 2 diabetes; however, the signs and symptoms of the two types are similar:

- high blood glucose levels
- glucose in the urine
- ketones in the urine
- frequency in passing urine (including waking at night)
- thirst
- increased appetite (usually type 1 only)
- weight loss (usually type 1 only)
- fatigue
- abdominal pain.

Type 2 diabetes can often be asymptomatic and only diagnosed on opportunistic screening or as a chance finding whilst the patient is being investigated or treated for other medical problems.

The signs and symptoms of diabetes are related to the high levels of glucose in the blood and the inability of the cells to utilise glucose due to a lack of insulin production or resistance to the effect of insulin in the body. Glucose is excreted by the renal tubules into the urine and this leads to increased urine production due to the osmotic effect of the glucose (water is drawn into and retained in the urine by the high levels of glucose). Thus, body levels of water are depleted and there is subsequent development of chronic thirst. The inability of the cells to use glucose as a primary fuel source leads to the metabolism of fats and amino acids and thus weight loss. Furthermore, the utilisation of fats and amino acids as fuel in the cells leads to the production of ketones (which are strong acids); these are excreted in the urine and as they are negatively charged they carry sodium and potassium ions with them, leading to electrolyte imbalance, a sign of which is abdominal pain (Marieb and Hoehn, 2010). Eventually, these processes can lead to an acute life-threatening hyperglycaemic event (Box 13.4).

Case study

David Arthur is a 63-year-old factory worker who lives with his wife and two teenage children. He has been admitted to hospital for a routine hernia operation. Whilst you are chatting to Mr Arthur, he states that he has been passing urine frequently, a fact that he puts down to his need to drink regularly. He also notes that he constantly feels tired. Further questioning reveals that he eats a high fat, high sugar diet and drinks 25–30 units of alcohol per week. He has been a smoker since the age of 15 and continues to smoke 20 cigarettes per day. He does no regular exercise. Mr Arthur states that he has no past medical history but that his father had heart disease and raised blood cholesterol levels.

Take some time to reflect on this case and then consider the following.

1. What risk factors does Mr Arthur have for developing diabetes mellitus?
2. What tests could be carried out to confirm your suspicion that Mr Arthur is suffering from diabetes mellitus?
3. What lifestyle advice would you give Mr Arthur?
4. What possible psychological effects could a diagnosis of diabetes mellitus have on Mr Arthur?
5. What is the potential significance of the father's past medical history if Mr Arthur is in fact suffering from diabetes mellitus?

Type 1 diabetes

Type 1 diabetes develops most commonly in childhood or early adulthood and comprises about 15% of the total incidence of diabetes in the UK; however, the rate of type 1 diabetes is increasing, particularly in children younger than 5 years of age (Royal College of Paediatrics and Child Health, 2009). Type 1 diabetes is normally caused by autoimmune destruction of the beta cells

Box 13.4   Endocrine emergency: hyperglycaemia.

Patients with either type 1 or type 2 diabetes are at risk of developing life-threatening hyper-glycaemia (Kearney and Dang, 2007).

Hyperosmolar hyperglycaemic state (HHS) is commonly associated with older patients with type 2 diabetes. The onset is usually over days to weeks and it may be the first indication that a patient is suffering from type 2 diabetes. HHS is characterised by a very high blood glucose (>33.3 mmol/L and often over 50 mmol/L), dehydration and confusion, but the absence of sig-nificant levels of ketones and therefore no acidaemia (reduced blood pH). Dehydration occurs due to excessive urine output, and low blood levels of sodium and potassium are common.

Diabetic ketoacidosis (DKA) is associated with type 1 diabetes and has a rapid onset (normally less than 24 hours). Patients present with hyperglycaemia (but usually not greater than 40 mmol/L due to the rapid onset of DKA), ketosis (ketones in the blood), acidaemia, dehydra-tion and reduced blood levels of sodium and potassium. The characteristic 'pear drop' or 'acetone' smell to the breath of a patient with DKA is produced by the excess of ketones in the blood.

The management of both HHS and DKA is similar and is aimed at replacing the lost fluid, reducing the blood glucose and correcting electrolyte imbalances. Large amounts of intrave-nous fluids are given (typically 1–1.5 L in the first hour), and potassium is usually added to subsequent fluids after the initial rapid fluid resuscitation. Low-dose intravenous insulin is com-menced to slowly reduce the blood glucose and the patient is closely monitored, including regular assessment of vital signs, blood glucose and electrolytes (Kearney and Dang, 2007).

387

of the pancreas and is therefore associated with a severe reduction in, or complete loss of, insulin production (Eizirik *et al.*, 2009).

The treatment of type 1 diabetes is the replacement of insulin, normally by subcutaneous injec-tion, although alternative methods of administration (including inhaled insulin, nasal administra-tion of insulin and oral insulin) are currently under investigation (Renard, 2009). Care must be taken to ensure that the insulin administered is balanced by a sufficient intake of food (particularly carbohydrates as sugars are quickly used in the body) to avoid low blood sugar levels (hypogly-caemia). Profound hypoglycaemia leads to the patient becoming mentally agitated, possibly aggressive; often the patient will be sweating profusely and will look pale. If the dose of insulin administered is not matched by sufficient intake of food, the patient will eventually become comatose and may die. Conscious patients may be given a sugary snack or drink and some form of carbohydrates; the patient will then require monitoring of their blood glucose until the crisis has passed. Unconscious patients require immediate medical assistance and the administration of an intramuscular injection of glucagon and potentially intravenous glucose (Kearney and Dang, 2007).

Type 2 diabetes

This is the most common form of diabetes and is traditionally thought to be a disease of people over the age of 40 years. Overall the number of patients developing type 2 diabetes is increasing and this increase is occurring across all age ranges, including in adolescents and young adults

(Royal College of Paediatrics and Child Health, 2009). The reasons for this increase are probably related to lifestyle factors, including the increase in the rates of obesity, overeating (particularly sugary foods) and a lack of exercise (Hossain *et al.*, 2007).

Type 2 diabetes is normally characterised by the development of resistance to the effects of insulin in the tissues, and a reduction in the ability of the beta cells to increase the production of insulin in response to this increased insulin resistance in the body. The resulting high blood levels of glucose lead to damage of the beta cells, thus further reducing the production of insulin. The treatment of type 2 diabetes varies depending on the severity of the condition. In some patients, weight reduction, increased exercise and reduced food intake can resolve the raised blood sugar levels. However, once the beta cell damage has occurred, the need for medications is increased. Current drug therapies for type 2 diabetes (oral hypoglycaemics) target several aspects of the disease, including reducing glucose production by the liver, enhancing insulin output from the pancreas or increasing the sensitivity of the muscle, fat and liver cells to the effects of insulin and thus reducing insulin resistance (Nathan *et al.*, 2006). Increasingly, a role is being seen for the use of insulin in type 2 diabetes (Farmer *et al.*, 2006).

Patients with both type 1 and type 2 diabetes will have similar educational needs in terms of their personal control of the diabetes. The aim of disease management is to alleviate the symptoms of diabetes and optimise the control of blood glucose levels, thus preventing long-term complications (Nair, 2007). Healthcare interventions include:

- Advice on appropriate diet – current advice emphasises the need for a healthy, balanced, diet. This includes reducing the amount of sugar and fat that is eaten, increasing the intake of fruit and vegetables, and substituting wholemeal bread and pastas for refined products such as white bread (Diabetes UK, 2011).
- Encouraging regular physical activity. However, strenuous exercise can reduce blood glucose levels and exercise regimens should be agreed with appropriate healthcare professionals.
- Advice and support for weight loss if required. Weight loss in overweight patients improves the control of diabetes as inactivity and obesity are strongly linked to insulin resistance (Hossain *et al.*, 2007).
- Advice and support on stopping smoking. Patients with diabetes have an increased risk of vascular diseases (including heart disease and stroke), and smoking further increases this risk.
- Education on how to monitor blood glucose levels using capillary blood glucose monitoring or urinalysis (as appropriate).
- The use and administration of medications, such as insulin injection techniques and adjusting insulin doses.

Poor control of diabetes often leads to hyperglycaemia and is associated with a range of long-term complications, including blindness or reduced vision, peripheral neuropathy, renal failure, cardiovascular disease, peripheral artery disease and foot ulcers (Box 13.5).

Box 13.5   Focus on diabetic foot ulcers.

Excluding accidents, diabetes is the leading cause of lower limb amputations in the UK (Vamos *et al.*, 2009); patients with diabetes have approximately a 15% lifetime risk of developing a foot ulcer (Lebrun *et al.* 2010).

The causes of diabetic foot ulcers are neuropathic, ischaemic or a mixture of both:

- Neuropathic – the reduced sensation in the feet of patients with peripheral neuropathy means that they are often unaware of the mechanical stresses being placed on their feet due to poorly fitting footwear or trauma (such as standing on a sharp object).
- Ischaemic – the reduced peripheral circulation in patients with long-term complications leads to easily damaged skin with a reduced ability to heal in response to damage.

Not all diabetic foot ulcers become infected, but when they do, the patient's limb and sometimes life can be in danger as the wound does not heal rapidly and infection can spread easily due to the reduction in the delivery of white blood cells to the peripheral tissues.

The treatment of diabetic foot ulcers may require surgical debridement of the wound to remove dead tissue which is a host for bacteria; appropriate wound dressings and antibiotics may also be necessary (Edwards and Stapley, 2010). Relief of pressure on the ulcer is critical to the success of treatment and referral to a podiatrist will be required for continued foot care and assessment for pressure-relieving shoes (Lavery *et al.*, 2010).

Conclusion

This chapter has introduced the physiology of both normal and disordered endocrine functioning and the treatment of the related disorders. The endocrine system has a wide and varied role in the maintenance of normal bodily functioning. Disorders of any of the endocrine organs can produce a variety of signs and symptoms and may even lead to a life-threatening crisis. The healthcare professional has a crucial role in the detection of endocrine conditions, the monitoring of disease progression and treatment effects, and the prevention and treatment of endocrine emergencies. Most patients with an endocrine disorder will take responsibility for the management of their own condition and it is essential that they are given appropriate advice and support. In order to carry out these roles, the healthcare professional must have a good understanding of the physiology and treatment of the endocrine disorders.

Test your knowledge

- What is the most common endocrine disorder in the community care setting?
- Why are patients with ischaemic heart disease started on lower doses of thyroxine?
- What is the difference between primary and secondary adrenal insufficiency?
- What is the function of glucagon in the regulation of blood glucose?
- Why should patients never suddenly stop taking steroid therapy?
- What are the signs and symptoms of hypoglycaemia?

Activities

Here are some activities and exercises to help test your learning. For the answers to these exercises, as well as further self-testing activities, visit our website at www.wiley.com/go/fundamentalsofappliedpathophysiology

Fill in the blanks

The pituitary gland is a pure _____ gland; it is located in the _____ below the _____ to which it is connected by the _____. The pituitary gland is split into two anatomical sections, the _____ and _____ lobes. The posterior lobe stores and releases _____ and _____ hormone (vasopressin) which are two hormones that are produced by the hypothalamus. The production and release of hormones from the anterior pituitary is mostly controlled by _____ and _____ hormones from the hypothalamus. The major cause of hypopituitarism is a _____ of the hypothalamus or _____ gland or nearby structures. The effects of hypopituitarism can be many and varied depending on the hormones that are affected. For instance, _____ is a condition where ADH production and release is _____ and this leads to excessive _____ output.

Choose from:
Urine; Posterior; Inhibiting; Reduced; Oxytocin; Brain; Infundibulum; Endocrine; Tumour; Diabetes insipidus; Releasing; Anterior; Hypothalamus; Pituitary; Antidiuretic

Label the diagram

From the list of words supplied, label the diagram.

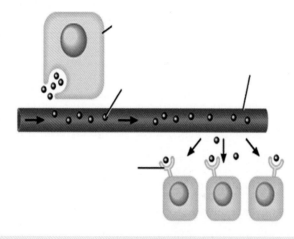

Endocrine cell; Circulating hormone; Distant target cells; Blood capillary; Receptors

Word search

A	G	P	R	N	S	T	H	Y	R	O	I	D	I	T	I	S	U	G	T
L	Z	L	I	E	X	H	A	Y	H	Y	U	I	S	Y	I	I	O	D	I
G	E	N	A	E	E	S	O	H	N	H	I	U	L	S	N	S	E	I	E
G	C	S	T	N	L	D	S	E	O	T	M	O	Y	I	L	Y	N	A	H
L	S	R	A	N	D	I	G	W	Y	A	I	H	L	E	L	H	H	B	Y
U	O	G	G	O	N	O	O	H	L	P	P	S	H	N	G	P	S	E	P
C	R	S	W	S	C	C	W	A	N	O	Y	T	B	U	R	O	P	T	O
O	S	S	U	Y	O	I	H	N	P	R	O	I	E	M	O	P	D	E	G
G	G	L	L	I	S	T	N	Y	R	U	E	M	T	M	T	Y	I	S	L
E	I	G	U	Z	O	R	H	E	L	E	P	U	A	I	P	H	A	M	Y
N	T	T	O	P	H	O	G	L	G	N	G	L	C	O	E	O	E	E	C
O	M	L	Y	D	N	C	N	L	L	I	S	U	E	T	C	R	O	L	A
L	L	H	K	E	T	O	N	E	S	E	R	S	L	U	E	U	T	L	E
Y	T	S	D	I	O	C	I	T	R	O	C	O	L	A	R	E	N	I	M
S	O	A	S	G	L	U	C	A	G	O	N	T	L	G	T	N	N	T	I
I	N	O	I	T	A	L	U	G	E	R	P	U	E	A	R	I	G	U	A
S	I	S	E	N	E	G	O	E	N	O	C	U	L	G	C	Y	O	S	S
P	Y	N	O	G	U	E	E	R	N	I	O	D	H	O	R	M	O	N	E
R	M	Z	O	I	A	O	N	K	O	M	E	D	U	L	L	A	B	U	N
C	O	T	C	U	I	C	O	Y	H	S	M	E	S	A	A	Y	T	L	R

391

Adenohypophysis	Glucogenolysis	Neurohypophysis
Autoimmune	Gluconeogenesis	Neuropathy
Betacell	Glycogen	Organ
Calorigenic	Hormone	Receptor
Cortex	Hypoglycaemia	Stimulus
Diabetesmellitus	Hypothalamus	Targetcell
Downregulation	Insulin	Thyroiditis
Gland	Ketones	Upregulation
Glucagon	Medulla	Zona
Glucocorticoids	Mineralocorticoids	

Further resources

Addison's Disease Self-Help Group

www.addisons.org.uk
The website of the only UK-based group specifically for those suffering from Addison's disease (adrenal insufficiency) is not only a good resource for patients diagnosed with Addison's disease, but also contains much information that is useful to the healthcare professional.

Diabetes UK

www.diabetes.org.uk
The website of the largest organization in the UK for people with diabetes has a large amount of information, including latest news regarding diabetes and guidance ranging from the clinical to the more practical (e.g. recipes for those with diabetes). The two 'Guides to diabetes' are a useful starting point for anyone wanting to know more about this condition.

EndocrineSurgeon.co.uk

www.endocrinesurgeon.co.uk
The personal website of surgical endocrinologist Mr John Lynn is hugely informative, with detailed sections on endocrine conditions, diagnostic tests and surgical procedures. It is interesting to note that this website is often highly recommended by other websites.

Pituitary Foundation

www.pituitary.org.uk
This website contains many useful resources. There is a comprehensive list of web links, reviews of pituitary-related disorders and proceedings from conferences (which are often hard to find).

The Endocrine Society

www.endo-society.org
This is the website of the world's largest society dedicated to the practice of endocrinology. It is worth viewing regularly as the news section is kept updated and there is a useful clinical guidelines section, including guidelines on some lesser known conditions such as Cushing's syndrome.

Glossary of terms

Acidaemia:	a state of relative acidity of the blood.
Adenoma:	a tumour of glandular tissue (usually benign).
Adenosine triphosphate (ATP):	a compound of an adenosine molecule with three attached phosphoric acid molecules. Essential for the production of cellular energy.

Adrenalitis:	inflammatory condition of the adrenal glands.
Amino acid:	the building block of proteins. The type of protein that is produced depends upon the number and types of amino acids that are used to construct it.
Arrhythmia:	a disorder of the normal heart beat.
Asymptomatic:	without symptoms.
Atrophy:	wasting away; a diminution in the site of a cell, tissue or organ.
Autoimmune:	immune response to the body's own tissues.
Benign:	causes no problem. In cancer, it means a growth that is not malignant.
Concordance:	current term for the person's adherence to a prescribed treatment.
Debridement:	removal of damaged tissues and cells.
Diuretic:	a drug that increases urine output.
Eclampsia:	a condition presenting in pregnancy that is characterised by high blood pressure, seizures and even coma.
Electrolyte:	a chemical element compound that includes sodium, potassium, calcium, chloride and bicarbonate.
Endocrine gland:	a ductless gland that secretes hormones into the bloodstream.
Euphoria:	an exaggerated state of well-being; the opposite of dysphoria.
Exocrine gland:	a gland that secretes hormones into ducts that carry the secretions to other sites (e.g. the intestine).
Exophthalmos:	excessive protrusion of the eyeballs.
Free T_4:	thyroxine in the blood that is not bound to proteins.
Gland:	any organ in the body that secretes substances not related to its own internal functioning.
Glycogen:	a carbohydrate (complex sugar) made from glucose. Excess glucose is stored as glycogen mainly in the liver.
Goitre:	pronounced swelling of the neck.
Homeostasis:	maintenance of relatively constant conditions within the body's internal environment despite external environmental changes.

Hormone:	a chemical substance that is released into the blood by the endocrine system, and that has a physiological control over the function of cells or organs other than those that created it.
Hyperglycaemia:	a high blood level of glucose.
Hyperkalaemia:	a high blood level of potassium.
Hypersecretion:	a high rate of secretion.
Hypertension:	raised blood pressure.
Hyperthermic:	high body temperature.
Hypoglycaemia:	a low blood level of glucose.
Hyponatraemia:	a low blood level of sodium.
Hyposecretion:	a low rate of secretion.
Hypotension:	low blood pressure.
Hypothermic:	low body temperature.
Hypovolaemia:	low level of fluid in the circulation.
Inotrope:	a drug used to increase the blood pressure in the critically ill.
Insulin resistance:	a condition where the usual body reaction to insulin is reduced.
Ion:	an atom or group of atoms that carries either a positive or a negative electrical charge.
Ischaemic heart disease:	a condition of the heart related to a lack of oxygen reaching the heart muscle.
Ketosis:	ketones in the blood.
Malignant:	invasive, has a tendency to grow and may spread to other parts of the body.
Neuropathy:	inflammation and degeneration of the nerves.
Opportunistic screening:	testing a person for particular diseases or conditions at a point in time they are accessing healthcare for other reasons.
Oral hypoglycaemic:	a drugs used in the treatment of diabetes that is taken by mouth and reduces the blood sugar level.
Osmosis:	the passive movement of water through a selectively permeable membrane from an area of high concentration of a chemical to an area of low concentration.

Osteoclast:	a type of cell that breaks down bone tissue and thus releases the calcium used to create bones.
Osteoporosis:	a condition characterised by reduced bone density and an increased risk of fractures.
Palpitations:	a feeling of pounding or racing of the heart.
Parasthaesia:	abnormal nerve sensations such as pins-and-needles, tingling or burning.
Peripheral artery disease:	disease of the arteries of the legs.
Podiatrist:	a healthcare professional who specialises in the diagnosis and treatment of disorders of the feet (also known as a chiropodist).
Postural hypotension:	inability of the body to maintain an adequate blood pressure when the person rises from sitting or lying to standing too rapidly. Usually characterised by dizziness or fainting if the person rises too quickly to a standing position.
Tachycardia:	fast heart beat (usually defined as above 100 beats per minute).
Tetany:	prolonged muscular spasms.
Thyroiditis:	an inflammatory condition of the thyroid gland.
Thyroid nodule:	the growth of thyroid tissue or fluid-filled cyst of the thyroid tissue.

References

Blanshard, H. (2011). Endocrine and metabolic disease. In: Allman, K.G. and Wilson, I.H. (eds). *Oxford Handbook of Anaesthesia*, 3rd edn. Oxford: Oxford University Press, pp. 155–190.

Boelaert, K. and Franklyn, J.A. (2005). Starling review: Thyroid hormone in health and disease. *Journal of Endocrinology*. 1(187): 1–15.

British Medical Association/Royal Pharmaceutical Society of Great Britain (2011). *British National Formulary*, 61st edn. London: British Medical Association/Royal Pharmaceutical Society of Great Britain.

Crilly, M. (2004). Correspondence: Thyroxine adherence in primary hypothyroidism. *The Lancet*. 363(9420): 1558.

Department of Health (2006). *Supporting People with Long Term Conditions to Self Care: A Guide to Developing Local Strategies and Good practice*. London: Department of Health.

Diabetes UK (2011). *Evidence-Based Nutrition Guidelines for the Prevention and Management of Diabetes*. London: Diabetes UK.

Edwards, J., Stapley, S. (2010) Debridement of diabetic foot ulcers. *Cochrane Database of Systematic Reviews*. Issue 1. Art. No.: CD003556. Eizirik, D.L., Colli, M.L. and Ortis, F. (2009). The role of inflammation in insulitis and B cell loss in type 1 diabetes. *Nature Reviews Endocrinology*. 5: 219–226.

Erichsen, M.M., Lovas, K., Skinningsrud, B. *et al.* (2009). Clinical, immunological, and genetic features of autoimmune primary adrenal insufficiency: Observations from a Norwegian registry. *Journal of Clinical Endocrinology and Metabolism.* 94(12): 4882–4890.

Farmer, A.J., Lasserson, D.S., Perera, R., Glasziou, P.P. and Holman, R. (2006). Different insulin regimens for type 2 diabetes mellitus (Protocol). *Cochrane Database of Systematic Reviews* Issue 4. Art No.: CD006299.

Feldt-Rasmussen, U. (2007). Treatment of hypothyroidism in elderly patients and in patients with cardiac disease. *Thyroid.* 17(7): 619–624.

Fraser, W.D. (2009) Hyperparathyroidism. *The Lancet.* 374(9684): 145–148.

Gardner, D.G. (2007). Endocrine emergencies. In: Gardner, D.G. and Shoback, D. (eds). *Greenspan's Basic and Clinical Endocrinology*, 8th edn. London: Lange books/McGraw-Hill, pp. 868–893.

Girling, J. and Martineau, M. (2010). Thyroid and other disorders in pregnancy. *Obstetrics, Gynaecology and Reproductive Medicine.* 20(9): 265–271.

Guyton, A.C. and Hall, J. (2010). *Textbook of Medical Physiology*, 12th edn. Philadelphia: Elsevier Saunders.

Hahner, S. and Allolio, B. (2009) Therapeutic management of adrenal insufficiency. *Best Practice and Research. Clinical endocrinology and Metabolism.* 23(2): 167–179.

Hahner, S., Loeffler, M., Bleicken, B. *et al.* (2009). Epidemiology of adrenal crisis in chronic adrenal insufficiency the need for new prevention strategies. *European Journal of Endocrinology.* 162: 597–602.

Hegedus, L. (2009). Treatment of Graves' hyperthyroidism: Evidence based and emergent modalities. *Endocrinology & Metabolism Clinics of North America.* 38(2): 355–371.

Hossain, P., Kawar, B. and El Nahas, M. (2007). Obesity and diabetes in the developing world – A growing challenge. *New England Journal of Medicine.* 356: 213–215.

Husebye, E. and Lovas, K. (2009) Pathogenesis of primary adrenal insufficiency. *Best Practice and Research. Clinical endocrinology and Metabolism.* 23(2): 147–157.

Kearney, T. and Dang, C. (2007). Diabetic and endocrine emergencies. *Postgraduate Medical Journal.* 83(976): 79–86.

Krishnan, P. and Randhir, S. (2011). Clinical perspectives of hypothyroidism. *Journal of Applied Pharmaceutical Science.* 01(05): 64–68.

Lavery, L.A., Hunt, N.A., La Fontaine, J., Baxter, C.L., Ndip, A. and Boulton, A.J.M. (2010) Diabetic foot prevention. A neglected opportunity in high risk patients. *Diabetes Care.* 33(7): 1460–1462.

Lebrun, E., Tomic Canic, M. and Kirsner, R.S. (2010) The role of surgical debridement in healing of diabetic foot ulcers. *Wound Repair and Regeneration.* 18(5): 433–438.

Marieb, E.N. and Hoehn, K. (2010). *Human Anatomy and Physiology*, 8th edn. San Francisco: Pearson Benjamin Cummings.

Medeiros-Neto, G., Romaldini, J.H. and Abalovich, M. (2011). Highlights of the guidelines on the management of hyperthyroidism and other causes of thyrotoxicosis. *Thyroid.* 21(6): 581–584.

Nair, M. (2007). Nursing management of the person with diabetes mellitus. Part 2. *British Journal of Nursing.* 16(4): 232–235.

Nathan, D.M., Buse, J.B., Davidson, M.B. *et al.* (2006). Management of hyperglycaemia in type 2 diabetes: A consensus algorithm for the initiation and adjustment of therapy. *Diabetes Care.* 29(8): 1963–1972.

Nieman, L.K., Biller, B.M.K., Findling, J.W. *et al.* (2008). The diagnosis of Cushing's disease: An Endocrine Society Clinical Practice Guideline. *The Journal of Clinical Endocrinology and Metabolism.* 93(5): 1526–1540.

Noble, K.A. (2006). Thyroid storm. *Journal of PeriAnesthesia Nursing.* 21(2): 119–125.

Okosieme, O.E., Belludi, G., Spittle, K., Kadiyala, R. and Richards, J. (2011). Adequacy of thyroid hormone replacement in a general population. *Quality Journal of Medicine.* 104: 395–401.

Renard, E. (2009). New developments in insulin administration. In: Stenhouwer, C.D.A. and Schaper, N.C. (eds) *Therapeutic Strategies in Diabetes*. Oxford: Clinical Publishing, pp. 39–66.

Rivkees, S.A. and Mandel, S.J. (2011) Thyroid disease in pregnancy. *Hormone Research in Paediatrics.* 76 (Suppl 1): 91–96.

Royal College of Paediatrics and Child Health (2009). *Growing Up with Diabetes: Children and Young People with Diabetes in England*. London: Royal College of Paediatrics and Child Health.

Schneider, H.J., Aimaretti, G., Kreitschmann-Andermahr, I., Stalla, G. and Ghigo, E. (2007). Hypopituitarism. *The Lancet.* 369(9571): 1461–1470.

Sharma, S.T. and Nieman, L.K. (2011) Cushing's syndrome: All variants, detection, and treatment. *Endocrinology & Metabolism Clinics of North America.* 40(2): 379–391.

Tortora, G.J. and Derrickson, B. (2011). *Principles of Anatomy and Physiology. Volume 1. Organisation, Support and Movement, and Control of the Human Body. International Student Version*, 13th edn. Hoboken, NJ: John Wiley and Sons Inc.

Vamos, E.P., Bottle, A., Majeed, A. and Millett, C. (2009). Trends in lower extremity amputations with and without diabetes in England, 1996–2005. *Diabetes Research and Clinical Practice.* 87(2): 275–282.

World Health Organization (2006). *Fact Sheet No 312 Diabetes.* Geneva: World Health Organization.

14

The reproductive systems and associated disorders

Ian Peate

Visiting Professor of Nursing, School of Nursing, Midwifery and Healthcare, Faculty of Health and Human Sciences, University of West London, Brentford, Middlesex, UK; Independent Consultant and Editor-in-Chief British Journal of Nursing

Contents

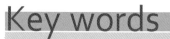

Key words

- Reproduction
- Hormones
- Cancer

Fundamentals of Applied Pathophysiology: An Essential Guide for Nursing and Healthcare Students, Second Edition. Edited by Muralitharan Nair and Ian Peate.

- Genitalia

- Ovulation

- Menstruation

- Self-esteem

- Puberty

- Prostaglandins

- Fertility

- Risk

- Reproductive tracts

Test your prior knowledge

- Describe the menstrual cycle.

- What are the functions of the prostate gland?

- How can issues associated with the reproductive tract impinge on an individual's self-esteem?

- Describe the role of the healthcare professional when caring for a person who has under-gone reproductive tract surgery.

- Outline the role of the healthcare professional in preventing sexually-transmitted infections.

Learning outcomes

On completion of this section the reader will be able to:

- Describe the main functions of the male and female reproductive tracts.

- List the organs of the female and male reproductive tracts.

- Discuss the normal and abnormal pathophysiological changes that can occur in association with the male and female reproductive tracts.

- Outline the care of people who have problems associated with the reproductive tract.

Don't forget to visit to the companion website for this book (www.wiley.com/go/ fundamentalsofappliedpathophysiology) where you can find self-assessment tests to check your progress, as well as lots of activities to practise your learning.

Introduction

Reproduction of the human species is a complex activity that requires a series of integrated ana-tomical and physiological events. The physiological and anatomical aspects of the reproductive tract are predominately associated with procreation; the psychological and social aspects of reproduction are also important, as too is the pleasure that is often provided by the reproductive organs. Ill health in relation to the reproductive tract can result in loss of life, and acute and chronic illness combined with physical and emotional distress.

The way an individual expresses themselves is a key aspect of reproductive health and this is often bound up in attitudes (the person's attitudes as well as those of the healthcare professional). Social norms and cultural upbringing will also impact on an individual's reproductive health; sexu-ality and sexual health are also closely linked to reproductive health.

This chapter provides an outline of the male and female reproductive tracts. A number of reproductive-related conditions and their associated care are discussed.

Reproductive health

Reproductive health (a complex term) should be a right for all men and women, and is a compo-nent of overall health throughout the life cycle regardless of the way the person chooses to express their sexuality; it is also an essential feature of human development. Reproductive health is defined by the United Nations (1994) as:

> A state of physical, mental, and social well-being in all matters relating to the reproductive system at all stages of life. Reproductive health implies that people are able to have a satisfying and safe sex life and that they have the capability to reproduce and the freedom to decide if, when, and how often to do so . . .

Despite the age of this definition it is evident that individuals have rights; these rights are enshrined in UK and international law. People have the right under the Human Rights Act 1998 (article 8) to respect for private and family life. Reproductive health also includes the reproductive processes and functions necessary to reproduce.

There have been a number of ground-breaking developments and the introduction of new technologies over recent years that are associated with reproduction; it could be suggested that these innovations have been in response to the national and global incidence of subfertility. For some members of our society, having children and bringing up a family are important aspects of their lives and for those who experience fertility problems, this can be devastating, denying them their opportunity to realise their aspirations and hopes.

Reproductive health also takes into account issues associated with sexual health and personal relationships. The role of the healthcare professional is multifaceted and one aspect of this role is to act as a health educator, promoting good reproductive health, preventing ill health and sup-porting people who may experience problems. In order to care for a person or couple who have reproductive health issues, and to be able to assess and plan care in an effective manner, the

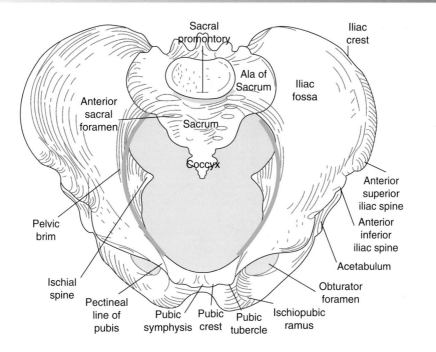

Figure 14.1   The female pelvis.

healthcare professional must be familiar with the anatomy and physiology of the reproductive tract.

The pelvis

The male and female pelve (singular pelvis) differ, with the female pelvis being wider and shallower than the male pelvis, so that the baby at birth can pass through it (Figure 14.1). The thickness of the bones of the pelvis also differs in the male and female. The female pelvic bones are thinner and more delicate than the male.

Generally, the pelvis is a ring of bone that supports the weight of the upper body. It can be described as a basin-shaped cavity. The bones of the pelvis are:

- the innominate bones
- the sacrum
- the coccyx.

There are two innominate bones and both are made up of:

- the ilium
- the pubic bone
- the ischium.

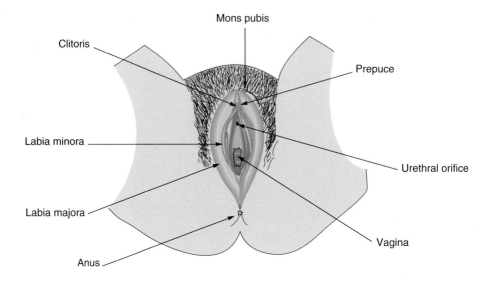

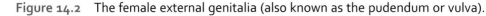

Figure 14.2   The female external genitalia (also known as the pudendum or vulva).

Towards the front of the pelvis (anteriorly), the bones join at the symphysis pubis. The sacrum and the coccyx come together at a joint that is moveable (inferiorly) – the sacrococcygeal joint. Strong connective tissues (ligaments) join the pelvis to the sacrum at the base of the spine. Large nerves and muscle pass through the pelvis, and there are a number of digestive and reproductive organs within it.

The female reproductive tract

Female external genitalia

The external genitalia, i.e. external to the vagina, are also known as the accessory structures of the female reproductive tract. Collectively, they are known as the vulva or pudendum and consist of the (Figure 14.2):

- mons pubis
- prepuce
- clitoris
- labia majora
- labia minora
- urethral orifice
- vagina
- Bartholin's glands.

There is a soft mound of fatty tissue covering the symphysis pubis at the front of the vulva – the mons pubis; post puberty this area is covered with pubic hair. The labia majora extend to both sides of the vulva and are covered with pubic hair – these are two longitudinal prominent folds of tissue. The outer surface of the labia majora is covered by a thin layer of skin containing hair follicles, sweat and sebaceous glands, and the inner surface is smoother, without pubic hair and contains a larger number of sebaceous follicles. Both the labia majora and minora are protective structures, protecting the inner structures of the vulva. Two soft folds of skin make up the labia minora within the labia majora and are situated either side of the opening of the vagina. The labia minora join close to the prepuce; these then cover the clitoris (the vulval vestibule) and extend backwards, enclosing the urethral and vaginal orifices. Connective, fatty and elastic tissues are what chiefly comprise the labia minora; there are no sweat glands or hair follicles as seen in the labia majora, but there are sebaceous glands present. The size and colour of the labia minora will change in response to sexual stimulation.

The clitoris (a sexual organ) is situated where the labia meet near the anterior folds of the labia minora; it is situated above the urethral and vaginal orifices. The clitoris is composed of erectile tissue; it is a small rounded area enclosed in fibrous membranes in layers. It is homologous to the penis and originates embryologically from the same tissue that forms the penis.

The clitoris becomes enlarged, erect and sensitive during sexual stimulation; it initiates and elevates sexual tension levels, and functions solely to bring about sexual pleasure. It is possible for female orgasm to occur when the clitoris is stimulated.

The Bartholin's glands are situated slightly below and to the left and right of the opening of the vagina (Marieb, 2010). As the female becomes sexually aroused, these glands secrete lubrication in the form of mucus; it is suggested that this can facilitate intercourse and allows for sexual stimulation, but the exact purpose is not fully understood. The secretions are known to contain pheromones; these are chemicals that can trigger a natural behavioural response in another person. Usually, the Bartholin's glands cannot be felt (palpated); however, in the event of obstruction, cyst formation can occur and the cysts may become infected, resulting in abscess formation. It must be noted that not all Bartholin's cysts are the result of an infection.

Female internal genitalia

The four organs of the female reproductive tract are the:

- fallopian tubes
- ovaries
- vagina
- uterus.

The uterus is a dense, muscular, pear-shaped hollow organ and is approximately 7.5 cm long. It is situated deep in the pelvic cavity between the urinary bladder and the rectum; it also touches the sigmoid colon and the small intestines. The uterus has three main parts (Figure 14.3):

- The fundus – the thick muscular region that is situated above the insertion of the fallopian tubes.
- The body (sometimes called the corpus) – the main aspect of the uterus joined to the cervix by an isthmus of tissue.
- The cervix – this is the narrower lower segment of the uterus, with an external os extending into the vagina.

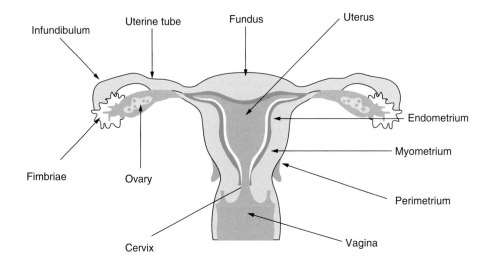

Figure 14.3   The uterus and associated structures.

The cavity of the uterus is continuous (laterally) with the lumen of the fallopian tubes and narrows as it reaches the cervix, creating a triangular, pear shape. The size of the uterus varies amongst women and during pregnancy, changes size, shape, structure and position. Postpartum, it usually returns to its normal shape and size within 6–8 weeks. The uterus has three layers (Figure 14.3):

- The perimetrium – this layer is the peritoneum and fascial outer layer. It supports the uterus within the pelvis. Sometimes it is called the parietal peritoneum.
- The myometrium – this layer is the middle layer and is composed of smooth muscle. The muscles in the myometrium stretch during pregnancy to allow for the growing fetus, and contract during labour. After delivery the myometrium contracts further to expel the placenta and control blood loss.
- The endometrium – this is the inner lining of the uterus and has a mucous lining. The surface is continuous with the vagina and the uterine tubes. During menstruation the layers of the endometrium slough away from the inner layer. During the menstrual cycle the endometrium thickens and becomes rich with blood vessels and glandular tissue.

A direct route exists from the vagina through the cervix, uterus and the fallopian tubes to the peritoneum as there is an opening of the uterus near the fundus into the lumen of the fallopian tubes.

The cervix (a Latin word for neck) is the lower constricted segment of the uterus; it is conical in shape and is a little wider in the middle than it is at the lower or upper ends; it joins to form the upper aspect of the vagina (Figure 14.4).

The ectocervix is the aspect of the cervix that projects into the vagina and has an epithelial surface. The opening of the cervix is known as the external os and it opens to the endocervical canal; the canal terminates at the internal os. The cervix provides a channel for discharge of the

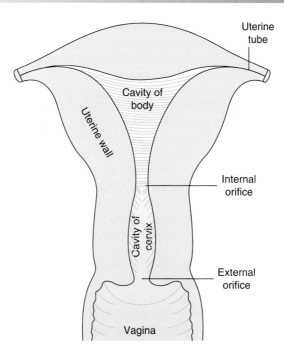

Figure 14.4   The cervix – ectocervix, internal os and external os.

menstrual fluid; it secretes secretions to assist in the transport of semen; during labour, it dilates to allow the passage of the fetus.

The fallopian tubes (also known as the salpinges) are two fine tubes that lead from the ovaries to the uterus; they range from 8 to 14 cm in length (Marieb, 2010). Collectively, the fallopian tubes, ovaries and support tissues are known as the adnexa. The key functions of the fallopian tubes are to provide a site for fertilisation and transport of the ovum to the uterus; this allows sperm and ova to meet for fertilisation in the tube. The ova are transported along the tube by the action of cilia and peristalsis. The fallopian tubes terminate at or near one ovary, becoming a structure called the fimbria (Figure 14.3).

The egg-producing organs are called the ovaries; they are the size and shape of a large almond and the two of them are situated on either side of the uterus. As well as being the reproductive organs, they are also endocrine glands. The ovaries are homologous to the testes in the male.

When a girl is born, each ovary will contain approximately 200 000–400 000 follicles – these are all the eggs that she will ever possess; the follicles are the shells of each egg. As the girl reaches puberty, the number of follicles will gradually decline, i.e. at puberty the number is between 100 000 and 200 000, and as the woman ages the number of follicles continues to decline.

The menstrual cycle

As a girl reaches puberty she begins to ovulate – her first menstruation is termed the menarche. Ovulation is the release of a ripe, mature egg from one of the ovaries every month until the menopause, a term used to describe the cessation of the menstrual cycle. Ovulation occurs as the body prepares the woman to become pregnant. If pregnancy does not occur, the woman has a menstrual period and the cycle begins again. The cycle is complex and is under the control of the reproductive hormonal system.

The cycle begins when a gland in the brain (the pituitary gland) releases a hormone called follicle-stimulating hormone (FSH); this hormone causes approximately 20 eggs to begin to grow and mature in the ovaries. The eggs grow within the follicle (its own shell) and FSH causes the follicle to produce oestrogen. As the levels of oestrogen (another hormone) increase, FSH production is stopped. Only one egg in the follicle will continue to grow and mature; the others die (Porth, 2010).

The next stage in the cycle occurs when the egg becomes mature; at this stage the pituitary gland produces another hormone called luteinising hormone (LH), and this causes the follicle to burst and the egg is released from the ovary. The follicle is now empty and becomes known as the corpus luteum; oestrogen continues to be produced by the corpus luteum and it then begins to produce another hormone called progesterone (Thibodeau and Patton, 2010). The role of progesterone at this stage is to begin to prepare the uterus to receive a fertilised egg.

The lining of the uterus (the endometrium) responds to the effects of oestrogen and progesterone and starts to thicken, resulting in a soft, nourishing environment for the fertilised egg. Implantation occurs as a result of the two hormones and the egg attaches itself to the endometrium. When implantation is successful, the egg then begins to divide by meiosis, forming cells and tissues that will eventually become a human being. Figure 14.5 gives a diagrammatic representation of the ovarian aspect of the menstrual cycle.

If fertilisation fails to occur (and there are many reasons why), then the egg will pass into the uterus and dissolve. When the hormone production slows down, the endometrial lining begins to break down and sloughs off; this then passes through the cervix and vagina and is known as menstruation. The menstrual cycle is said to begin from the first day of one menstrual period until the start of another one, and is on an average from 22 to 45 days (Monga and Dobbs, 2011).

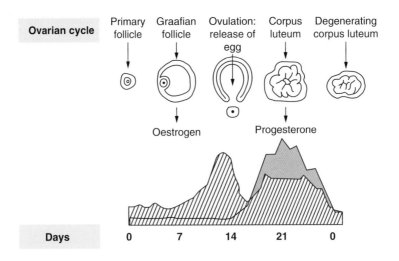

Figure 14.5   The menstrual cycle (ovarian).

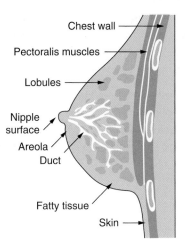

Figure 14.6 A cross-sectional of the female breast.

The female breast

The female breasts are usually considered as accessory organs of reproduction and play a key role in nurturing the young by producing milk. Structurally, the male breast is identical to the female breast but less prominent; male and female breasts develop embryologically from the same tissue (Marieb, 2010). Figure 14.6 shows a cross-section of the female breast.

The breast is composed of lobes. The lobes contain glandular tissue and fat; breasts are modified sweat glands that produce milk (lactation). The hormone prolactin is produced by the pituitary gland at the end of pregnancy and stimulates the glandular tissue to lactate (Marieb, 2010). The glandular tissue is further stimulated when the infant suckles at the breast, resulting in contraction and milk is transported via the ducts to the nipple. The breasts are covered with skin and each breast contains a nipple surrounded by a pink to dark brown tissue called the areola. The areola contains a number of sebaceous glands. Marieb and Hoehn (2012) suggests that the role of sebum produced by the sebaceous glands is to reduce chapping and cracking of the skin of the nipple.

During the menstrual cycle, some women may experience changes in their breasts; they may become enlarged and tender. In the premenstrual period, in response to the increasing levels of oestrogen and progesterone, the breasts may enlarge and become tender or nodular. After menstruation this growth reverts.

Menstrual disorders

Some women may experience problems with their menstrual cycle and these include:

- irregular periods
- excessive pain
- excessive bleeding.

This section addresses some of these problems.

Chapter 14

Case study

Miss Alice Oyelow is 22 years old. She has no children and presents with painful periods. Miss Oyelow informs the doctor that she has had painful periods since she started menstruating aged 13 years. The pain is becoming very bad. Her periods are regular with a 4–5/28 day cycle. She is not on the contraceptive pill and uses condoms for safer sex activity; she says recently she has been finding sexual intercourse painful. Miss Oyelow is otherwise well with no other complaints; her mother has a history of painful periods that necessitated a hysterectomy when she was aged 28 years.

Take some time to reflect on this case and then consider the following.

1. What do you think is the most likely diagnosis?
2. What other information would you need from Miss Oyelow to ensure you had a full history?
3. What investigations may be required?
4. What might the treatment options be?

Dysmenorrhoea

Dysmenorrhoea is defined as pain that occurs during menstruation (Monga and Dobbs, 2011). During the menstrual cycle, the woman may experience pain in the abdomen, and the pain can be so severe that it can impinge on her ability to perform the activities of daily living, such as going to work; often it is because the woman is unable to carry out these activities that she may seek help. Jones (2004) states that approximately 40–50% of menstruating women experience dysmenorrhoea and that it is the most common cause of absenteeism amongst young women.

Prior to the menstrual period beginning, the breasts may feel large and ache. Some pain during the menstrual period is normal but extreme pain is not; women can experience pain prior to and during the menstrual period, and it tapers off towards the end of the period. The pain can be sharp, intermittent or a dull ache, and is felt predominantly in the pelvic region/lower abdomen; it may also be felt in the back and thighs and can be described as 'dragging'. The abdomen may become distended and can be tender to touch, and constipation can occur. The woman experiences severe blood loss and can become incapacitated.

Two types of dysmenorrhoea have been described:

- primary dysmenorrhoea
- secondary dysmenorrhoea.

Table 14.1 outlines the differences between primary and secondary dysmenorrhoea.

Primary dysmenorrhoea

This refers to menstrual pain that is a result of physiological activities of menstruation accompanied by muscle contraction. This type of pain exists in women who are otherwise healthy (Morrow, 2009). Women in the younger age bracket (late teens to early 20s) experience primary dysmenorrhoea more than older women do.

Table 14.1   Primary and secondary dysmenorrhoea – distinctions.

	Primary dysmenorrhoea	Secondary dysmenorrhoea
Age at symptom onset	Adolescence	Mid to late 20s
Pain at other times of menstrual cycle	First 2–3 days of period	Persists beyond first 2–3 days of period
Other types of pain?	No	Dyspareunia

Adapted from Mazza (2011).

Secondary dysmenorrhoea

In contrast to primary dysmenorrhoea, secondary dysmenorrhoea is attributed to some form of organic pelvic disease (underlying pelvic pathology). In secondary dysmenorrhoea, there is evidence of an underlying disease process or some form of structural abnormality within or outside of the uterus. Secondary dysmenorrhoea is uncommon before the age of 25 years (Monga and Dobbs, 2011). The most common cause is endometriosis.

Risk factors

Increased risk is associated with those who are in the younger age group and if they have a past medical history (Andrews and Steele, 2005):

- early age of menarche
- nulliparous
- obesity
- cigarette smoking
- alcohol consumption
- family history of dysmenorrhea
- pelvic infection (i.e. pelvic inflammatory disease)
- history of (or current) sexually-transmitted infection
- endometriosis
- leiomyomas
- use of an intrauterine device.

Pathophysiology

Prostaglandins are released by the uterus during menstruation due to the breakdown of the endometrial cells and the release of their contents. Excessive levels of prostaglandin are closely related to dysmenorrhea. The increased production of prostaglandins by the uterus results in intense uterine contractions (uterine hypercontractility); the uterus can go into spasm and the muscle (the endometrium) becomes ischaemic, producing uterine pain that is similar to the pain experienced in angina (see Chapter 5). The excessive amount of prostaglandin can also cause the women to experience:

- nausea
- vomiting
- diarrhoea
- faintness
- headache
- lower backache.

The reason why some women produce excessive prostaglandin is unknown (Linhart, 2007); prostaglandin levels have been found to be much higher in those women with excessive menstrual pain as opposed to those who feel moderate to no pain. Andrews and Steele (2005) point out that there may be other causes of dysmenorrhoea, e.g. congenital abnormalities, and these may need to be investigated.

Diagnosis

Diagnosis is made by taking a full health and medical history from the woman. The healthcare professional should pay particular attention to the type of pain the woman describes, the duration and what (if any) remedies she uses to alleviate the pain.
Diagnosis may be confirmed by:

- ultrasound
- hysterosalpingogram
- laparoscopy
- laparotomy.

Care and management

Controlling the pain associated with dysmenorrhoea is a primary care intervention. Medications including non-steroidal anti-inflammatory drugs (NSAIDs), such as ibuprofen, mefenamic acid and naproxen, are very effective in the treatment of the pain that is associated with dysmenorrhoea. NSAIDs are able to inhibit the synthesis of prostaglandin (Monga and Dobbs, 2011). The healthcare professional must be aware that some patients are unable to take NSAIDs as they can cause:

- gastrointestinal bleeding
- nephrotoxicity
- nausea
- vomiting
- dyspepsia
- headache.

It must also be remembered that these drugs are contraindicated in patients who have:

- aspirin-induced asthma
- peptic ulcer
- renal disease
- clotting disorders.

NSAIDs in this context are used to prevent pain rather than acting as an analgesic, and the woman should be told that she should take the NSAID as soon as she knows that the period is imminent or as soon as the bleeding begins; the medication should be taken on a regular basis for the first 1–3 days of the period as it prevents pain.

The oral contraceptive pill is an effective first-line agent for the treatment of primary dysmenorrhoea when NSAIDs have failed (Harel, 2006). In those women in whom the oral contraceptive pill or NSAIDs do not work (approximately 10–20%), transdermal glyceryl trinitrate patches may be of benefit (Jones, 2004). The patches (containing glyceryl trinitrate) can cause relaxation of uterine contractions (French, 2005).

Oral contraceptives may be effective in treating primary dysmenorrhoea as they have the potential to block ovulation and reduce blood flow to the uterus. Another prostaglandin inhibitor is vitamin E.

The aim of treatment in secondary dysmenorrhoea is to identify and correct the underlying organic cause. Pelvic inflammatory disease (PID) is a cause of secondary dysmenorrhoea, and if this is the case, then the PID should be treated to relieve the symptoms associated with secondary dysmenorrhoea.

In rare cases, surgical intervention may be required for some women. Hysterectomy can be a success in terms of relieving women of their presenting symptoms. This procedure should be performed once childbearing is complete.

There are a number of non-pharmacological treatments that may help the women. Transcutaneous electrical nerve stimulation (TENS) can help with or without pharmacological analgesics (Wang *et al.*, 2009). Acupuncture may be of value; however, there is insufficient evidence to determine the effectiveness of acupuncture on the abdomen in reducing pain. Some women may find comfort in the use of a hot water bottle. Exercise can have the effects of releasing endogenous endorphins – these are the body's own analgesic.

Amenorrhoea

Amenorrhoea, the absence of periods, can occur:

- prior to the menarche
- after the menopause
- during pregnancy
- postoperatively
- post treatment.

Primary amenorrhoea occurs prior to the menses happening and secondary amenorrhoea occurs when menstruation has previously taken place but has stopped for at least 6 consecutive months in a woman who has had regular periods.

The most common cause of secondary amenorrhoea is pregnancy. Other causes according to the Royal College of Obstetricians and Gynaecologists (2007) include:

- polycystic ovary syndrome
- hypothalamic causes – due to excessive weight loss (anorexia) or excessive exercise
- hyperprolactinaemia – an elevated level of prolactin in the blood; in women this may be caused by a prolactinoma
- contraception – the contraceptive pill and depot injection.

Diagnosis

The healthcare professional must undertake a full health, medical and menstrual history, including:

- sexual history in order to rule out pregnancy
- family history to determine if there are any genetic abnormalities
- the presence of any associated illness such as hypothyroidism or diabetes mellitus
- emotional upsets
- changes in body weight
- increase in exercise
- drug history, e.g. contraceptive pill/injection, chemotherapy
- previous surgery.

In all women who present with amenorrhoea, it may be advisable to perform a pregnancy test. In secondary amenorrhoea, a number of blood tests may be carried out in order to assess levels of hormones, such as FSH and LH, as well assessment of thyroid function. Prolactin levels will also need to be assessed to determine if there is any evidence of hyperprolactinaemia. A pelvic ultrasound can demonstrate the presence of polycystic ovaries (enlarged ovaries), and magnetic resonance imaging (MRI) or computer tomography (CT) scans can identify a pituitary tumour; if these are suspected a hysteroscopy may be required.

412

Care and management

The role and function of the healthcare professional is to provide the women with emotional as well as physical support, and information that she is able to understand in order to make informed decisions about her treatment options. Healthcare professionals are ideally placed to discuss lifestyle issues with the women, such as smoking and alcohol consumption, and stress-reducing activities, and to provide information about diet and weight gain (if needed), and the balance between excessive and therapeutic levels of exercise. The woman may need support in relation to the perceived threat to her self-esteem and with concerns associated with fertility as a result of amenorrhoea. Explanations should be provided about the type of investigations that may be required and the reason why they are being performed. The treatment required will depend on the cause. Surgical intervention or hormone replacement therapy may be needed.

Menorrhagia

The term menorrhagia is defined as bleeding in excess of 80 mL (Andrews and Steele, 2005); on average, women lose approximately 35 mL of blood with each period (Mazza, 2011). Some people refer to menorrhagia as heavy periods. The heavy period can interfere with a woman's physical, social, emotional and/or material quality of life.

Diagnosis

A full healthcare history and menstrual history will need to be undertaken in order to offer the woman appropriate and effective treatment. The aim of any intervention should be to improve the woman's quality of life. Questions to be asked include:

- How much bleeding occurs (how often are tampons/sanitary pads changed)?
- Are there any blood clots?
- How long do periods last?
- Does bleeding occur after sex?
- Is there any pelvic pain?

- Is there any bleeding between periods?
- Are there any other related symptoms?

A physical examination will need to be undertaken and this can include an internal examination as well as an external abdominal examination (palpation). The person carrying out the examination can identify, for example, if there are any indications of fibroids.

There are a variety of tests and investigations that may be undertaken in order to determine why the woman is experiencing menorrhagia. Blood testing will determine if the women is anaemic or has a blood clotting disorder. Assessment of thyroid function and other aspects of the endocrine system may be required.

An ultrasound scan may be required as this can determine if there are any structural abnormalities. In some instances, a biopsy may be needed to exclude any potential disorders, e.g. endometrial cancer. If the ultrasound demonstrates that there are abnormalities (or it is inconclusive), then hysteroscopy can be performed to aid diagnosis or to determine the exact location of the fibroid.

Care and management

If the ultrasound examination and the biopsy demonstrate that there are no obvious problems with the uterus, then a pharmacological approach to treatment may be considered. Table 14.2 outlines the different kinds of drugs that may be used in the treatment of menorrhagia. The woman must be provided with all the information she requires to make an informed decision;

Table 14.2   Drugs that may be used in the treatment of menorrhagia.

Drug	What it is?	How it works?	Possible side effects	Comments
Levonorgestrel – a hormone	A small plastic device that is placed in the uterus, slowly releasing progestogen	The hormone prevents the lining of the uterus from growing too quickly	Irregular bleeding Breast tenderness Acne Headaches Amenorrhoea	This is also a contraceptive First-line treatment
Tranexamic acid	Tablet format The medication is taken from the start of the menstrual period for up to 4 days	Promotes clot formation within the uterus; this reduces the amount of bleeding	Indigestion Headaches Diarrhoea	If symptoms do not improve within 3 months, treatment should be stopped Considered as second-line treatment

Continued |

Table 14.2   *Continued*

Drug	What it is?	How it works?	Possible side effects	Comments
Non-steroidal anti-inflammatory drugs (NSAIDs)	Tablet format Medication to be taken from the start of the menstrual period or just before and until heavy bleeding stops	Prostaglandin production is reduced	Indigestion Diarrhoea	If symptoms do not improve within 3 months, treatment should be stopped
Combined oral contraceptives	Pill format that contains the hormones progestogen and oestrogen One pill is taken for 21 days, then stopped for 7 days, and the cycle is repeated	Prevents the menstrual cycle from occurring	Mood change Headache Nausea Fluid retention Breast tenderness	This is also a contraceptive Considered as second-line treatment
Oral progesterone (norethisterone)	Tablets taken 2–3 times per day from the 5th to 26th day of the menstrual cycle	Prevents the lining of the uterus from growing too quickly	Weight gain Bloating Breast tenderness Headache Acne	This is also a contraceptive Considered as third-line treatment
Injected or implanted progesterone	The hormone progestogen is injected or implanted. The implant releases the hormone slowly for 3 years	Prevents the lining of the uterus from growing too quickly	Weight gain Bloating Breast tenderness Headache Acne Irregular bleeding Amenorrhoea Bone density loss can occur	This is also a contraceptive Considered as third-line treatment
Gonadotrophin-releasing hormone analogue	An injection that stops the body producing oestrogen and progesterone	Prevents the menstrual cycle from occurring	Menopause-like symptoms (hot flushes, increased sweating, vaginal dryness)	Considered as third-line treatment

Adapted from National Institute of Health and Clinical Excellence (2007).

Table 14.3   Potential surgical treatments for women with heavy periods.

Proposed surgical intervention	What it is?	Possible side effects	Comments
Endometrial ablation: Thermal balloon endometrial ablation (TBEA) Impedance-controlled bipolar radiofrequency ablation Microwave endometrial ablation (MEA) Free fluid thermal ablation	A device is inserted in all techniques through the vagina and cervix into the uterus When the device is *in situ*, several methods can be used to heat the device, e.g. by using radio energy microwaves. The purpose is to destroy the lining of the uterus	Vaginal discharge Increased pain during the menstrual period Infection	In some women, the procedure may need to be repeated as the lining of the uterus can grow back This procedure is not suitable if the woman wishes to become pregnant
Uterine artery embolisation (UAE)	This procedure aims to block the blood supply to the uterus Small particles are injected into the blood vessels that take blood to the uterus with the aim of blocking any blood supply to fibroids in the expectation that they shrink	Vaginal discharge Pain Nausea Vomiting	There may be need for further surgery Women undertaking this procedure may be able to become pregnant
Myomectomy	Surgical removal of a fibroid can be performed either through an abdominal incision or via the vagina. The vaginal route necessitates the use of a hysteroscope	Adhesions and as a result a possibility of pain and impaired fertility Infection Perforation of the uterus	Women having this procedure may be able to become pregnant
Hysterectomy	There are two main methods of performing a hysterectomy – vaginally or abdominally In total hysterectomy the uterus and cervix are removed, whereas in subtotal hysterectomy only the uterus is removed	Haemorrhage during or after surgery Infection Damage to adjacent organs, e.g. bowel or urinary tract Urinary/faecal dysfunction	Women wishing to have a hysterectomy will not be able to become pregnant Removal of the uterus means the women will no longer have a menstrual period

however, for some women hormonal contraception as a form of treatment may be unacceptable, e.g. religious reasons or the wish to conceive. The woman may need to be treated with hormone replacement; she might also require other interventions such as counselling.

When the pharmacological approach fails or is unacceptable, surgical intervention may be recommended after the woman has been given the opportunity to review and agree any treatment decision. Ensure that sufficient time has been provided and appropriate support given to the women during the decision-making process. There are several interventions that need to be considered (Table 14.3).

If surgical intervention is required, the woman (and her family) will need support; this can be physical and psychological support as well as socioeconomical support. It is important to organize service provision and a co-ordinated multidisciplinary approach is advocated with the women at the centre of it.

The information offered to the woman must be provided in a format she understands, and it must also be relevant to her circumstances; this may mean that the information may need to be translated into her mother tongue. Information has to point out the risks and benefits of the various treatments and procedures being offered, and opportunity must be provided for the woman to ask questions. It must be emphasised that she can change her mind if she wishes, and she is entitled to a second opinion.

The male reproductive tract

The male reproductive tract is designed to produce spermatozoa and deposit these inside the female vagina; this contributes to reproduction. The spermatozoa are responsible for the fertilisation of the female egg. Unlike the female genitalia, male genitalia are found outside of the body (Figure 14.7).

Male genitalia

The penis and scrotum comprise the male external genitalia. Within the scrotal sac, a loose bag-like sac of skin, suspended by the spermatic cord in between the thighs, are the testes. They are approximately the size of a walnut – 4.5 cm in length, 2.5 cm in breadth and 3 cm in diameter; they feel smooth and move freely within the scrotal sac (Thibodeau and Patton 2010). While the testes are found outside of the abdominal cavity in the scrotum, they begin their development in the abdominal cavity and normally descend into the scrotal sac during the last 2 months of fetal development. The testes traverse the inguinal canal and inguinal rings and move into the scrotum where they are suspended.

It is normal for one testis to hang lower than the other. As the cremasteric muscle contracts, the spermatic cord (to which it is attached) shortens and the testes moves up towards the abdomen; the result of this is that it provides the testes with more warmth. For effective development of sperm, the testes must be at a lower temperature than the body; this is the reason the testes are situated outside of the body.

The testes have two functions – to secrete the hormone testosterone, which is responsible for the development of the male secondary sex characteristics (deep voice, beard growth, body hair), as well as the function of the male reproductive system in the production of spermatozoa (Tortora, 2011). The testes are the essential male organs of reproduction.

The composition of the testes, contained under a membranous shell, is glandular tissue that is composed of several lobules differing in size according to their location. The lobule consists of

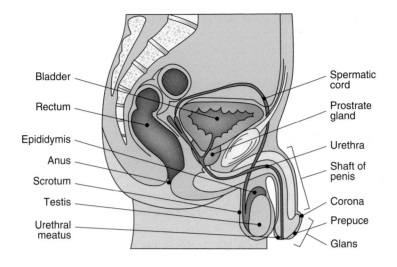

Bladder

Rectum

Epididymis

Anus

Scrotum

Testis

Urethral
meatus

Spermatic
cord

Prostrate
gland

Urethra

Shaft of
penis

Corona

Prepuce

Glans

Figure 14.7   The male reproductive system.

417

approximately 660–1200 seminiferous tubules that are small convoluted structures, responsible for the production of sperm. The spermatozoa develop in different stages in different parts of the tubules. The tubules form sperm continuously; in a young man, sperm is produced at the rate of 120 million per day. The sperm travel from the seminiferous tubules to the rete testes, to the efferent ducts onwards to the epididymis where spermatogenesis takes place and newly created mature sperm cells are formed. Spermatogenesis is complex and can be divided into three phases:

- mitotic proliferation to produce a large number of cells
- meiotic division to produce genetic diversity
- maturation, preparing sperm for transit and penetration of the oocyte in the female tract.

The sperm cells are then moved on to the vas deferens and expelled through the urethra as a result of rhythmic contractions.

Situated between the seminiferous tubules are cells called the Leydig cells, where testosterone and other androgens are formed. The physical changes in the male related to testosterone are:

- increase in penile size
- enlargement of the scrotum
- growth in the size of the testes
- enlargement of the larynx and deepening of the voice
- increase in muscle mass
- increase in basal metabolic rate
- increase in sebaceous glands
- thickening of the bones.

The penis is an external male reproductive organ, and within the penis is the urethra. The penis provides a route for the elimination of ejaculate and urine via the urethral orifice situated at the tip of the penis; the enlarged aspect is called the glans penis. The glans penis is homologous with the female clitoris.

The penis is made up of three columns of erectile tissue:

- two corpora cavernosa
- one corpus spongiosum.

The end of the corpus spongiosum is the bulbous glans penis; the glans is covered with a thin layer of skin that allows for erection and, in uncircumcised males, the skin at the glans folds over on itself to form the prepuce or foreskin; the area where the foreskin is attached, underneath the penis, is called the frenulum, which is homologous with the female clitoral hood. The urethra, the terminal end of the urinary tract, lies on the tip of the glans and is known as the urethral meatus. Erection requires complex vascular activity – dilation of the arteries supplying blood to the penis and sympathetic nervous system activity.

The prostate gland is approximately 2.5 cm in length and lies at the base of the urinary bladder surrounded by the upper part of the urethra (Marieb and Hoehn, 2012). The function of the prostate gland is not well understood. The gland is described as chestnut-shaped and is made up of 20–30 compound tubular–alveolar glands; these glands are embedded in a mass of smooth muscle and dense connective tissue. A thin milky fluid is secreted, adding bulk to semen on ejaculation. Prostatic fluid accounts for approximately one-third of semen volume. During orgasm, sperm cells are transmitted from the urethra via the ejaculatory ducts that are situated in the prostate gland, and smooth muscle within the prostate gland contracts during ejaculation, helping to expel semen.

Male reproductive disorders

This section discusses four common male reproductive tract disorders:

- phimosis
- paraphimosis
- hydrocele
- benign and malignant prostate cancer.

It is not possible in a chapter of this size to outline in depth all of the details associated with these disorders. The reader is advised to delve deeper into the subject in order to gain more comprehensive insight into the care and management of men with reproductive tract disorders.

Case study

Mr Joseph Wilson is a 56-year-old university lecturer who is married with three children. He presented with a left-sided uncomfortable scrotal swelling. Mr Wilson was acutely embarrassed when he arrived at the general practitioner's surgery. The swelling has grown to such an extent he was embarrassed to go out and to go to work. He reported that he and his wife no longer had intimate relationships and he said he was feeling depressed and had stopped going to the gym and swimming. Mr Wilson gave past health and medical history informing the doctor that as a child he was born with an undescended testes and has on two occasions, aged 5 and 7, had minor left-sided hydroceles; they resolved of their own accord. A physical examination was carried out by shining a light underneath the scrotum; this illuminated a fluid-containing sac and an ultrasound scan was booked to confirm the diagnosis of hydrocele.

Take some time to reflect on this case and then consider the following.

1. How might you help to relieve Mr Wilson of his embarrassment?
2. What treatment options might be available for Mr Wilson?
3. What advice would you give a man with regards to testicular self-examination?
4. Are there any complications associated with hydrocele?

Phimosis

Phimosis occurs when the opening of the foreskin (or prepuce) is unable to be retracted behind the glans penis; the foreskin is too tight for retraction. Phimosis can be congenital or it can occur as result of infection, inflammation or trauma (Warshaw, 2007); it is most frequently due to a condition known as balanitis xerotica obliterans (BXO), the cause of which is unknown. BXO (sometimes called lichen sclerosis) is a fibrosing condition resulting in thick (sclerosing) scaring of the skin of the penis, because of which the skin becomes discoloured.

Diagnosis

As the foreskin cannot be retracted, this may result in poor hygiene and the man with phimosis may present with balanoposthitis. The glans penis becomes infected (balanitis) as does the foreskin (posthitis); the patient may complain of itching and irritation, pain, discomfort, bleeding on sexual intercourse or masturbation, white discharge (smegma) and there may be dysuria and retention of urine due to restriction of the foreskin. Urethral stenosis and inflammation can also occur.

Care and management

A holistic assessment of individual needs is required along with appropriate health promotion activity by teaching the patient how to ensure, and reinforcing the need for, good personal hygiene. If infection is present, then prescribed antibiotic therapy is the first line of treatment along with an antifungal preparation (if required); analgesia will also be required. Hot baths may also aid in reducing the swelling caused by infection. The healthcare professional must ascertain if the man is sexually active; if this is the case, his partner may also require treatment. If a barrier method of contraception is not being used, then the use of a condom for sexual intercourse should be advocated to prevent transmission of infection.

In severe cases of foreskin restriction, e.g. when urinary retention occurs, an emergency circumcision may need to be performed. Postcircumcision, wound healing must be promoted; a non-adherent dressing and patient education focusing on ways to reduce inflammation are required. The man should be taught how to perform personal hygiene associated with the genitalia. The penis should be bathed at least daily in warm soapy water and the non-adherent dressing reapplied in order to prevent clothing disturbing wound healing. Explain to the man what the signs of infection are; he should be told that if excessive bleeding occurs, he needs to contact his general practice or accident and emergency department. Sexual intercourse and masturbation should cease until after the wound has healed.

Paraphimosis

Conversely, paraphimosis occurs when the foreskin is retracted over the glans penis and forms a constriction near the base of the glans. The cause is usually related to failure of the foreskin to return to its usual position covering the glans penis after manipulation has occurred. The band of foreskin that is retracted becomes swollen and can cause compression of the blood vessels supplying the glans – as circulation is reduced, pain can occur. Ghory and Sharma (2009) suggest that paraphimosis can be classed as a medical emergency as gangrene of the penis can occur.

In an attempt to relieve the swelling, cold compresses can be applied to the penis and the foreskin may be able to be manipulated back over the glans penis. Analgesia, oral and/or topical, can be applied to help with manipulation. If manipulation fails, then a dorsal slit may be made in the foreskin, and circumcision may be advised at a later date as recurrence can occur.

When assisting those men who are unable to carry out the activities of daily living independently, e.g. when assisting with personal hygiene or performing catheter care, ensure that the foreskin (in uncircumcised men) is fully retracted to cover the glans penis. The same can also apply to those men who may be confused or those who have decreased sensation in the penis.

Hydrocele

A hydrocele occurs when there is collection of fluid in the membranous sac that surrounds the testes within the scrotum; typically a hydrocele appears unilaterally. A hydrocele can occur spontaneously and the cause may be unknown, or it can be the result of inflammatory conditions such as epididymitis or orchitis – inflammation of the epididymis or testes respectively; trauma may also cause hydrocele. In some cases, the cause may be a testicular tumour.

Diagnosis

A detailed healthcare and medical history will need to be taken, asking the patient about any recent injury or trauma, other medical conditions and sexual history. The scrotum can swell to a considerable size and it is usually painless (asymptomatic), but the excessive swelling can cause discomfort. It becomes painful when the fluid surrounding the testes becomes infected. The patient may seek help because the size of the swelling can prevent him from enjoying and taking part in social activities such as swimming, running, walking and sexual activity. The swelling can progress and cause the blood supply to the testes to become compromised.

Examination of the contents of the scrotal sac reveals a dullness when the sac is percussed; the swelling feels smooth and is usually located in front of the testes. A hydrocele and tumour can be differentiated using of illumination, i.e. a light source (transillumination): a hydrocele allows the light to pass through, whereas a tumour is dense and prevents this from occurring. Ultrasound may be required to determine if there is any underlying cause, e.g. testicular cancer.

Care and management

Elevation of the scrotum by the wearing of a scrotal support may reduce the swelling. In most cases, however, the fluid will need to be drained off with a small trocar and cannula, as aspiration of the fluid carries with it the risk of infection. If the fluid is infected, then the man will need to be prescribed antibiotics.

Hydrocelectomy (also known as hydrocele repair) is a surgical procedure that is used to correct a hydrocele; this can be performed with the patient attending the hospital on an outpatient basis. Postoperatively, the patient will be observed for any signs of haemorrhage, and there is a risk of infection; however, this is rare. Damage may occur to the spermatic vessels, but again this is rare.

Benign and malignant prostate cancer

As a man ages his prostate gland becomes larger, and as ageing progresses the gland atrophies and connective tissue accumulates. Cancer of the prostate gland (benign and malignant) occurs slowly and as such the symptoms may occur over many years. This accumulation of connective tissue and atrophy is not usually due to cancer and is known as benign prostatic hyperplasia (BPH). BPH is the most common neoplastic growth in men; over 50% of men aged 60 years will have BPH and, according to Thorpe and Neal (2003), not all of those men will have symptoms (they may be classed as asymptomatic).

Diagnosis

When symptoms are present, they are the same for BPH and malignant prostate cancer and include:

- dysuria
- frequency of micturition
- urgency
- nocturia
- hesitancy.

There may be a history of recurrent urinary tract infection and increasing urinary obstruction can cause back pressure leading to renal impairment. Acute urinary retention can occur if the prostate gland becomes enlarged and is further complicated if the gland is also infected (prostatitis). Pathological changes as a result of abnormal enlargement of the prostate gland or cell multiplication in either benign or malignant prostate cancer can occur; the key change is pressure caused by the enlarged gland on the prostatic urethra, which can (as discussed) lead to impeded urinary outflow. Over time urinary retention can impair urinary function and prostatic obstruction can result in:

- obstruction of the urethra
- diverticulum of the bladder
- hydroureter
- hydronephrosis
- infection
- renal failure.

After a detailed medical history has been undertaken, diagnosis may be confirmed by digital rectal examination (DRE), transrectal ultrasound (TRUS), assessment of prostate-specific antigen (PSA) and other blood tests, such as measurement of serum acid phosphatase. Biopsy of the prostate gland may be undertaken whilst the TRUS is happening. A general physical examination is usually undertaken, the abdomen is palpated and the lymph glands are examined.

The malignant cancer cells of the prostate gland can spread to other parts of the body (metastasise) and this occurs in particular to the bones as well as the lymph glands and lungs.

Care and management

The care and management of the man with prostate cancer is complex and will depend on the individual. There are a number of factors that must be given consideration and a key element of the healthcare professional's role is to provide the man with the information he requires and in a format that he understands in order to make an informed decision. The staging of the cancer will reveal its size and how far it has spread. The treatment options for a cancer that is small and has not spread far will be different from those for a cancer that is large and has spread widely. The cells of the cancer are also examined under the microscope and this then allows it to be graded. The more abnormal the cells, the higher the grade is likely to be; low-grade cancers usually spread more slowly. Other factors that need to be taken into account include the age of the man and the results of the PSA, DRE and TRUS.

The following treatment options are available and they require discussion with the man and the urology team. Treatment depends on the wishes of the individual man and whether or not the cancer has spread (National Institute for Health and Clinical Excellence, 2008):

- watchful waiting
- surgery
- laser therapy
- transurethral ablation
- transurethral microwave therapy
- brachytherapy.

Chemotherapy, radiotherapy and hormone therapy can also be considered, again depending on the individual man.

Surgical intervention may be required to remove the whole gland or the part of the gland that is causing the obstruction. The most common surgical procedure used for BPH is transurethral resection of the prostate gland (TURP). When TURP is performed, a cystoscope is passed into the bladder to visualise the interior of the urinary bladder; a rectoscope is then passed and resection begins by chipping away small sections of the gland tissue that is compressing the urethra and the neck of the bladder.

Postoperatively, a three-way urethral catheter is *in situ* and the urinary bladder is continuously flushed out with a non-electrolyte solution to prevent blood clots from forming.

There are potential complications that can arise in association with surgery on the prostate gland, e.g.:

- haemorrhage
- infection
- clot retention
- deep vein thrombosis
- urethral stricture
- incontinence
- erectile dysfunction
- retrograde ejaculation.

The healthcare professional is required to ensure that the patient is kept pain free postoperatively. It is vital that a strict fluid balance is maintained and that catheter care is carried out, making every effort to prevent infection. The patient should be encouraged to mobilise as soon as possible as his condition permits. If the patient is to be discharged home with his catheter *in situ*, he will need to be taught how to care for this, and referral will need to be made to the community nurse.

Conclusion

Reproduction of the human species is complex with the key function of the male and female reproductive tracts being associated with procreation. Whilst the physiological functions associated with reproduction are important, it is also essential to remember that there is pleasure associated with the reproductive tract and that this component of a human being can also be important for many.

This chapter has provided insight into the normal and abnormal anatomy and physiology as well as providing discussion on a number of pathological changes that may occur in the male and female reproductive tracts. Emphasis has been placed on the provision of sound information in a format that the person understands in order to make complex decisions concerning treatment options and care pathways.

Test your knowledge

- List three causes of menstrual dysfunction.

- Explain how the healthcare professional can improve the self-esteem of an individual who has experienced reproductive health problems.

- Explain how an enlarged prostate gland can cause difficulties with urinary output.

- Define the term infertile and list the possible causes.

- What advice would you give to a woman who is experiencing heavy and painful bleeding during her menstrual periods?

Activities

Here are some activities and exercises to help test your learning. For the answers to these exercises, as well as further self-testing activities, visit our website at www.wiley.com/go/fundamentalsofappliedpathophysiology

Fill in the blanks

The _____ tubes are small tubes that carry _____ from the _____ to the uterus. The uterus is a pear-shaped organ with three distinct aspects; these are the _____, the body and the _____. The cervix is the narrower lower segment of the uterus, with an external os extending into the vagina. The uterus has three layers: the _____, the _____ and the _____. During _____ the layers of the endometrium slough away from the inner layer. During the menstrual cycle the endometrium _____ and becomes rich with blood vessels and _____ tissue. Eggs placed here are _____. The walls of the _____ are elastic, allowing them to _____ during child birth.

Choose from:
Fertilised; Myometrium; Fundus; Ovaries; Fallopian; Cervix; Thickens; Eggs; Endometrium; Perimetrium; Expand; Vagina; Glandular; Menstruation

Label the diagram

From the list of words supplied, label the diagram.

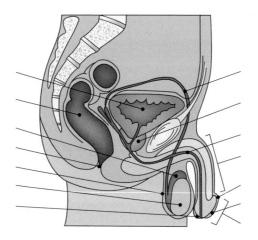

Bladder; Rectum; Anus; Scrotum; Testis, Urethral meatus; Spermatic cord; Prostrate gland; Urethra; Shaft of penis; Corona; Prepuce; Glans; Epididymis

Word search

F	Y	E	Y	S	N	Y	L	Y	Y	U	D	B	L	T	N
O	A	O	A	V	S	S	R	O	R	P	I	V	O	R	N
Y	S	L	A	V	U	A	A	C	N	M	S	C	M	S	A
S	I	S	L	C	V	L	F	S	I	E	U	P	N	I	X
H	N	P	I	O	O	T	V	T	P	L	I	T	E	L	P
O	E	A	R	R	P	N	S	A	P	L	R	S	C	R	U
R	P	N	L	N	O	I	T	A	L	U	C	A	J	E	M
M	I	I	Z	G	T	T	A	R	E	O	L	A	S	D	R
O	D	G	H	Y	L	E	I	N	A	R	E	I	A	D	E
N	I	A	M	A	M	I	E	L	T	C	B	R	R	A	T
E	D	V	O	R	H	E	T	A	C	U	T	C	A	L	V
S	Y	M	P	H	Y	S	I	S	P	U	B	I	S	B	A
E	M	U	U	T	E	R	U	S	S	C	I	E	O	A	E
X	I	V	R	E	C	N	N	E	R	V	E	S	S	N	N
I	S	L	P	R	S	O	P	B	A	M	N	A	N	R	R
I	Y	N	O	U	M	M	T	O	R	E	R	H	D	R	V

Areola	Enzyme	Rectum
Urethra	Ejaculation	Ovary
Sperm	Contraction	Nipple
Penis	Vulva	Mons pubis
Nerves	Vagina	Clitoris
Hormones	Cervix	Fallopian tubes
Epididymis	Uterus	Bladder
Glans	Symphysis pubis	Breast

Further resources

National Institute for Health and Clinical Excellence (NICE)

http://www.nice.org.uk/
NICE provides guidance, sets quality standards and manages a national database to improve people's health and prevent and treat ill health. There are many excellent resources on this website that can help guide and inform practice.

Men's Health Forum

http://www.menshealthforum.org.uk/
This is a charity that provides an independent and authoritative voice for male health in England and Wales, and tackles the issues and inequalities affecting the health and well-being of men and boys. The site is packed with data and a numerous links to other sites and resources.

Sexual Advice Association

http://www.sda.uk.net/
This is the website of a charitable organization with the aim of helping to improve the sexual health and well-being of men and women and to raise awareness of the extent to which sexual conditions affect the general population. It also has a helpline that can be used to discuss concerns that people feel they cannot discuss with their doctor.

Verity

http://www.verity-pcos.org.uk/home
A self-help group for women with polycystic ovary syndrome. Verity organises conferences and conducts research.

Everyman

http://www.everyman-campaign.org/index.shtml
Everyman's mission is to stamp out testicular and prostate cancer. It raises awareness of prostate and testicular cancers by making everyone recognise the tell-tale signs and understand the importance of treating them.

Women's Health Forum Royal College of Nursing

http://www.rcn.org.uk/development/communities/rcn_forum_communities/womenshealth
This forum provides nurses and others with up to date information and news associated with women's health. The forum organises a number of events, conferences and meetings. The site has a variety of useful links and other resources.

Glossary of terms

Ablation:	to destroy (e.g. endometrial ablation means to destroy the layer of the cells that lines the uterus).
Asymptomatic:	without symptoms.
Atrophy:	wasting away; a diminution in the size of a cell, tissue or organ.
Bartholin's glands:	two small round structures on either side of the vaginal opening. Secretions from these glands provide vaginal lubrication. The exact purpose of the fluid secreted is not fully understood.
Benign:	causes no problem. In cancer, it means a growth that is not malignant.
Brachytherapy:	in prostate cancer, implantation of tiny radioactive seeds under anaesthetic directly into the prostate gland.
Cilia:	small hair-like structures on the outer surface of some cells; used to propel liquids.
Clitoris:	a small body of tissue that is highly sexually sensitive; it is protected by the prepuce. Becomes enlarged and erect during sexual stimulation.
Cystoscope:	a thin tube with a light and eye piece attached to it, allowing the user to see the inside of the urinary bladder.
Diverticulum:	a pouch or sac opening from a tubular or saccular organ (e.g. the urinary bladder).
Dorsal:	pertaining to the back; the rear aspect.
Dyspareunia:	pain with intercourse.
Fibroid:	a non-cancerous growth in the uterus.
Hydronephrosis:	an abnormal enlargement of the kidney that may be due to ureteral obstruction.
Hydroureter:	distension of the ureter with urine as a result of blockage.
Hysterosalpingogram:	X-ray examination of the uterus and uterine tubes after radio-opaque dye has been injected.
Ischaemia:	a low oxygen state in a part of the body. Usually the result of an obstruction to the blood supply to tissues.
Labia majora:	the inner layers of the vulva – thinner than the labia minora; protects the urethra, vagina and clitoris.
Labia minora:	the outer layers of the vulva, covered with pubic hair and containing sweat and sebaceous glands. Situated on either side of the vagina.

Laparoscopy:	the passage of a laparoscope into the abdominal cavity via the abdominal wall to allow the cavity to be viewed.
Laparotomy:	a surgical procedure that requires an incision to be made into the abdomen.
Lumen:	the inside space of a tubular structure.
Malignant:	invasive, has a tendency to grow and may spread to other parts of the body.
Mons pubis:	also known as the mons veneris (Latin for the Hill of Venus, the Roman Goddess of love). Fatty tissue covering the symphysis pubis.
Nulliparous:	never having given birth to a viable infant.
Os:	mouth; a term applied to an opening in a hollow organ such as the cervix.
Peristalsis:	a wave-like contraction.
Prepuce:	a loose fold of skin covering the glans penis and glans clitoris .
Prolactin:	a hormone primarily associated with lactation. Secreted by the anterior pituitary gland.
Prolactinoma:	a prolactin-producing tumour of the anterior pituitary gland; a slow-growing benign swelling.
Prostaglandin:	complex unsaturated fatty acid produced by the mast cells and acting as a messenger substance between cells. Intensifies the actions of histamine and kinins. They cause increased vascular permeability, neutrophil chemotaxis, stimulation of smooth muscle (e.g. the uterus) and can induce pain.
Slough:	dead tissue that has separated from the living structure.
Trocar:	a sharp-pointed surgical instrument that fits inside a tube (cannula).
Unilateral:	affecting only one side as opposed to bilateral affecting both sides.

References

Andrews, G. and Steele, J. (2005). Common gynaecological problems. In: Andrews, G. (ed) *Women's Sexual Health*, 3rd edn. Edinburgh: Elsevier, pp. 513–546.

French, L. (2005). Dysmenorrhoea. *American Family Physician.* 71(2): 285–291.

Ghory, H. and Sharma, R. (2009) Phimosis and Paraphimosis. *eMedicine*. http://emedicine.medscape.com/article/777539-overview last accessed May 2011

Harel, Z. (2006). Dysmenorrhea in adolescents and young adults: Etiology and management. *Journal of Pediatric and Adolescent Gynecology.* 19(6): 363–371.

Jones, A.E. (2004). Managing the pain of primary and secondary dysmenorrhoea. *Nursing Times*. 100(10): 40–43.

Linhart, J. (2007). Female reproductive problems. In: Monahan, F.D., Sand, J.K., Neighbors, M., Marek, J.F. and Green, C.J. (eds). *Phipps' Medical Surgical Nursing: Health and Illness Perspectives*, 8th edn. St. Louis: Mosby, pp. 1685–1720.

Marieb, E.N. (2010). *Human Anatomy and Physiology*, 8th edn. San Francisco Park: Pearson.

Marieb, E.N. and Hoehn, K. (2012). *Human Anatomy and Physiology*. New Jersey: Pearson.

Mazza, D. (2011). *Women's Health in General Practice*. Edinburgh: Elsevier.

Monga, A. and Dobbs, S. (2011). *Gynaecology by Ten Teachers*, 19th edn. London: Hodder.

Morrow, C. (2009) Dysmenorrhea. In: Heidelbaugh, J.J. (ed). *Primary Care: Clinics in Office Practice*. Philadelphia: Saunders, pp. 19–32.

National Institute for Health and Clinical Excellence (2007). *Treatment and Care for Women with Heavy Periods*. London: NICE.

National Institute for Health and Clinical Excellence (2008). *Prostate Cancer*. London: NICE.

Porth, C.M. (2010). *Pathophysiology: A Concepts of Health States*, 8th edn. Philadelphia: Lippincott.

Royal College of Obstetricians and Gynaecologists (2007). *Long Term Consequences of Polycystic Ovary Syndrome: Guidance Number 23*, 2nd edn. London: RCOG.

Thibodeau, G.A. and Patton, K.T. (2010). *The Human Body in health and Disease*, 5th edn. St. Louis: Elsevier.

Thorpe, A. and Neal, D. (2003). Benign prostatic hyperplasia. *Lancet*. 361(9366): 1359–1367.

Tortora, G.J. (2011). *Principles of Anatomy and Physiology*, 13th edn. New York: Wiley.

United Nations (1994). *International Conference on Population and Development*. Report of the International Conference on Population and Development: Cairo, New York: United Nations.

Wang, S-F., Lee, J.P. and Hwa, H-L. (2009). Effect of transcutaneous electrical nerve stimulation on primary dysmenorrhea. *Neuromodulation*. 12(4): 302–309.

Warshaw, M.K. (2007). Male reproductive problems. In: Monahan, F.D., Sand, J.K., Neighbors, M., Marek, J.F. and Green, C.J. (eds). *Phipps' Medical Surgical Nursing: Health and Illness Perspectives*, 8th edn. St. Louis: Mosby, pp. 1721–1749.

15

Pain and pain management

Anthony Wheeldon

Senior Lecturer, Department of Adult Nursing and Primary Care, School of Health and Social Work, University of Hertfordshire, Hatfield, Hertfordshire, UK

Contents

Fundamentals of Applied Pathophysiology: An Essential Guide for Nursing and Healthcare Students, Second Edition. Edited by Muralitharan Nair and Ian Peate.
© 2013 John Wiley & Sons, Ltd. Published 2013 by John Wiley & Sons, Ltd.

Key words

- Acute pain
- Chronic pain
- Neuropathy
- Opioid
- Ascending pain pathway
- Descending pain pathway
- Nociceptors
- Somatic pain
- Analgesia
- Gate control theory
- Non-opioid
- Visceral pain

Test your prior knowledge

- What is the difference between acute and chronic pain?
- How would you assess a patient's pain?
- Discuss the pain pathway.
- List five non-pharmacological methods of pain control.

Learning outcomes

On completion of this section the reader will be able to:

- Describe the physiology of pain transmission and sensation.
- Explain the difference between acute and chronic pain.
- Discuss the impact of psychosocial issues on the individual with pain.
- Explain the principles of the gate control theory of pain.

Don't forget to visit to the companion website for this book (www.wiley.com/go/fundamentalsofappliedpathophysiology) where you can find self-assessment tests to check your progress, as well as lots of activities to practise your learning.

Introduction

Pain is an integral part of life. Everyone experiences it at various times throughout their lifetime; indeed, pain is the most common reason for an individual to seek medical advice. Yet, despite its prevalence, it remains difficult to define. One common definition states that 'Pain is whatever the experiencing person says it is, existing when he says it does' (McCaffery, 1979, p. 11). Pain is not only an unpleasant or uncomfortable sensation that occurs as a result of injury, strain or disease, it can also be an emotional experience unrelated to tissue damage. For example, pain is a term used to describe feelings relating to loss, grief and even unrequited love. Pain is also an individual and personal experience. The way someone expresses and deals with their pain will be determined by their culture, life experiences and personality.

Unresolved pain can have an adverse effect on the cardiovascular, respiratory, gastrointestinal, neuroendocrine and musculoskeletal systems. It can also promote anxiety and sleeplessness (MacIntyre and Ready, 2001). The management of pain is often associated with the administration of analgesia; however, there are a wide range of non-pharmacological methods of pain control available. Because it is an emotional as well as physiological phenomenon, the successful assessment and control of pain is reliant upon an individualised holistic plan of care, which utilises both pharmacological and non-pharmacological treatments.

The physiology of pain

The physiology of pain is complex and in some instances not fully understood. However, the generation of pain follows a basic three-step process (Figure 15.1).

1. An irritation or injury, such as a cut or burn, is detected in the peripheral nervous system by special nerve cells called nociceptors.
2. A nerve impulse is then generated, sending a pain impulse towards the central nervous system.
3. This message is received by the brain where the extent and significance of the irritation or injury is interpreted and pain is sensed.

Nociceptors

Nociceptors are free nerve endings present in every tissue in the body, except for the brain. They are activated by noxious stimuli, of which there are three broad types – thermal, mechanical and chemical. As the name suggests, thermal stimuli are sensations of severe heat or cold. Mechanical stimuli on the other hand are produced by tissue damage caused by trauma or disease, including:

- damage to tissue due to trauma or minor injury
- lack of blood flow and oxygen, i.e. ischaemia and hypoxia
- ulceration
- infection

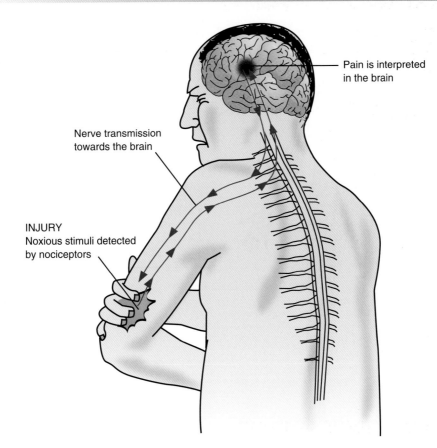

- Pain is interpreted in the brain

Nerve transmission towards the brain

INJURY
Noxious stimuli detected by nociceptors

Figure 15.1   Pathway of pain transmission and interpretation.

- nerve damage
- inflammation.

   Chemical stimuli detect the presence of chemicals such as histamine, kinins and prostaglandins, which are released as a result of tissue damage and inflammation.

   The actions of nociceptors are not clear; however, two types have been identified – polymodal nociceptors, which detect mechanical, thermal and chemical stimuli, and mechanoceptors, which sense intense mechanical stimuli only.

The ascending pain pathway

Nociceptor stimulation leads directly to the transmission of a pain impulse along special sensory fibres towards the thalamus and somatosensory cortex within the brain, where the severity and meaning of the pain is analysed. This line of communication is called the ascending pain pathway. It consists of three linked neurons called first-, second- and third-order neurons depending on their place in the pathway. The first-order neurons travel from the nociceptors to the spine;

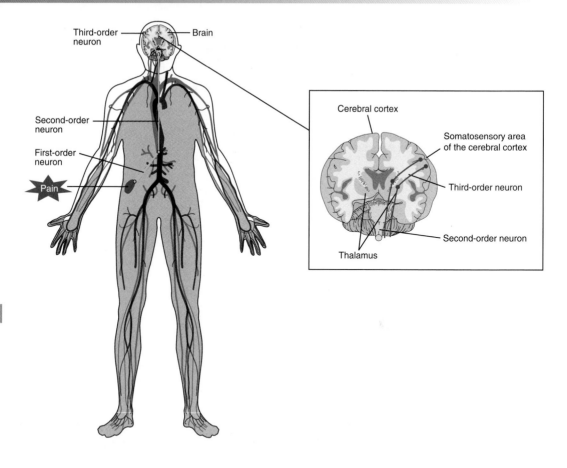

Figure 15.2   The ascending pain pathway.

second-order neurons travel upwards through the spinal cord towards the thalamus in the brain; and third-order neurons run from the thalamus through the brain towards the somatosensory area of the cerebral cortex (Figure 15.2). The line of communication between the first-, second- and third-order neurons is maintained by a number of neurotransmitters, such as substance P and serotonin (MacLellan, 2006).

The two first-order neurons responsible for the transmission of the pain impulse between the nociceptors and the spinal cord are A-delta (Aδ) fibres and C fibres. The speed of this transmission depends upon the diameter of the fibre and whether or not the fibre is myelinated. The axons of myelinated fibres are surrounded by a sheath of myelin, which electrically insulates them and increases the speed of nerve conduction (Figure 15.3). Aδ fibres are thicker and are myelinated, and therefore transmit pain impulses faster than C fibres, which are thinner and non-myelinated (Table 15.1).

Pain is often described as having two phases, referred to as first and second pain. First pain is described as a sharp or pricking pain, whereas second pain is the dull, burning or aching pain that follows. Aδ fibres are thought to receive input from mechanoceptors and also generate the first pain sensation. C fibres on the other hand are thought to receive input from polymodal nocicep-

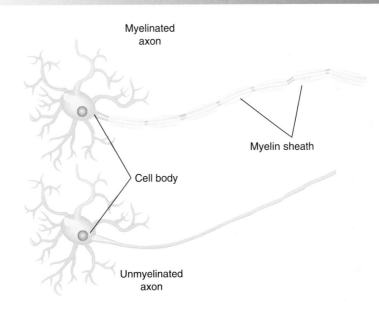

Figure 15.3   Basic structure of myelinated and unmyelinated nerve fibres.

Table 15.1   Size and speed of first-order sensory fibres.

Sensory fibre	Diameter (µm)	Myelinated	Speed of conduction (m/s)
A-beta (Aβ) fibres	6–12	Yes	35–75
A-delta (Aδ) fibres	1–5	Yes	5–35
C fibres	0.2–1.5	No	0.5–2

tors and are more likely to produce second pain. Pain impulses follow the same pathway as touch and mild heat and cold. The sensory fibres responsible for these sensations are A-beta (Aβ) fibres. Aβ fibres are myelinated and are thicker than both Aδ fibres and C fibres and therefore can transmit signals much faster. Stimulation of Aβ fibres, by rubbing a mild injury, for example, can alleviate the pain.

The first-order neurons enter the spinal cord at a location called the dorsal horn (Figure 15.4). Here they synapse (connect) with second-order neurons, of which there are two types – nociceptive-specific (NS) and wide dynamic range (WDR) neurons. Both respond to noxious stimuli; however, WDR neurons also react to non-noxious input, such as those transmitted by Aβ fibres, i.e. touch, heat and cold. Both NS and WDR neurons cross over the spinal cord into white matter, where they continue to rise up the spinal cord towards the thalamus along a pathway called the spinothalamic tract (Figure 15.5).

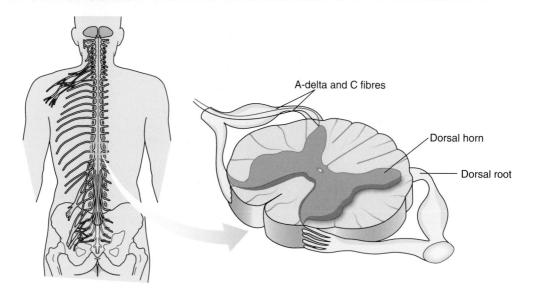

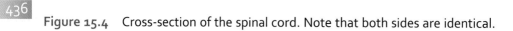

Figure 15.4   Cross-section of the spinal cord. Note that both sides are identical.

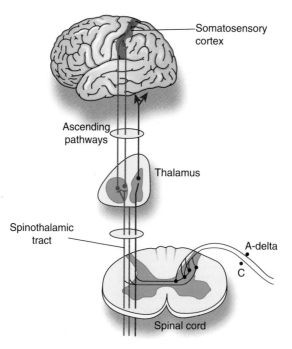

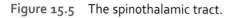

Figure 15.5   The spinothalamic tract.

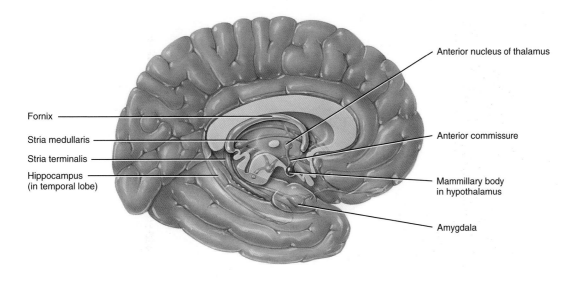

Anterior nucleus of thalamus

Fornix

Stria medullaris

Stria terminalis

Hippocampus
(in temporal lobe)

Anterior commissure

Mammillary body
in hypothalamus

Amygdala

Figure 15.6   The limbic system.

437

Pain interpretation

The spinothalamic tract ends at the thalamus, where second-order neurons meet third-order neurons. Third-order neurons travel through the brain towards the somatosensory cortex, a part of the brain that allows the individual to locate pain and describe it. As well as locating the pain, the brain will also generate an emotional response, be it anger or distress or mild irritation. The area of the brain thought to influence this emotional response is the limbic system (Figure 15.6). Often referred to as the 'emotional brain', the limbic system deals with feelings of pain, pleasure, affection and anger. An individual's response is not predictable as it is dependent upon their personality, life history and culture. The limbic system also evaluates the seriousness of the pain and helps the individual to remember why the pain occurred. Over time people learn to avoid painful stimuli, such as sharp objects and broken glass, and thus protect themselves from injury (Godfrey, 2005a). However, this protective element has its limits, e.g. individuals may deliberately expose themselves to potential injury and pain if it means rescuing a loved one from a perilous situation, i.e. from a house fire (Johnson, 2005).

Reflex arcs

Because pain is not sensed until pain messages from nociceptors have been interpreted by the brain, there is a minute fraction of time between the initial injury and pain sensation. Reflex arcs aim to reduce the amount of tissue damage by forcing the body away from the source of the injury quickly and before the brain processes the inevitable pain messages. Stepping on a pin provides a good example of a reflex arc in action. After stepping on a pin, reflex arcs ensure that the foot involuntarily moves up and away from the pin before pain is sensed, thus reducing the amount of tissue damage. Reflex arcs work by collecting pain impulses from first-order neurons and then immediately sending impulses, via interneurons, along motor nerves back towards skeletal muscle (Figure 15.7).

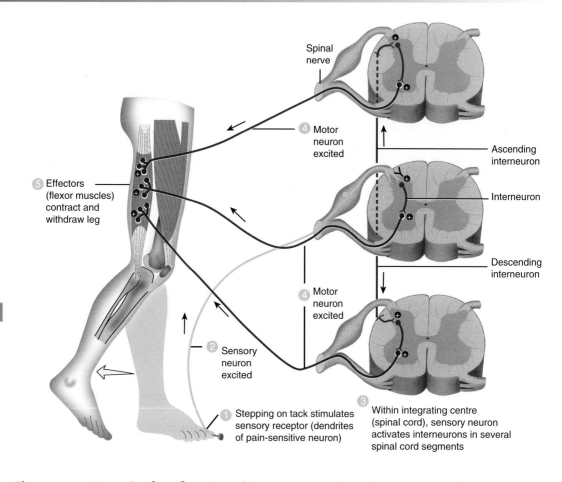

Figure 15.7   Example of a reflex arc working in response to pain.

Descending pain pathways

Descending pain pathways seek to inhibit the sensation of pain. They involve the release of special neuropeptides that have analgesic properties. They bind with opiate receptors, which are present throughout the central nervous system, and block the action of the neurotransmitter, substance P. Because of their analgesic effect these neuropeptides are often referred to as endogenous or natural opiates. There are three groups of endogenous opiate – endorphins, encephalins and dynorphins, and there are four major categories of opiate receptor – mu (μ), kappa (κ), sigma (σ) and delta (δ). Levels of endorphins, encephalins and dynorphins increase during periods of stress and pain. However, stimulation of opiate receptors also promotes feelings of euphoria and well-being, and it is endogenous opiates such as endorphins that are associated with the pleasant sensations experienced during excitement, sexual activity and even exercise.

Pain classification

Transient, acute and chronic pain

Pain is classified according to its duration. A short episode of pain, as a consequence of a stubbed toe or a cut finger, for example, is classified as transient pain. The injured individual, despite perhaps becoming momentarily upset, will consider the pain to be of no consequence and not seek medical attention.

Acute pain is associated with a severe sudden onset; however, unlike transient pain, it is prolonged and continues until healing begins. Acute pain is intense and can be an intolerable experience; in response areas of the brain seek to restore homeostasis by initiating an autonomic response. The thalamus, hypothalamus and reticular formation (Figure 15.8), for example, promote diaphoresis, tachycardia, hypertension and tachypnoea in response to acute pain.

The term chronic pain is used to describe pain that continues even though healing is complete. Although the pain may remain as intense as acute pain, there is little or no autonomic response. Acute pain is a symptom of an associated medical condition or injury. Chronic pain, on the other hand, exists after the injury or disease has ceased. For this reason, chronic pain is often considered to be a syndrome – a medical condition in its own right (Melzack and Wall, 1988).

439

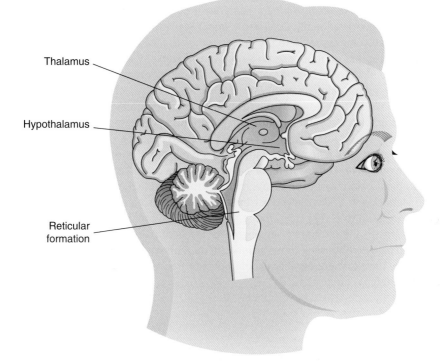

Figure 15.8   Location of the thalamus, hypothalamus and reticular formation.

Superficial and deep pain

Pain is categorised according to location and is often called deep or superficial. Superficial pain occurs due to nociceptor stimulation in the skin. Because there are large numbers of nociceptors in skin, pain can be easily located. Acute superficial pain is often described as a sharp, pricking sensation. Deep pain, on the other hand, is dull and prolonged. Deep pain can be either somatic or visceral. Somatic pain emanates from structures such as bones, muscles, joints and tendons. Visceral pain is produced when nociceptors in organs such as the kidneys, stomach, gallbladder and intestines are stimulated. Unlike the skin, these organs and others like them have far fewer nociceptors, and therefore it is often difficult for an individual to describe the exact location of their pain (MacLellan, 2006).

The pain experience

The term pain threshold is often used to describe an individual's response to pain, e.g. a patient may be said to have a high or low pain threshold. Pain threshold is the point at which an individual will report pain. It is generally accepted that all humans have a similar pain threshold. People nonetheless express pain in a variety of ways. This is because the expression of pain is influenced by emotional state, personality, past experience, culture and social status, rather than a personal pain threshold.

The limbic system, which processes emotional responses to pain, interacts closely with the frontal lobes, which are responsible for cognitive thought. This explains why people in acute pain may at times behave irrationally. Conversely, people can often control their emotions if pain occurs when it is socially unacceptable to cry out or complain (Marieb and Hoehn, 2007). The person's state of mind also has an influence on pain intensity. Anxiety and depression, for example, have been shown to increase pain levels (Carr et al., 2005), whereas reducing anxiety levels through education can reduce pain (Lin and Wang, 2005).

An individual's attitude towards pain can also affect its intensity. Attitudes towards pain are often influenced by the meaning of the pain experience. For example, patients having undergone elective surgery report less pain than patients involved in sudden traumatic accidents. This may be because postsurgical pain may be viewed as a symptom of surgery and healing, and therefore as something positive. The meaning of pain can change and alter pain perception. For instance, mild abdominal pain may become severe when the individual learns that it may be something serious (Melzack and Wall, 1988). Past experiences are also a contributing factor. Patients who have been exposed to severe pain during a prior medical procedure may become anxious about future treatments and ultimately sense greater levels of pain. People also learn how to express and react to pain by observing those around them. A person's attitude towards their pain may be influenced by the experiences of family members or their ethnicity and culture (Briggs, 2010; Bell and Duffy, 2009).

Pain theories

Most pain theories acknowledge that the pain experience is both emotional and psychological. The specificity theory hypothesises that pain is experienced when specific nerve endings are stimulated. Information is then carried to a pain centre in the brain. It is the characteristics of the stimulus that determines the intensity of the pain, rather than the brain. Pattern theory, on the other hand, suggests that no separate system for pain sensation exists. Rather pain is interpreted by the brain when intense peripheral nerve stimulation occurs. Such theories do not explain why pain can occur as a result of a gentle stimulus, i.e. neuralgia, or when no tissue damage exists. Neither do they explain why two people with the same injury may experience different levels of pain. For this reason, Melzack and Wall's gate control theory is more widely accepted as the most important pain theory.

Gate control theory of pain

The gate control theory of pain proposes that pain impulses must pass through a theoretical 'gate' at the dorsal horn of the spinal cord before ascending towards the brain (Figure 15.9). Pain

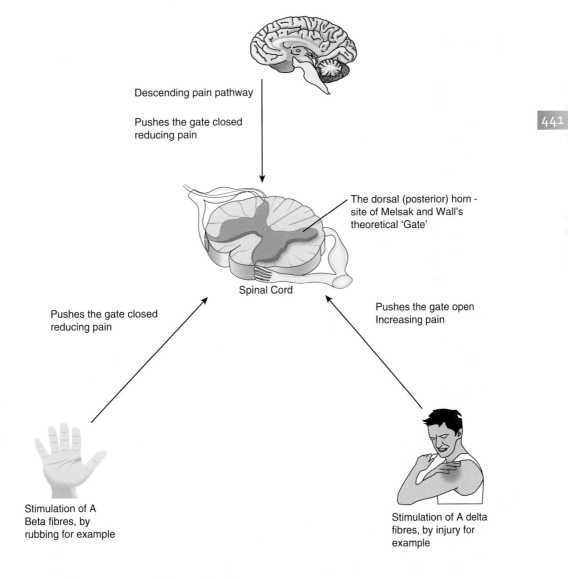

Descending pain pathway

Pushes the gate closed
reducing pain

The dorsal (posterior) horn -
site of Melsak and Wall's
theoretical 'Gate'

Spinal Cord

Pushes the gate closed
reducing pain

Pushes the gate open
Increasing pain

Stimulation of A
Beta fibres, by
rubbing for example

Stimulation of A delta
fibres, by injury for
example

Figure 15.9   The gate control theory of pain.

messages from Aδ and C fibres will push open the gate. However, the actions of Aβ fibres and the descending pain pathway will push the gate closed. The intensity of an individual's pain, therefore, is determined by a balance between noxious stimuli and Aβ fibre or descending brain activity. The wider the gate opens, the more intense the pain; if the gate closes, the pain ceases (McCaffery et al., 2003).

Stimulation of the larger Aβ fibres with touch or heat can inhibit pain transmission via Aδ and C fibres. This helps explain how rubbing mild injuries, acupuncture and transcutaneous electrical nerve stimulation (TENS) may reduce pain levels. Increased activity in the descending pain pathway also seeks to close the gate to pain. This may explain why a person's emotional state, personality and culture may determine how pain is expressed. For example, increased levels of endogenous opiates can push the gate closed. The gate control theory also proposes that pain intensity is influenced by the action of transmission cells and substantia gelatinosa cells, which are found within the dorsal horn of the spinal cord. Transmission (T) cells transmit pain messages towards the brain. Substantia gelatinosa (SG) cells, on the other hand, inhibit T-cell activity and thus push the gate to pain closed. The activity of both T cells and SG cells are enhanced by the descending pain pathway and therefore the individual's state of mind. In depressive and anxious states, T-cell activity is enhanced, pushing the gate open and increasing pain intensity. However, in relaxed and contented states, SG cell action is increased, pushing the gate closed and decreasing pain levels (Melzack and Wall, 1988; Figure 15.10).

Pain pathophysiology and management

Learning outcomes

On completion of this section the reader will be able to:

- Discuss the pathophysiology of a range of pain disorders.
- Discuss the impact of postoperative pain, neurogenic pain and oncology pain.
- Identify an effective range of pain assessment strategies.
- Explain the difference between opioid and non-opioid analgesics.
- List a range of effective non-pharmacological pain control interventions.

Pathophysiology

Referred and phantom limb pain

Referred pain occurs when tissue damage in one area of the body leads to pain elsewhere, e.g. pain as a result of angina. Although the tissue damage arises in the coronary arteries, pain is also felt radiating down the left arm. Despite sensing intense pain, the tissue there remains healthy. Referred pain happens because the damaged or inflamed organ and the area where pain is felt are served by nerves from the same segment of the spinal cord. Other examples include pain due

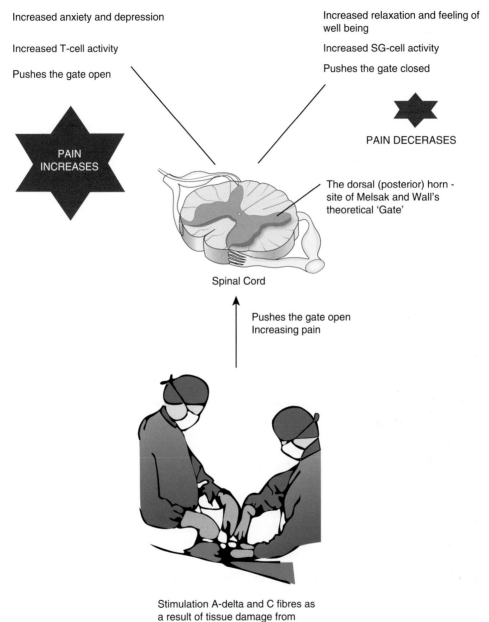

Increased anxiety and depression

Increased T-cell activity

Pushes the gate open

Increased relaxation and feeling of well being

Increased SG-cell activity

Pushes the gate closed

PAIN
INCREASES

PAIN DECERASES

The dorsal (posterior) horn - site of Melsak and Wall's theoretical 'Gate'

Spinal Cord

Pushes the gate open
Increasing pain

Stimulation A-delta and C fibres as a result of tissue damage from surgery

Figure 15.10 The gate control theory and the influence of T (transmission)- and SG (substantia gelatinosa)-cell activity.

443

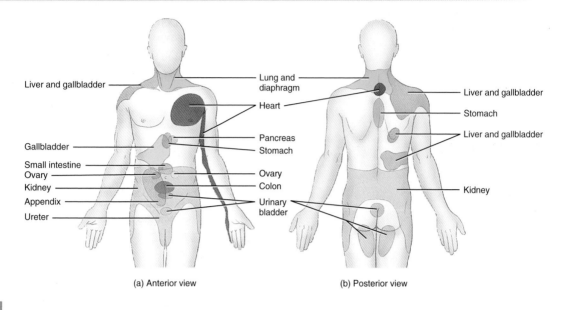

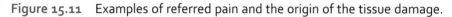

(a) Anterior view   (b) Posterior view

Figure 15.11   Examples of referred pain and the origin of the tissue damage.

to liver or gallbladder inflammation being sensed in the right shoulder. Figure 15.11 highlights the main instances of referred pain (Tortora and Derrickson, 2011).

The term phantom limb pain describes the pain sensed by amputees where the removed limb once was. The pain is often described as tingling, numbness, itching or tickling and it has been reported by the majority of trauma and surgical amputees (Richardson et al., 2006). The precise pathophysiology is unknown. However, there are two possible explanations. First, the brain interprets pain impulses from damaged fibres in and around the site of amputation (the stump) as pain signals for the whole (now non-existent) limb. Another possibility is that the brain contains neurons that produce an awareness of body shape and that the neurons that processed information from the removed limb are still active (Richardson, 2008).

Neuropathy

Neuropathic pain occurs when the nociceptors and neurons are damaged. There are many conditions that lead to the development of neuropathic pain:

- entrapment (trapped nerves)
- causalgia (sensory nerve damage)
- scar tissue
- thoracotomy
- amputation
- diabetes
- herpes
- ischaemia.

Neuropathies produce pain that is described as a burning, electric or tingling, and the pain can be continuous or spasmodic. The nervous tissue in the ascending pain pathways is said to be plastic, meaning it can change in response to psychological and physical stimuli. This includes changes to the sensitivity of nociceptors, which can begin to generate pain impulses in response to ordinary feelings of touch. The patient may complain of pain when slight pressure is exerted on the site of injury, a phenomenon called allodynia. Damaged neural tissue also leads to increased sensitivity to painful stimuli and the individual will feel pain that is out of proportion to the level of tissue damage. This increase in pain sensitivity is referred to as hyperalgesia (Scadding, 2003).

Postoperative pain

Almost all patients undergoing surgery experience pain afterwards, with up to 80% of patient reporting severe pain (Manias, 2003). A significant contributory factor to postoperative pain is anxiety, which can increase pain intensity. Anxiety and depression prior to surgery lead to high levels of anxiety postoperatively (Carr et al., 2005). In order to reduce postoperative pain, carers should invest in preoperative care strategies that minimise preoperative anxiety, such as patient education (Johansson et al., 2005). Carers are also ideally placed to minimise postoperative pain as they are responsible for the administration and evaluation of prescribed analgesics.

Unresolved pain leads to a complicated postsurgical recovery. Pain in the chest or abdomen, for example, can affect respiration. People in pain tend to breathe shallowly and avoid coughing. Painful movement can also render patients reluctant to mobilise. Pain also slows down gastric emptying and reduces intestinal motility, probably due to the activation of a reflex arc. Prolonged pain also increases levels of anxiety. Indeed, pain and anxiety are intertwined problems as during the postoperative period one inevitably leads to the other. The effects of unresolved anxiety can have a severe detrimental effect on the patient's postoperative recovery. Prolonged anxiety will lead to a stress response as the body attempts to maintain homeostasis. During stress the neuroendocrine system releases numerous hormones that increase blood pressure, pulse and metabolism. Epinephrine (adrenaline), for example, increases heart rate and aldosterone increases blood pressure. Cortisol and glucagon, on the other hand, liberate more glucose for the production of energy. Cortisol also decreases immune function (MacIntyre and Ready, 2001). The combination of unresolved pain and anxiety affects many major body systems, which can lead to chest infection, impaired wound healing and deep vein thrombosis among other complications (Table 15.2).

Cancer pain

There is a high prevalence of pain in patients with cancer. Indeed, in some studies up to 96% of patients with cancer experience pain, more than those with HIV (80%), heart disease (77%), renal disease (77%) and chronic obstructive pulmonary disease (50%) (Solano et al., 2006). The causes of cancer pain are wide and varied, but the most common cancer pain is that caused by bone metastases. Cancer pain can be classified as being either nociceptive or neuropathic. Table 15.3 lists the common causes and descriptions of cancer pain.

The aim of palliative care is to minimise pain and its associated distressing symptoms (World Health Organization, 2002). Cancer pain is therefore classified according to when it occurs or if it becomes more intense and unmanageable. There are three classifications of cancer pain:

- Breakthrough pain – pain that is more intense than normal.
- Incident pain – pain caused by specific activities, i.e. walking, lifting, etc.
- End of dose failure pain – occurs if effects of analgesia subside before the next dose is due.

Table 15.2   The effects of pain and stress on four major body systems.

System	Response	Consequence
Respiratory system	Hypoventilation	Hypoxaemia
	Decreased cough	Hypoxia
	Tachypnoea	Retained sputum
		Chest infection
Cardiovascular system	Tachycardia	Elevated heart workload
	Hypertension	Deep vein thrombosis
	Reduced venous return	Pulmonary embolism
	Coronary vasoconstriction	
Musculoskeletal system	Reduced mobility	Prolonged postoperative recovery
	Muscle atrophy	Deep vein thrombosis
		Pulmonary embolism
Gastrointestinal system	Delayed gastric emptying	Nausea and vomiting
	Intestinal motility	Reduced nutrition
		Poor wound healing
Renal system	Increased retention of sodium and water	Lower urine output
Pancreas	Increased glucagon	Increased blood sugar levels
	Decreased insulin	

Adapted from Cousins and Power (2003); Macintyre and Ready (2001).

Table 15.3   Types of cancer pain, their source, causes and descriptions.

Type of pain	Structures affected	Causes	Patient description
Somatic nociceptor	Muscle and bone	Bone metastases	Aching, sharp, gnawing or dull
		Surgical incisions	Easily located
Neuropathic	Nerves	Chemotherapy	Burning, itching, numbness, tingling, shooting
		Tumour	
Visceral nociceptor	Organs of the abdomen, pelvis and thorax	Tumour	Crampy, colicky, aching, deep, squeezing, dull
			Less easily located

Listed in order of prevalence. Most patients have a combination of somatic and visceral nociceptor pain.
Adapted from Kochhar (2002).

447

Breakthrough and incident pain are common even in patients whose pain is well controlled. End of dose pain, however, is an indicator that the patient's current pain control may need reviewing (Hayden, 2006).

Case study

Chloe is a 34-year-old teacher. She was brought into accident and emergency by her husband after complaining of severe abdominal pain for the past 2 hours. She states that on a scale of 1 to 10, where 10 is the worst pain imaginable, her pain scores 9. The pain is constant and intense. On examination she is cold and clammy to touch, her pulse is 120 beats per minute and her blood pressurs is 155/110 mmHg. The medical team decides to admit Chloe for further investigations and she is booked in for an emergency laparotomy.

Take some time to reflect on this case and then consider the following.

1.   What type of pain is Chloe suffering from, and how would you classify and categorise this kind of pain?
2.   Chloe is going for surgery. How do you think she will feel prior to the surgery and how might her level of pain impact on postoperative pain?
3.   Which analgesia may be prescribed for Chloe and what are their major side effects?

Pain assessment

Effective pain assessment allows the practitioner to best select appropriate pharmacological and non-pharmacological interventions. However, pain is a complex multifaceted phenomenon and

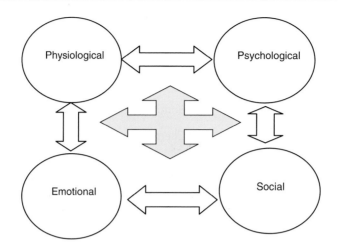

Figure 15.12   Four dimensions of the pain experience. (Adapted from Manias *et al.*, 2002.)

its assessment can be challenging. The pain experience involves four dimensions, all of which are interlinked (Figure 15.12). Any health assessment must pay attention to physiological, psychological, emotional and social aspects of pain if effective holistic care is to occur (Manias *et al.*, 2002). Furthermore, pain is a subjective experience and the healthcare professional must rely on the patient's own description of the pain. However, many patients are often unable to verbalise or describe their pain. For this reason, non-verbal cues are of particular importance.

A description of pain is rarely enough to determine appropriate treatment. Further information on the location, duration and onset of pain can aid healthcare professionals in managing the patient's pain. Every pain assessment must also include the following:

- Location of pain – where is the pain, does it radiate anywhere?
- Duration of pain – how long has the patient had the pain?
- Onset – when did the pain start and what was the patient doing at the time?
- Frequency – how often does the pain occur?
- Intensity – how painful is it; does the level of pain change?
- Aggravating factors – what makes the pain worse?
- Relieving factors – what makes the pain feel better?
- Other symptoms – does the patient feel dizzy, nauseous, sweaty or short of breath?
- Sleep patterns – does the pain keep the patient awake? (Godfrey, 2005b; MacLellan, 2006)

Further information on the patient's psychological and emotional response to their pain should also be gathered. For example:

- the patient's expectations of any potential treatments
- the patient's concerns of the cause of their pain
- any personal or spiritual beliefs
- acceptable pain levels

- pain levels that will allow the patient to return to work
- feelings of stress and anxiety
- any coping mechanisms
- the patient's preferences regarding treatment options. (MacLellan, 2006).

Acute pain also produces an autonomic response and often patients will present with hypertension, tachycardia and changes in respiratory rate. Pain assessment should therefore include measurement of blood pressure, pulse, temperature and respiration rate. However, chronic pain may not have an adverse effect on these vital signs; therefore, the patient's description of the pain should remain the principal indicator of pain intensity.

Formal structured pain assessment tools can facilitate pain assessment. There is a variety of pain assessment tools at the carer's disposal, ranging from simple single-dimension scales to comprehensive pain questionnaires. The most common single-dimension scales are the verbal rating scale, the visual analogue rating scale and the numerical rating scale. Verbal rating scales ask the patient to select which adjective from a list best describes their pain (Figure 15.13), and with a numerical scale the patient assigns a number to match the pain intensity (Figure 15.14). The visual analogue scale is much simpler. The patient is shown a basic continuum running from no pain to worst pain possible. The patient can point or state whereabouts on the continuum their pain is (Figure 15.15). The main advantage of simple rating scales is their ease of use. They can be utilised swiftly and do not overburden the acutely sick person. Nevertheless, they only assess one aspect of pain, its intensity, and there is an assumption that the patient will be literate (MacLellan, 2006).

The most common multidimensional pain assessment tool is the McGill Pain Questionnaire (Figure 15.16). This comprehensive assessment tool contains a series of adjectives that patients

449

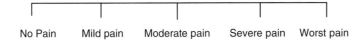

No Pain   Mild pain   Moderate pain   Severe pain   Worst pain

Figure 15.13   An example of a verbal rating scale.

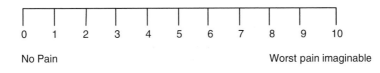

0   1   2   3   4   5   6   7   8   9   10

No Pain   Worst pain imaginable

Figure 15.14   An example of a numerical rating scale.

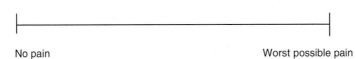

No pain   Worst possible pain

Figure 15.15   An example of a visual analogue scale.

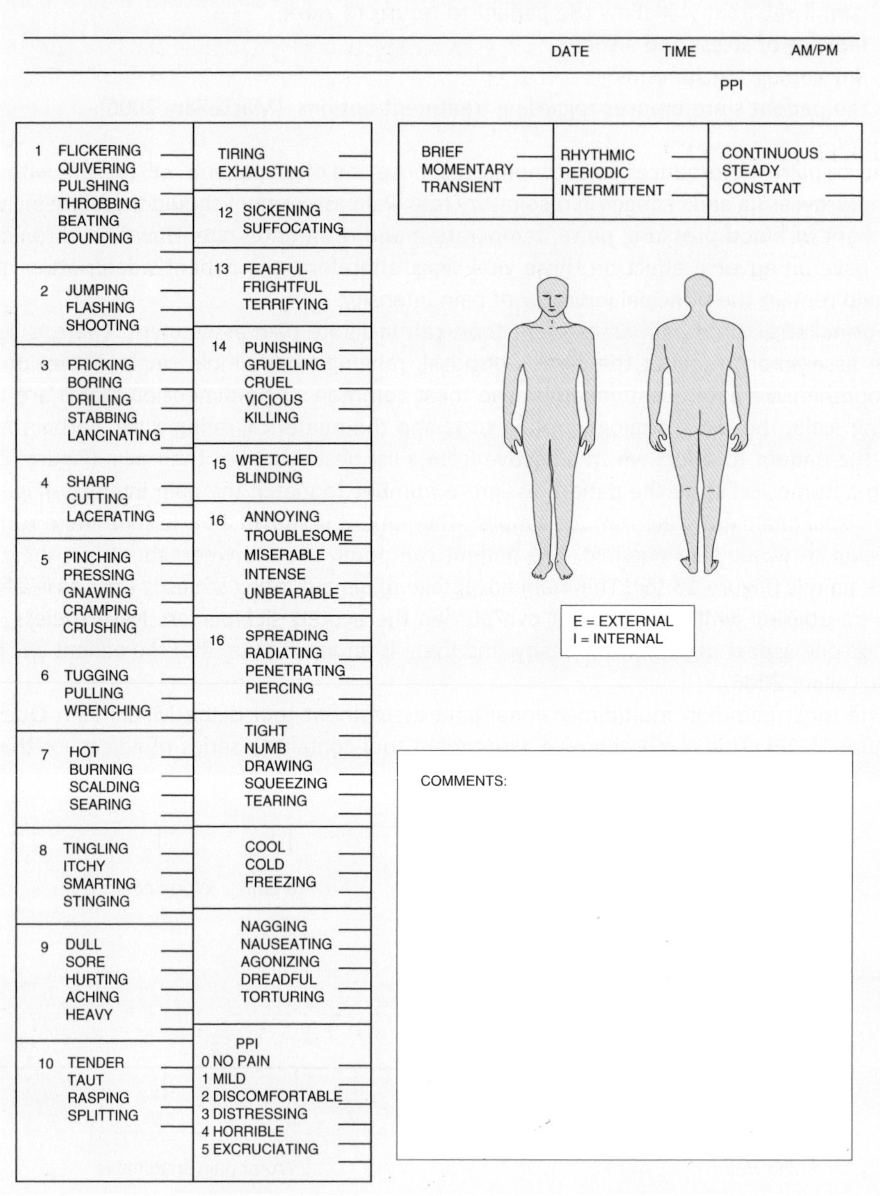

DATE TIME AM/PM

PPI

1 FLICKERING
QUIVERING
PULSHING
THROBBING
BEATING
POUNDING

2 JUMPING
FLASHING
SHOOTING

3 PRICKING
BORING
DRILLING
STABBING
LANCINATING

4 SHARP
CUTTING
LACERATING

5 PINCHING
PRESSING
GNAWING
CRAMPING
CRUSHING

6 TUGGING
PULLING
WRENCHING

7 HOT
BURNING
SCALDING
SEARING

8 TINGLING
ITCHY
SMARTING
STINGING

9 DULL
SORE
HURTING
ACHING
HEAVY

10 TENDER
TAUT
RASPING
SPLITTING

TIRING
EXHAUSTING

12 SICKENING
SUFFOCATING

13 FEARFUL
FRIGHTFUL
TERRIFYING

14 PUNISHING
GRUELLING
CRUEL
VICIOUS
KILLING

15 WRETCHED
BLINDING

16 ANNOYING
TROUBLESOME
MISERABLE
INTENSE
UNBEARABLE

16 SPREADING
RADIATING
PENETRATING
PIERCING

TIGHT
NUMB
DRAWING
SQUEEZING
TEARING

COOL
COLD
FREEZING

NAGGING
NAUSEATING
AGONIZING
DREADFUL
TORTURING

PPI
0 NO PAIN
1 MILD
2 DISCOMFORTABLE
3 DISTRESSING
4 HORRIBLE
5 EXCRUCIATING

BRIEF
MOMENTARY
TRANSIENT

RHYTHMIC
PERIODIC
INTERMITTENT

CONTINUOUS
STEADY
CONSTANT

E = EXTERNAL
I = INTERNAL

COMMENTS:

Figure 15.16 The McGill Pain Questionnaire (Melzack and Torgerson, 1971).

can use to describe their pain. The descriptive words are divided into three classes – sensory, affective and evaluative. The questionnaire also utilises a rating scale that runs from 0 – no pain to 5 – excruciating. The assessment of pain is based on three measures – the pain rating index (PRI), which is based on the numerical values assigned to each number; the number of words selected; and the rating scale or present pain index (PPI). The McGill Pain Questionnaire also has line drawings of the human body that can facilitate the location of the pain. The McGill Pain Questionnaire is now widely used to assess chronic pain and has been shown to be very effective when measuring pain in arthritis (Grafton *et al.*, 2005).

Pain management

Pain management or control can be either pharmacological or non-pharmacological. Pharmacological pain management involves the administration of drugs. Drugs that are used for pain control are referred to as analgesia or analgesics. There are two main types of analgesia – opioids (or opiates) and non-opioids. As the name suggests, non-pharmacological pain management does not involve any drugs. As pain is a total experience, effective pain control is often achieved through a combination of both approaches (Hader and Guy, 2004).

Opioids

Opioid drugs are used for moderate to severe pain. They work by mimicking the body's own endogenous opiates by binding to opiate receptors in the central nervous system. Opiate receptors such as μ, κ and δ block the action of substance P when stimulated. However, unlike endogenous opiates such as endorphins, opioids are not rapidly broken down by the body. Therefore, their analgesic effects are powerful and long-lasting. In addition to analgesia the stimulation of opiate receptors produces many other physiological changes (Table 15.4), which the healthcare professional needs to be aware of:

451

- respiratory depression
- constipation
- nausea and vomiting
- drowsiness
- bradycardia
- hypotension.

Opioids are controlled drugs governed by the Misuse of Drugs Act 1971 (Her Majesty's Stationery Office, 1971). Opioid drugs are classified as either weak or strong. Despite their name, weak opioids are very effective analgesics. The main weak opioids are used in combination with non-opioid analgesia such as paracetamol or aspirin. Such combinations are prescription only rather than controlled drugs (Her Majesty's Stationery Office, 1968). Tables 15.5 and 15.6 summarise the main weak and strong opioids used in the NHS.

In some instances patients can administer their own opioid drugs via a system known as patient-controlled analgesia (PCA). The patient is attached to a small syringe driver that contains an opioid drug. The syringe is operated by a button, which when pressed by the patient delivers a set dosage. To protect against overdose, after each dose the syringe driver locks for a short time and no drug can be delivered, even if the button is pressed. Patient-controlled analgesia has been routinely and safely used for the past 30 years (Layzell, 2008).

Non-opioid drugs

Non-opioid analgesia is used for mild to moderate pain and is rarely effective in acute or postoperative pain. However, it can enhance the effect of opioid drugs, and when used in combination with opioids can reduce opioid use by 20–40% (MacIntyre and Ready, 2001). The most common

Table 15.4 Actions of opiate receptors.

Receptor	Physiological effects
Mu (μ)	Analgesia
	Euphoria
	Respiratory depression
	Bradycardia
	Nausea and vomiting
	Inhibition of gut motility
	Miosis
	Pruritus
	Smooth muscle spasm
	Physical dependence
Kappa (κ)	Analgesia
	Sedation
	Dysphoria
	Respiratory depression
	Physical dependence
Delta (δ)	Analgesia
	Euphoria
	Respiratory depression
	Miosis
	Inhibition of gut motility
	Smooth muscle spasm
	Physical dependence

non-opioid drug is paracetamol (acetaminophen). The precise action of paracetamol remains controversial; however, it is widely thought to suppress the production of prostaglandins. Prostaglandins are hormone-like substances that increase inflammation and also stimulate nociceptors and promote pain. Paracetamol is an effective analgesic; however, it rarely acts for longer than 4 hours and therefore may not be appropriate for prolonged pain. Despite its relative safety, paracetamol can cause liver failure even in small overdoses.

Table 15.5   Common weak opiates and their routes of delivery.

Drug	Preparations	Route
Codeine	Codeine phosphate	Oral – tablet, syrup
		Injection (controlled drug)
	Co-codamol (Paracodol®)	Oral – capsule and dispersible tablets
	Codeine phosphate 8 mg or 30 mg with 500 mg paracetamol	
	Co-codaprin®	Oral – dispersible tablets
	Codeine phosphate 8 mg with 400 mg aspirin	
Dihydrocodeine	Dihydrocodeine (DF118®)	Oral – tablet
		Injection (controlled drug)
	Co-dyramol	Oral – tablet
	Dihydrocodeine 10 mg with 500 mg paracetamol	
Tramadol	Tramadol (Zydol®)	Oral – capsule
		Injection
	Tramacet®	Oral – tablet
	Tramadol 37.5 mg with 325 mg paracetamol	

Prostaglandins are derived from arachidonic acid, which is released from damaged cells. The production of prostaglandins from arachidonic acid is accelerated by the presence of an enzyme called cyclo-oxygenase-2 (COX-2) (Figure 15.17). Analgesics that suppress prostaglandin production are collectively known as non-steroidal anti-inflammatory drugs (NSAIDs). There are many different NSAIDs used in the UK (Box 15.1); however, the main ones are aspirin, ibuprofen, diclofenac, indomethacin and naproxen. In addition to the suppression of COX-2, NSAIDs can also suppress another enzyme, cyclo-oxygenase-1 (COX-1), which promotes prostaglandin production in the stomach where it performs an important protective role by inhibiting gastric acid. A major side effect of NSAIDs is, therefore, the development of gastric irritation and ulcers (Gilron *et al.*, 2003). NSAIDs are also associated with hypersensitive reactions in patients with asthma (Jenkins *et al.*, 2004).

Non-opioid analgesics have actions other than pain control, e.g. temperature control and prophylaxis of heart disease. Because prostaglandins promote fever as well as inflammation, NSAIDs and paracetamol may reduce core body temperature and are often used solely to reduce pyrexia. Aspirin also has antiplatelet properties. Used in small doses, it has been shown to reduce the risk of cardiovascular disease.

Table 15.6   Common strong opiates and their routes of delivery.

Drug	Examples	Route
Morphine	Morphine	Injection
		Suppository
	Oramorph®	Oral – liquid, tablet
	Sevredol®	Oral – tablet
	MST Continus®	Oral – tablet, suspension
Diamorphine	Diamorphine	Oral – tablet
		Injection
Oxycodone	Oxynorm®	Oral – tablet, liquid
		Injection
	Oxycontin®	Oral – tablet
Fentanyl	Fentanyl	Patch
		Injection
	Durogesic	Patch
	DTrans®	
Pethidine	Pethidine	Oral – tablets
		Injection
	Pamergan	Oral – tablets
	P100®	Injection

The analgesic ladder

The World Health Organization (WHO) produced the analgesic ladder in 1986 to help combat cancer pain. However, it is now widely used to manage many different types of pain (Godfrey, 2005b). The ladder has three steps, each containing a recommended level of pharmacological treatment (Figure 15.18). If pain persists, the patient's treatment should be moved up to the next step. The goal is for the patient to be pain free at the lowest point on the ladder. Step one involves the use of non-opioid drugs, step two recommends adding a weak opioid and the final step advocates the use of strong opioids. Each step also suggests the use of an adjuvant. Adjuvants are a range of drugs that have analgesic effects despite being normally prescribed for other conditions. Antidepressants, anticonvulsants, muscle relaxants, corticosteroids and local anaesthetics have all been shown to reduce pain when used in conjunction with opioid and non-opioid drugs.

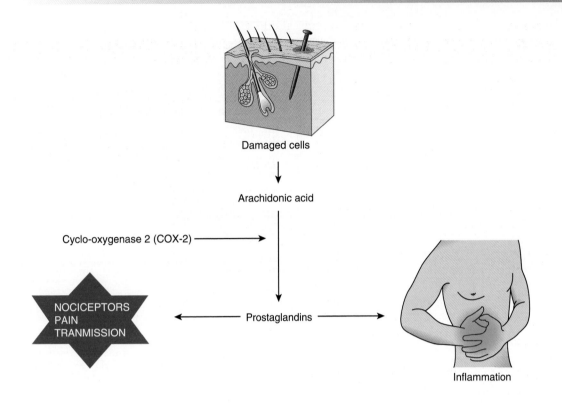

Figure 15.17   The prostaglandin-enhancing action of cyclo-oxygenase-2 (COX-2) enhancing prostaglandin action.

Box 15.1   Common NSAIDs (trade name).

Aceclofenac (Preservex®)
Acemetacin (Emflex®)
Aspirin (Caprin®)
Azapropazone (Rheumox®)
Celecoxib (Celebrex®)
Dexibuprofen (Seractil®)
Dexketoprofen (Keral®)
Diclofenac (Volterol®)
Etodolac

Etoricoxib (Arcoxia®)
Fenbufen (Fenbufen®)
Fenoprofen (Fenopron®)
Flurbiprofen (Froben®)
Ibuprofen (Brufen®)
Indometacin (Rimacid®)
Ketoprofen (Orudis®)

Mefenamic acid (Ponstan®)
Meloxican (Mobic®)
Nabumetone (Relifex®)
Naproxen (Arthroxen®)
Piroxicam (Brexidol®)
Sulindac (Clinoril®)
Tenoxicam (Mobiflex®)
Tiaprofenic acid (Surgam®)

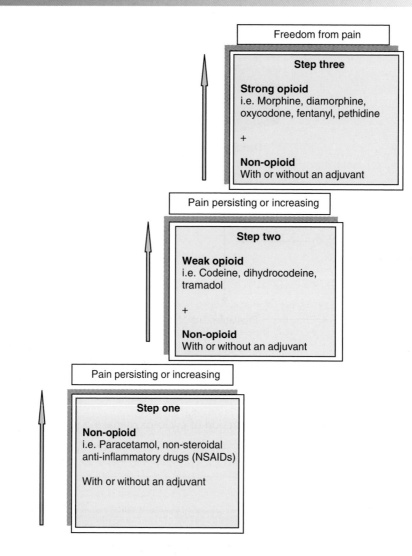

Figure 15.18   The World Health Organization analgesic ladder (WHO, 1986).

Non-pharmacological pain management

There are many different forms of non-pharmacological pain management interventions available in the UK:

- cognitive behavioural therapy
- transcutaneous electric nerve stimulation (TENS)
- application of heat and cold substances
- acupuncture
- Alexander technique
- aromatherapy

- massage
- chiropractic treatment
- hypnosis
- homeopathy
- meditation
- osteopathy
- reflexology
- relaxation
- shiatsu. (Wigens, 2006)

There is only evidence of effectiveness for a small number of techniques, e.g. massage and cognitive behavioural therapy (Furlan *et al.*, 2002; Eccleston *et al.*, 2009). As a result, the use of non-pharmacological pain control is controversial, with many healthcare professionals being sceptical of their effectiveness (Wigens, 2006).

Physical interventions

Many non-pharmacological pain control techniques have a physiological basis. A transcutaneous electric nerve stimulation (TENS) machine, for example, sends a constant stream of small electrical impulses through the skin (Figure 15.19). These impulses are thought to reduce pain in two ways. First, they may stimulate the large diameter Aβ fibres and interrupt the pain impulse travelling along the smaller Aδ and C fibres, i.e. the same effect as rubbing a mild injury. Second, the continuous electrical stimulation may increase levels of endogenous opiates such as endorphins (Sluka and Walsh, 2003). TENS machines are widely used for the treatment of postoperative pain, chronic pain, back pain and pain during labour and childbirth; however, evidence of its effectiveness remains inconclusive (Nnoaham and Kumbang, 2008).

Acupuncture is the insertion of fine needles at strategic points around the body. It too is thought to stimulate the release of endogenous opiates (Lundeberg and Stener-Victorin, 2002). Acupuncture is widely used and is accepted as an effective analgesia in many countries; however, there is very little evidence to suggest that it is effective (Lee and Ernst, 2005).

The stimulation of large diameter Aβ fibres also helps explain the therapeutic effects of pressure- and touch-based interventions such as osteopathy, reflexology and shiatsu. The most widely

457

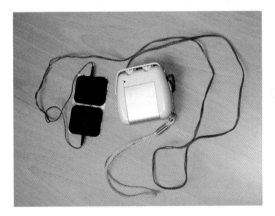

Figure 15.19   Transcutaneous electrical nerve stimulation (TENS) machine.

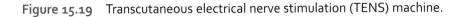

used touch- and pressure-based intervention is massage. Massage has been shown to be potentially effective in patients with low back pain (Furlan *et al*., 2002). As well as sensing pressure and touch, Aβ fibres also respond to sensations of heat and cold. The therapeutic effects of mild heat and ice packs on injuries are well known. Heat can also be used to alleviate menstrual pain as well as joint and muscle strains. However, there is little evidence for the use of heat and cold substances in the clinical setting (French *et al*., 2005).

Psychological interventions

Pain is a holistic experience and the psychological aspects of the pain experience are an integral aspect of pain sensation. The gate control theory of pain suggests that descending pain pathways from the brain influence pain intensity. Furthermore, anxiety, stress and low mood states are significant factors that can increase pain sensation. Any non-pharmacological method that can alleviate anxiety, stress or help an individual to cope with their pain could be beneficial. It is not surprising therefore that psychological-based non-pharmacological pain control methods are being increasingly utilized by chronic pain sufferers (Dopson, 2010).

Psychological-based pain control interventions range from simplistic methods such as relaxation and distraction to more alternative therapies such as meditation, Alexander technique and hypnotherapy. A more intense psychological approach is cognitive behavioural therapy (CBT). CBT involves a series of structured, patient-focused sessions that aim to address the individual's psychological and emotional experience of their pain and enable them to self-manage and control their anxiety and therefore their pain. CBT should complement rather than replace traditional pharmacology-based therapies. As a pain control method for those in chronic pain, CBT has proved effective (Eccleston *et al*., 2009).

Case study

Derek is 38 years old and has been suffering from pain in his shoulder and right arm for the past 6 months. The intensity has gradually increased over recent months. Although he cannot remember injuring his shoulder, he has a very physical job working for a removals firm and believes continual muscle strain is the cause. Derek has been taking non-steroidal anti-inflammatory drugs for the pain but finds they provide little relief. The pain is such that he finds it difficult to sleep, concentrate or socialise. Today he has visited his GP for more advice. Derek is recently divorced and his ex-wife and their children now live 100 miles away.

Take some time to reflect on this case and then consider the following.

1. What type of pain is Derek suffering from, and how would you classify and categorise this kind of pain?
2. How do non-steroidal anti-inflammatory drugs work and what are their main side effects?
3. What further treatment options are at the GP's disposal and what advice would you provide?

Conclusion

Pain is a personal experience. The brain plays a fundamental role in the interpretation of pain and therefore a patient's state of mind, personality, background and culture will all shape the way in which an individual expresses or verbalises their pain. Acute pain affects the function of many body systems and left unresolved can become prolonged chronic pain. Pain control therefore is essential if homeostasis is to be maintained. There are many forms of analgesia that can be used to control pain; however, as pain is an emotional as well as physiological phenomenon, non-pharmacological methods should also be utilised, especially for the patient in chronic pain. Because pain is individualized, the selection of appropriate pharmacological and non-pharmacological pain management strategies is reliant upon a comprehensive and holistic assessment. Healthcare professionals are therefore ideally placed to provide effective care for the patient with pain.

Test your knowledge

- List the structures involved in the ascending pain pathway and describe their functions.

- Explain why two different people with the same injury may have different pain experiences.

- Explain the purpose of a reflex arc

- What are the main differences between acute and chronic pain?

- What are the major side effects of opioid analgesia and explain why they may occur?

- Using the gate control theory of pain, explain why a patient may find non-pharmacological methods of pain control effective.

Activities

Here are some activities and exercises to help test your learning. For the answers to these exercises, as well as further self-testing activities, visit our website at www.wiley.com/go/fundamentalsofappliedpathophysiology

Fill in the blanks

Pain is classified according to its _____. Pain of a short duration is called _____ pain. _____ pain is severe and associated with a _____ onset. It stimulates an _____ response and patients can often present with _____, _____, _____ and _____. Pain that continues even after healing has occurred is _____ pain. Pain is also categorized according to its _____. Superficial pain originates from the _____ and deep pain emanates from body tissue. Deep pain can be _____, meaning pain from _____, or _____, meaning pain from _____, _____ and _____. Superficial pain is _____ to locate, whereas locating deep pain is _____. This is because the skin has a higher concentration of _____.

Choose from:
Somatic; Sudden; Transient; Duration; Location; Autonomic; Nociceptors; Organs; Tachycardia; Diaphoresis; Acute; Chronic; Hypertension; Joints; Difficult; Visceral; Tachypnoea; Easy; Skin; Muscles; Bones

Label the diagram

Using the list of words supplied, label the diagram.

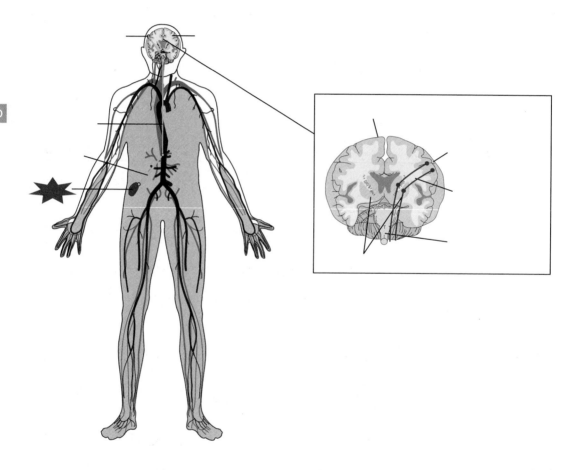

Cerebral cortex; Second-order neuron; Thalamus; Third-order neuron; Second-order neuron; Somatosensory area; Brain; First-order neuron; Cerebral cortex; Third-order neuron

Word search

A	B	N	E	U	R	O	P	A	T	H	Y	I	E	C	K
N	P	A	S	B	E	N	I	H	P	R	O	M	A	I	D
A	W	P	V	Q	D	S	T	U	E	U	E	R	L	L	F
L	N	Y	A	J	S	K	A	C	U	T	E	G	L	N	M
G	B	E	N	K	L	U	M	P	S	K	X	E	O	I	D
E	C	O	N	R	E	I	P	Y	F	S	U	T	D	R	B
S	S	R	G	I	O	T	S	E	R	D	L	P	Y	I	V
I	C	A	D	P	H	C	H	O	R	C	P	E	N	P	I
A	T	F	I	S	I	C	T	N	I	F	A	E	I	S	S
F	G	A	I	B	H	P	A	T	C	B	I	D	A	A	C
F	T	P	M	B	E	G	A	M	Z	I	W	C	O	G	E
E	J	I	R	C	R	M	H	R	S	D	N	C	I	M	R
B	L	S	I	J	O	E	P	O	E	N	F	O	C	A	A
S	P	C	G	S	T	N	S	F	P	E	E	F	R	A	L
I	O	A	H	C	P	L	K	A	W	H	C	T	S	H	S
N	H	G	U	O	R	H	T	K	A	E	R	B	D	V	C

461

Nociceptors	Acute	Diamorphine
Analgesia	Opiate	Neuropathy
Deep	Somatic	Kappa
C fibres	Chronic	Breakthrough
TENS machine	Superficial	Visceral
Allodynia	Limbic system	Aspirin

Further resources

British Pain Society

http://www.britishpainsociety.org
This website contains publications, newsletters and information for patients, all of which can inform your care of patients with chronic pain and help you in your academic work.

Pain Concern

http://www.painconcern.org.uk
This website also hosts regular radio programmes and podcasts, which could be helpful to you in your academic work. Its discussion sites also provide insight into how individuals cope with chronic pain.

Pain Talk

http://www.pain-talk.co.uk/
This is a useful website for students studying chronic pain. Once registered, viewers can gain access to discussion forums, news, pain search engines, information on study days and conferences, and details of other useful pain websites.

The Pain Association

http://test.painassociation.com
This website provides support and guidance on how to manage chronic pain, with advice on everyday issues such as dealing with anxiety, breathing exercises and promotion of sleep. It also contains access to books and CDs for patients with pain. This information may prove useful in your academic studies.

NHS Choices

http://www.nhs.uk/Conditions/Back-pain
This website provides guidance to help you care for patients in pain. It gives access to advice on back pain, as well as a host of other pain conditions.

London Pain Consortium

http://www.lpc.ac.uk/html/
This website gives the latest research into pain physiology, and London Pain Consortium publications, as well as links to other pain websites and journals. This site provides an excellent resource for students studying chronic and acute pain.

🔍 Glossary of terms

Aldosterone:
a hormone that increases blood pressure by increasing re-absorption of water and sodium by the kidneys.

Alexander technique:
a method of teaching people how to improve their body posture and thereby avoid muscle tension.

Allodynia:
pain in response to stimuli that should not cause pain.

Amputation:
surgical removal of a limb.

Analgesic:
pain killer.

Angina:
central crushing chest pain that occurs as a result of reduced blood flow through the coronary arteries.

Antiplatelet:
a substance that reduces the clotting action of platelets.

Arachidonic acid:
a substance found in the cell membrane which can produce prostaglandins.

Aromatherapy:
the use of odours and fragrances to alter an individual's mood.

Autonomic:
pertaining to the autonomic nervous system; associated with the maintenance of homeostasis.

Axon:
the long part of a nerve cell that carries nerve impulses.

Bone metastases:
cells from a tumour that have spread to bone tissue.

Bradycardia:
having a slow heart beat (usually defined as less than 60 beats per minute).

Central nervous system:
the brain and spinal cord.

Cerebral cortex:
the outer surface of the brain.

Chiropractice:
the manipulation and realignment of the spine.

Controlled drug:
a therapeutic preparation governed by the Misuse of Drugs Act (1971).

Coronary artery:
supplies oxygenated blood to the heart.

Coronary vasoconstriction:
constriction of coronary blood vessels.

Cortisol:
a hormone released by the adrenal glands, which increases resistance to stress.

Cyclo-oxygenase-2:   an enzyme which speeds up the production of prostaglandins from arachidonic acid.

Deep vein thrombosis: the formation of a blood clot in the veins of the legs.

Diaphoresis: excessive sweating.

Dorsal horn: the section of grey matter found on either side of a cross-section of the spinal cord.

Dynorphin: a neuropeptide found in the central nervous system.

Dysphoria: low mood; opposite of euphoria.

Endorphin: a neuropeptide found in the central nervous system. Counteracts pain sensation by inhibiting substance P.

Enzyme: a protein that speeds up chemical reactions.

Epinephrine (adrenaline): hormone released during times of stress.

Frontal lobe: area of the cerebrum (outer part of the brain).

Glucagon: a hormone released by pancreas, which increase blood sugar levels.

Histamine: a substance that causes constriction of smooth muscle, dilates arterioles and capillaries, and stimulates gastric juices. See serotonin.

Homeopathy: treatment based on the principle that 'like can be cured with like'.

Hyperalgesia: increased or heightened pain sensation.

Hypertension: raised blood pressure.

Hypothalamus: a small region of the brain found in the diencephalon; important regulatory organ of the nervous and endocrine systems.

Hypoventilation: slow and shallow breaths.

Hypoxaemia: reduced levels of oxygen in arterial blood.

Hypoxia: reduced levels of oxygen in the tissues.

Interneuron: short neuron that connect nearby neurons in the brain and spinal cord.

Ischaemia: a low oxygen state in a part of the body. Usually the result of obstruction to the blood supply to tissues.

Kinin:	a substances released during inflammation that causes vasodilation and increased capillary permeability; also attracts phagocytes. The primary kinin is bradykinin.
Limbic system:	part of the forebrain. Sometimes called the emotional brain, the limbic system controls feelings of emotion and behaviour.
Miosis:	contraction of the pupils.
Motor nerve:	a nerve that travels from the brain and spinal cord out to an organ, muscle or gland.
Muscle atrophy:	muscle wasting.
Myelin:	an electrically insulating phospholipid.
Myelinated:	covered by a protected sheath of myelin.
Neuron:	a nerve cell.
Neuropeptide:	a substance found in the nervous system that counteracts the effects of neurotransmitters.
Neurotransmitter:	a molecules that transmits messages from one nerve to another at a junction called the synapse.
Nociceptor:	a special cells that detects damage and irritants that cause pain.
Non-steroidal anti-inflammatory drug (NSAID):	a non-opioid pain killer that reduces inflammation.
Opiate:	a powerful analgesic agent that stimulates opiate receptors within the central nervous system.
Opiate receptor:	a receptor found in the central nervous system that is stimulated by neuropeptides and opiate drugs.
Osteopathy:	the manipulation of bones and joints to diagnose and treat illness.
Patient-controlled analgesia:	a method of self-administration of intravenous analgesia.
Peripheral nervous system:	the nervous system outside of the central nervous system.
Prostaglandin:	a complex unsaturated fatty acid produced by the mast cells and acting as a messenger substance between cells. Intensifies the actions of histamine and kinins. They cause increased vascular permeability, neutrophil chemotaxis, stimulation of smooth muscle (e.g. the uterus) and can induce pain.

465

Pruritis:	itchy sensation on the skin.
Pulmonary embolism:	reduced blood flow through the lungs due to a blood clot.
Pyrexia:	elevated temperature associated with fever .
Reflex arc:	nervous pathway from sensory nerve to motor nerve via the spinal cord.
Reflexology:	the manipulation of various areas of the feet and hands in order to promote well-being.
Reticular formation:	a network of neurons found in the central part of the brainstem.
Sensory fibre:	a special nerve fibre that transmits sensations of pain, heat, cold and touch.
Serotonin:	a neurotransmitter found in the central nervous system that is released from platelets in response to injury, trauma or infection. Along with other substances, such as histamine, it causes temporary, rapid constriction of the smooth muscles of large blood vessel walls and dilation of the small veins (venules). This results in increased blood flow and increased vascular permeability. Associated with pain sensation.
Shiatsu:	finger pressure applied to various areas of the body in order to stimulate the internal energy of the body and thus promote healing.
Somatosensory cortex:	a region of the cerebral cortex that processes feelings of touch, pain, heat, cold and muscle and joint position.
Spinothalamic tract:	the sensory pathway that transmits messages of pain, temperature, touch and pressure upwards along the spinal cord.
Substance P:	a neurotransmitter found in sensory nerves, spinal cord and brain; associated with the sensation of pain.
Substantia gelatinosa:	a part of the spinal cord's grey matter; it is composed of large amounts of small nerve cells.
Synapse:	the junction where two neurons meet or where a neuron meets tissue.
Syndrome:	a collection of symptoms that characterises a specific disorder.

Tachycardia:	a fast heart beat (usually defined as above 100 beats per minute).
Tachypnoea:	a rapid and usually shallow respiration rate, greater than 20 breaths per minute.
Thalamus:	a pair of oval masses of grey matter which accounts for 80% of the diencephalon area of the brain.
Thoracotomy:	incision in the chest.
Transcutaneous electrical nerve stimulation (TENS):	a method of pain control which stimulates Aβ, Aδ and C fibres with small electrical currents.
Ulceration:	the erosion of skin or an internal surface.
Venous return:	the volume of blood entering the right atrium.
White matter:	the tissue of the spinal cord that surrounds the grey matter.

467

References

Bell, L. and Duffy A. (2009). Pain assessment and management in surgical nursing: a literature review. *British Journal of Nursing*. 18(3): 153–156.

Briggs, E. (2010). Understanding the experience and physiology of pain. *Nursing Standard*. 25(3): 35–39.

Carr, E.C.J., Thomas, V.N. and Wilson-Barnet, J. (2005). Patient experiences of anxiety, depression and acute pain after surgery: A longitudinal perspective. *International Journal of Nursing Studies*. 42: 521–530.

Cousins, M. and Power, I. (2003). Acute and postoperative pain. In: Melzack, R. and Wall, P.D. (eds). *Handbook of Pain Management: A Clinical Companion to Wall and Melzack's Textbook of Pain*. Edinburgh: Churchill Livingstone.

Dopson, L. (2010). Role of pain management programmes in chronic pain. *Nursing Standard*. 25(13): 35–40.

Eccleston, C., Williams, A. Morley, S. (2009). Psychological therapies for the management of chronic pain (excluding headache) in adults (review). *The Cochrane Library*. Issue 2.

French, S.D., Cameron, M., Walker, B.F., Reggars, J.W. and Esterman, A.J. (2005). Superficial heat or cold for low back pain. *The Cochrane Database of Systematic Reviews*. Issue 1.

Furlan, A.D., Brosseau, L., Imamura, M. and Irvin, E. (2002). Massage for low back pain. *The Cochrane Database of Systematic Reviews*. Issue 2.

Gilron, I., Milne, B. and Hong, M. (2003). Cyclooxygenase-2 inhibitors in postoperative pain management. *Anaesthesiology*. 99(5): 1198–1208.

Godfrey, H. (2005a). Understanding pain, part 1: Physiology of pain. *British Journal of Nursing*. 14(16): 846–852.

Godfrey, H. (2005b). Understanding pain, part 2: Pain management. *British Journal of Nursing*. 14(17): 904–909.

Grafton, K.V., Foster, N.E. and Wright, C.C. (2005). Test-retest reliability of the short-form McGill pain questionnaire. *Clinical Journal of Pain*. 21(1): 73–82.

Hader, C.F. and Guy, J. (2004). Your hand in pain management. *Nursing Management.* 35(11): 21–28.

Hayden, D. (2006). Pain management in palliative care. In: MacLellan, K. (ed). *Expanding Nursing and Health Care Practice: Management of Pain.* Cheltenham: Nelson Thornes.

Her Majesty's Stationery Office (1968). *The Medicine's Act.* London: HMSO.

Her Majesty's Stationery Office (1971). *The Misuse of Drugs Act.* London: HSMO.

Jenkins, C., Costello, J. and Hodge, L. (2004). Systematic review of prevalence of aspirin induced asthma and its implications for clinical practice. *British Medical Journal* 328: 434–440.

Johansson, K., Nuutila, L., Virtanen, H., Katajisto, J. and Salantera, S. (2005). Preoperative education for orthopaedic patients: Systematic review. *Journal of Advanced Nursing.* 50(2): 212–223.

Johnson, M. (2005). Physiology of chronic pain. In: Banks, C. and Mackrodt, K. (eds). *Chronic Pain Management.* London: Whurr Publishers.

Kochhar, S.C. (2002). Cancer pain. In: Warfield, C.A. and Fausett, H.J. (eds). *Manual of Pain Management,* 2nd edn. Philadelphia: Lippincott Williams & Wilkins.

Layzell, M. (2008). Current interventions and approaches to post-operative pain management. *British Journal of Nursing.* 17(7): 414–419.

Lee, H. and Ernst, E. (2005). Acupuncture analgesia during surgery: A systematic review. *Pain.* 114(3): 511–517.

Lin, L. and Wang, R. (2005). Abdominal surgery, pain and anxiety: Preoperative nursing intervention. *Journal of Advanced Nursing.* 51(3): 252–260.

Lundeberg, T. and Stener-Victorin, E. (2002). Is there a physiological basis for the use of acupuncture in pain? *International Congress Series.* 1238: 3–10.

MacIntyre, P.E. and Ready, L.B. (2001). *Acute Pain Management: A Practical Guide,* 2nd edn. London: W.B. Saunders.

MacLellan, K. (2006). *Expanding Nursing and Health Care Practice: Management of Pain.* Cheltenham: Nelson Thornes.

Manias, E. (2003). Pain and anxiety management in the postoperative gastro-surgical setting. *Journal of Advanced Nursing.* 41(6): 585–504.

Manias, E., Botti, M. and Bucknall, T. (2002). Observation of pain assessment and management – the complexities of clinical practice. *Journal of Clinical Nursing.* 11: 724–733.

Marieb, E. and Hoehn, K. (2007). *Human Anatomy and Physiology,* 7th edn. San Francisco: Pearson Benjamin Cummings.

McCaffery, M. (1979). *Nursing Management of the Patient with Pain,* 2nd edn. New York: J.B. Lippincott Company.

McCaffery, R., Frock, T.L. and Garguilo, H. (2003). Understanding chronic pain and the mind–body connection. *Holistic Nursing Practice.* 17(6): 281–287.

Melzack, R. and Torgerson, W.S. (1971). On the language of pain. *Anesthesiology.* 34(1): 50–59.

Melzack, R. and Wall, P. (1988). *The Challenge of Pain,* 2nd edn. London: Penguin.

Nnoaham, K.E. and Kumbang J. (2008). Transcutaneous electrical nerve stimulation (TENS) for chronic pain (review). *The Cochrane Library, Issue 1.*

Richardson, C. (2008). Nursing aspects of phantom limb pain following amputation. *British Journal of Nursing.* 17(7): 422–426.

Richardson, C., Glenn, S,. Nurrmikko, T., Horgan, M. (2006). Incidence of phantom phenomena including phantom limb pain 6 months after major lower limb amputation in patients with peripheral vascular disease. *The Clinical Journal of Pain.* 22(4): 353–358.

Scadding, J.W. (2003). Peripheral neuropathies. In: Melzack, R. and Wall, P.D. (eds). *Handbook of Pain Management: A Clinical Companion to Wall and Melzack's Textbook of Pain.* Edinburgh: Churchill Livingstone.

Sluka, K.A. and Walsh, D. (2003). Transcutaneous electrical nerve stimulation: Basic science mechanisms and clinical effectiveness. *The Journal of Pain.* 4(3): 109–121.

Solano, J.P., Games, B. and Higginson, I.J. (2006). A comparison of symptom prevalence in far advanced cancer, AIDS, heart disease, chronic obstructive pulmonary disease (COPD) and renal disease. *Journal of Pain and Symptom Management* 31(1): 58–69.

Tortora, G.J. and Derrickson, B. (2011). *Principles of Anatomy and Physiology Organisation, Support and Movement, and Control Systems of the Human Body Volume 1*, 13th edn. New York: John Wiley and Sons.

Wigens, L. (2006). The role of complementary and alternative therapies in pain management. In: MacLellan, K. (ed) *Expanding Nursing and Health Care Practice: Management of Pain*. Cheltenham: Nelson Thornes.

World Health Organization (1986). *Cancer Pain Relief*. Geneva: WHO.

World Health Organization (2002). *National Cancer Control Programmes: Policies and Management Guidelines*, 2nd edn. Geneva: WHO.

16

The musculoskeletal system and associated disorders

Ian Peate

Visiting Professor of Nursing, School of Nursing, Midwifery and Healthcare, Faculty of Health and Human Sciences, University of West London, Brentford, Middlesex, UK; Independent Consultant and Editor-in-Chief British Journal of Nursing

Contents

Fundamentals of Applied Pathophysiology: An Essential Guide for Nursing and Healthcare Students, Second Edition. Edited by Muralitharan Nair and Ian Peate.

Key words

- Muscles
- Tendons
- Joints
- Mobility
- Independence/dependence
- Fracture
- Ligaments
- Inflammation
- Degeneration
- Osteoporosis
- Cartilage

471

Test your prior knowledge

- How many bones are there in the human body?
- Describe the role of osteoclasts and osetoblasts.
- Discuss a range of factors that can impinge on a person's ability to mobilise independently.
- What are the key functions of the skeleton?
- How can healthcare professionals help people gain independence after sustaining a fall?

Learning outcomes

On completion of this chapter the reader will be able to:

- Discuss the development and growth of healthy bone.
- Describe the function of the musculoskeletal system.
- Describe some of the pathophysiological changes that may occur to the musculoskeletal system.
- Outline the care of people who have problems associated with the musculoskeletal system.

Don't forget to visit to the companion website for this book (www.wiley.com/go/ fundamentalsofappliedpathophysiology) where you can find self-assessment tests to check your progress, as well as lots of activities to practise your learning.

Introduction

Every activity that an individual performs is associated with movement, e.g. non-verbal communication in the form of facial expression, which allows another person to interpret or begin to interpret what we are attempting to communicate. In order to function in an optimal manner, a fully functioning musculoskeletal system is required. Mobility is required for the life-sustaining activity of breathing and the exchange of gases. It is the musculoskeletal system that allows these activities to occur. Mobility is an intrinsic aspect of living.

When injury or disease affects the musculoskeletal system, it can result in the person becoming dependent on another person (nurse/carer); the independence usually enjoyed by the person becomes a dependency. Davis (2006) states that diseases of the musculoskeletal system are a major cause of health problems and for the older population they are the biggest, non-neurological threat to health and well-being.

The protection of internal structures is also the responsibility of the musculoskeletal system. Support is provided to the various internal structures, e.g. the ribs protect and support the lungs, the heart and the kidneys.

In order to provide safe and effective care (for both the patient and the healthcare professional), the healthcare professional needs to understand the fundamental issues related to the musculoskeletal system and how this works. This chapter outlines how the musculoskeletal system operates in order to enable an individual to mobilise. The reader is provided with an overview of the musculoskeletal system and a number of musculoskeletal-related conditions are outlined alongside their associated care.

The healthcare professional's role is to prevent or reduce further injury, identify and reduce the risk of complications, assist in the promotion of healing, and promote and maximise independence. If there is a need for rehabilitation, then the healthcare professional will also be involved in this.

The musculoskeletal system

The musculoskeletal system is also known as the locomotor system.

There are 206 bones in the adult human, of various shapes and sizes; babies are born with 300 bones, but as humans age a number of bones fuse to become bigger bones. A baby's bones are primarily made up of cartilage and over time most of this cartilage turns into bone through a process called ossification (Figure 16.1). Half of the bones in the adult are in the feet and hands.

The presence of joints in the limbs (i.e. the elbow and knee joints) allows movement; if there were no joints, then there could be no movement, and the skeleton would be rigid. Cartilage, a type of cushion, provides protection for those joints that are exposed to force that is generated during movement. Ligaments help to provide joint strength and are either incorporated into the joint capsule or they may be independent of it. Movement at the joint is achieved by contraction of muscles that pass across it.

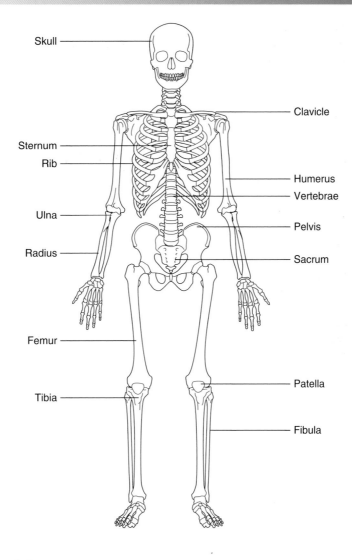

Skull

Clavicle

Sternum

Rib

Humerus

Vertebrae

Ulna

Pelvis

Radius

Sacrum

Femur

Patella

Tibia

Fibula

Figure 16.1   The skeleton.

The skeleton, the joints and skeletal muscle work together to provide basic functions that are essential to life:

- protection for internal organs and to provide support to soft tissue
- support – maintain an upright posture
- blood formation – in red bone marrow, haemopoiesis
- mineral homeostasis, storage and release of minerals as the body requires them. The bones store most of the body's calcium requirement
- storage – fat and minerals in the yellow bone marrow
- leverage, working with the muscles, and the bones in the upper and lower limbs pull and push, allowing for movement.

Bone structure

Bone is a collagen-based matrix with minerals laid upon it; its strength depends on both components. The mineral aspect is composed primarily of calcium, magnesium and phosphorus, and the collagen fibres help with the tension and compression the bone is subjected to. The collagen fibres and the minerals are densely packed together, resulting in a hardening of bone. Vitamin D, parathyroid hormone and calcitonin are important factors in bone mineralization.

Bone formation is controlled by osteoblastic and osteoclastic activity. Osteoblasts control bone formation and osetoclasts are responsible for bone destruction. Throughout life, bone continues to reform and remodel itself – it is firm, rigid, elastic and dynamic. Bone is more than a rigid structure, and it constantly changes and remodels itself.

The way an individual moves, the amount and type of exercise taken and the diet eaten and drunk will all influence bone structure (Figures 16.2 and 16.3).

The skeleton is the body's supporting framework and there are four types of bone:

- long, i.e. the femur
- short, i.e. tarsal bones
- flat, i.e. ribs
- irregular, i.e. the mandible.

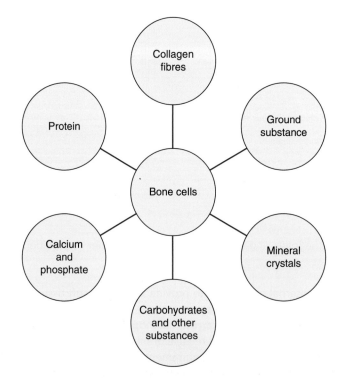

Figure 16.2   Bone production. (Adapted from Davis, 2006.)

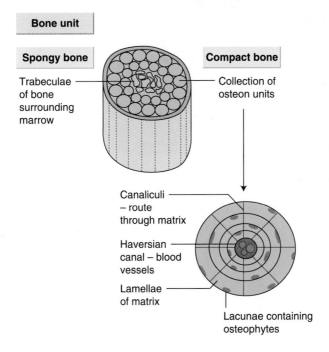

Figure 16.3   Bone structure.

Joints

Where one bone meets another is a joints. There are three type of joint:

- those that allow free movement (i.e. diarthrosis)
- those that are fixed (i.e. synarthrosis)
- those that permit limited movement (amphiarthroses).

Joints are classified as follows:

- synostotic
- cartilaginous
- fibrous
- synovial.

The synovial joint allows free movement. Bony surfaces (the ends of the bones) are covered by articular cartilage and are connected by ligaments; the types of synovial joints include:

- pivotal joints (i.e. the joint between the humeral radius and the ulna)
- ball and socket joints (i.e. the hip joint)
- hinge joints (i.e. the interphalangeal joints of the fingers).

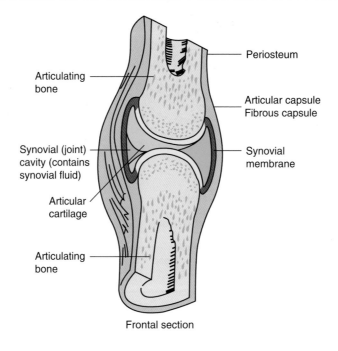

Frontal section

Figure 16.4   A synovial joint.

In synovial joints (Figure 16.4), a space exists between the bone surfaces, which allows movement of one bone against the other. Synovial fluid present in the synovial joint provides nutrition for the articular cartilage and lubrication for the joint surfaces. Throughout life, synovial joints are subjected to wear and tear as a result of the stress placed upon them. The wear and tear is usually seen in the cartilage at the end of one bone where the end of another bone rubs against it; when this occurs it can cause an inflammatory process, which can bring with it pain and loss of movement.

Muscle

Skeletal muscle has the ability to contract and relax. A motor neuron innervates 100–1000 skeletal muscle fibres and when contraction of the muscle occurs, the impulse that travels from the nerve to the muscle does so across the neuromuscular junction. The electrical activity causes thin actin-containing filaments to shorten, resulting in contraction of muscle. Removal of this actin-rich stimulus results in relaxation of the muscle (Figure 16.5). Electrical activity is discussed later.

Muscles are often arranged in pairs associated with two or more bones and a joint. Those muscles that are associated with movement are to be found within the skeletal region where movement is caused by leverage. The pair of muscles has opposing functions: one muscle acts as the flexor (contracting and flexing) and the other as the extensor (relaxing and extending). The muscles that are attached to the bones provide the necessary force to move an object.

Body mechanics is a term used to incorporate the following co-ordinated efforts of the musculoskeletal and nervous systems:

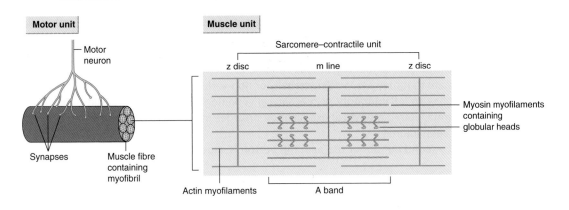

Figure 16.5 Muscle.

- to maintain balance
- to provide posture
- to ensure body alignment.

The muscles associated with posture are primarily the muscles of the trunk, neck and back. They converge obliquely at a common tendon, are short and featherlike in appearance. Working together, they provide stability and support body weight, thus allowing a sitting or standing posture to be maintained.

The nervous system

Movement and posture are both regulated by the nervous system. There is an area in the brain (the cerebral cortex) that houses the voluntary motor area. A specific area in the cerebral cortex – the precentral gyrus or motor strip – sends impulses down the motor strip to the spinal cord during voluntary movement. Muscles are stimulated after a variety of very complex neural and chemical activities take place and movement occurs.

Movement can be impaired by a number of disorders that impede neural and chemical activity; if the muscles cannot be stimulated, movement will not occur. The concept – mobility – is complex, and there are various texts available that will explain in more detail this multifaceted activity. This aspect of the chapter has merely touched on the complexities associated with the activity – mobility. Suffice it to say that in order to care for a patient with problems related to mobility, the healthcare professional needs to have a sound understanding of the many principles underpinning it.

Assessing the patient with a musculoskeletal disorder

In order to help people who present with altered pathophysiology of the musculoskeletal system, the healthcare professional needs to take an in-depth health and medical history; combined with a physical examination, this can help the healthcare professional help the patient. Further diagnostic tests may be needed to confirm diagnosis and aid in the management of care.

Taking a history requires excellent effective communication skills. The competent healthcare professional will be able to identify serious conditions that need urgent attention. Many patients will communicate that they are in pain (verbally or non-verbally). The type of pain will determine if the patient has an inflammatory or mechanical condition (Bulstrode and Swales, 2010; Conaghan and Sharma, 2009); a physical examination provides information about what aspect of the anatomy has been injured.

Much can be found out about the pain the person is experiencing by asking three questions:

- Where is the pain?
- What is the type of pain?
- What makes the pain better or worse?

Table 16.1 highlights some important issues associated with pain in relation to the musculoskeletal system.

Examining the patient provides much information in relation to the anatomical site. When examining the person with a musculoskeletal problem, the person undertaking the examination is generally able to make a comparison with the unaffected side of the body; usually it is advised that the unaffected side be examined first to determine what is normal for the patient. See Table 16.2 for some issues associated with physical examination and the musculoskeletal system.

Table 16.1   Pain and its possible causes in association with the musculoskeletal system.

Characteristic	Possible meaning
Numb, burning shooting, 'pins and needles'	May be neurological in nature
Pain that is relieved by rest is known as claudication pain	May mean that there is arterial insufficiency
Pain that is worse on movement or when weight bearing and is relieved by rest	Likely to be associated with damage to articular structures
Some types of pain that are associated with a joint but in a vague way; when examined the joint seems normal; pain that is unceasing even at night	May be due to referred pain or a bone lesion
Multiple painful joints, morning stiffness that improves with exercise. The patient may also be feeling unwell, has a pyrexia and experienced weight loss	May be signs of inflammation. Could be the result of rheumatoid arthritis
Short duration of morning stiffness, with little or no pain at rest. The pain may become worse during or after sustained exercise and particularly if there is no evidence of systemic disease (e.g. the patient feels unwell, has a pyrexia and has lost weight)	Can suggest local mechanical problems, e.g. osteoarthritis, a sprain or strain

Table 16.2   Issues associated with the examination of the musculoskeletal system.

Characteristic	Possible meaning
Warmth over the joint, e.g. the elbow	Can indicate an inflammatory process
Swelling of the joint, e.g. the knee	There may be joint effusion, enlargement of the bone or synovial thickening
Reduced range of movement with tenderness	Soft tissue injury or muscle injury
Unable to move the limb independently or with help	Structurally abnormal joint
Crepitus with pain	Could suggest damage to articular surfaces
Knee or ankle muscle weakness (unstable)	Ligament tear

When the history has been taken and a physical examination performed, there may be a need for further investigations, such as blood tests, X-rays and various other imaging procedures, e.g. magnetic resonance imaging (MRI) and computed tomography (CT).

479

Disorders of the musculoskeletal system

There are many conditions that may result in a disorder of the musculoskeletal system:

- congenital anomalies
- infection
- inflammation
- degenerative processes
- trauma
- cancer
- vascular disease
- metabolic disorders.

Musculoskeletal conditions can usually be divided into acute or chronic (long-term) conditions, and the care and treatment required will reflect this. Acute conditions are often the result of injury or over-use and are treated according to the acronym **RICE**:

Rest until the swelling and the worst of the pain has settled down.
Ice packs can reduce the swelling, but be careful that the patient does not suffer ice burns to the skin.
Compression and compassion – support in the form of a Tubigrip may be required and care must be taken when applying it so as not to cause the person any more pain. Acknowledge the person's pain.
Elevation – swelling can be reduced by elevating the limb.

Pain relief may be required and this can be prescribed; however, some patients will buy over-the-counter medications such as ibuprofen or paracetamol. The person should be encouraged to mobilise as soon as possible; this may be gradual and should be non-weight bearing. Referral to a physiotherapist or sports physiotherapist can be arranged as they can provide expert advice on how to return to normal functioning in a safe way.

Musculoskeletal problems are the main reason for short- and long-term work absence according to the Chartered Institute for Personnel Development (2009). This absence from work has an economic and emotional impact on individuals and society.

A long-term condition is one that cannot currently be cured and does not resolve of its own accord, but can be controlled with the use of medication and/or other therapies (Department of Health, 2010). Osteoarthritis is an example of a chronic musculoskeletal condition.

Fractures and bone healing

Many patients refer to fractures as 'broken bones': fractures are defined as a break in the continuity of bone and this can be the result of direct or indirect trauma, underlying disease or repeated stress on a bone. Those fractures that are caused by underlying disease are known as pathological fractures and those by repeated stress are called stress fractures (Langstaff, 2000).

It has already been stated that one of the unique functions of bone is its ability to regenerate; it is able to produce new cells and remove those cells that have died. Tortora and Grabowski (2006) suggest that the balance of calcium is a critical element in bone growth and repair; this is affected by the level of vitamin D in the body as well as renal and intestinal functioning, parathyroid gland functioning and the ability of the adrenal glands to work effectively.

Osteology is the scientific study of bones. While bone has the ability to heal by itself, this can be aided by making the broken bone immobile, restricting movement or surgical intervention. A well-balanced diet will also aid bone healing. A well-balanced diet includes foods from the five main food groups:

- bread cereal and potatoes
- fruit and vegetables
- meat and fish
- milk and dairy foods
- fat and sugar.

Fibroblasts (cells that take part in bone healing) originate within the connective tissue of the periosteum; therefore, the more damage that occurs to the periosteum, the more difficult it will be for the bone to heal (Tortora and Grabowski, 2006). McRae (2006) describes the bone-healing process and states that it can take months for full bone healing to take place. There are several stages involved in the bone healing process (Table 16.3).

Fracture of the bone can occur for a variety of reasons; however, the most common type of fractures are those sustained by the older population as result of osteoporosis, with most fractures occurring near the proximal aspect of the head of the humerus (Docherty, 2007). The type of fracture sustained can be classified as follows (Figure 16.6):

- hairline – usually only affects the outer bone
- simple – bone damage but little or no soft tissue injury
- incomplete (also known as greenstick) – commonly seen (but not exclusively) in children; only one side of the bone is fractured
- comminuted – more than two fragments of bone have been broken; the bone has broken off
- compound – a very complicated type of fracture where the bone breaks through the skin.

Table 16.3 Osteology.

Time scale	Bone activity
Within the first 6 hours	As result of the blood vessels in the bone becoming ruptured; a haematoma forms
6–48 hours	The inflammatory process begins and cytokines are released; this causes fibroblasts to migrate to the haematoma and tissue granulation begins
2–7 days	As granulation tissue begins to form, it becomes denser and more stable, and joins with infiltrating cartilage tissue. Macrophages begin to work on the haematoma and osteoclasts resorb the damaged bone
Weeks	Callus formation occurs – this is where the structure surrounding the fracture area becomes hard. This harder woven bone is eventually remodelled and becomes lamellar bone
Months	The callus, over time, becomes smaller as the bone is reconstructed

Adapted from McRae (2006).

481

There is a high risk of haemorrhage and infection when this type of fracture is sustained.

The aim of bone healing is to restore the normal anatomy and function of the fractured bone. The healthcare professional also has a responsibility to reduce the complications that can occur as a result of immobility. Some of the complications associated with immobility are:

- deep vein thrombosis
- pulmonary embolism
- increased cardiac workload
- orthostatic hypotension
- decreased cardiac output and reduced tissue perfusion
- chest infection
- renal stones
- incontinence
- muscle wasting
- joint contractures
- loss of self-esteem
- frustration
- boredom
- isolation.

Bone loss and muscle atrophy can occur as a result of long-term bed rest. Spray (2011) report that in adult patients who are confined to bed rest there is evidence of bone loss as immobility leads to bone resorption when the bone tissue becomes less dense. The loss of bone over several

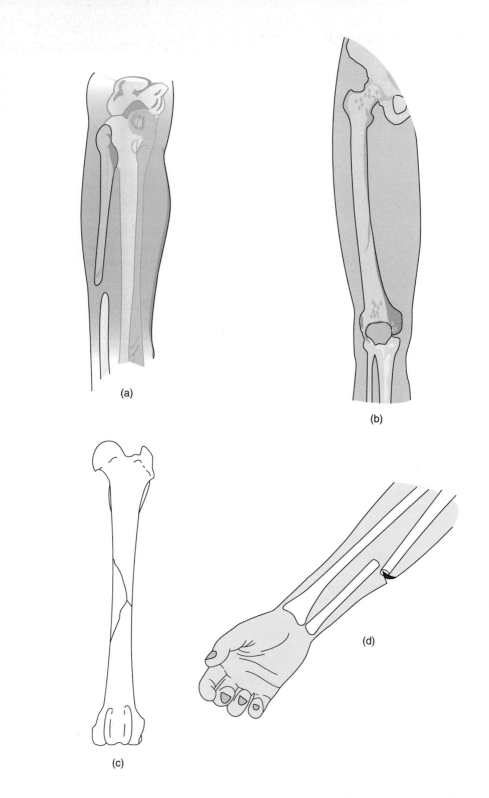

Figure 16.6 The four types of fractures: (a) simple, (b) incomplete (greenstick), (c) comminuted and (d) compound.

weeks is a concern and can put the person at risk of a pathological fracture. It can be seen that bed rest is not without serious complications. The healthcare professional must be aware of these actual and potential complications, such as constipation and chest infection, and be proactive when planning care interventions to prevent or reduce the harmful consequences of bed rest.

Bed rest, however, is a therapeutic intervention that will help achieve several objectives (Perez, 2011) such as:

- the provision of rest for those patients who are exhausted
- decreased oxygen consumption
- reduced pain and discomfort.

These objectives also link with the key role of the healthcare professional:

- to act as a preventative agent
- to educate
- to provide comfort.

Although there are good reasons for bed rest, however it can be counterproductive to the patient's recovery. The healthcare professional has a key role in helping to promote independence and to provide the patient with a sense of well-being. In some instances, there may be a need to move the person when they are unable to do so themselves. Brown and McLennan (2007) suggest that it may be necessary for one, two or more staff using mechanical aids to move a patient; safe moving and handling techniques must be implemented to help prevent injury to themselves as well as the patient.

Osteoarthritis

The most common disorder to affect the joints is osteoarthritis (Conaghan and Sharma, 2009); as a person ages, its frequency increases, causing pain and disability. Osteoarthritis is the single most important cause of locomotor disability. The following joints can be affected:

- the small joints of the hands
- the neck
- the lower back
- the big toe
- the knee
- the hip.

Osteoarthritis is a degenerative disease (due to wear and tear) of articular cartilage; it is now suggested that the cause of osteoarthritis is also a result of metabolic disease. The disease causes damage to the cartilage surfaces of synovial joints. In more severe cases, the joint space narrows and osteophytes form. The patient tends to seek help because of the pain caused by osteoarthritis and the way it interferes with their ability to mobilise. There are known risk factors associated with the disease (Davies *et al.*, 2006):

- age 45 years and over (uncommon in younger people)
- female sex
- black or Asian ethnicity

- genetic predisposition
- overweight and obesity
- poor muscle function
- some occupations
- previous fracture
- menisectomy.

Signs and symptoms

The patient presents with joint pain and there is a history of joint stiffness. On examination there may be evidence of creptius, swelling and muscle weakness and wasting; often the person becomes increasingly immobile – loss of function can occur. Most commonly the patient complains of pain in the hands, hip or knee.

Diagnosis

History and examination are vital. X-ray analysis may demonstrate a reduced joint space, osteophyte formation and other abnormalities (Figure 16.7). Other investigations are needed to exclude other causes of pain, e.g. blood tests to rule out inflammatory disease such as inflammatory arthritis.

Care and management

The role of the healthcare professional is to reduce pain, increase mobility and independence and minimise progression of the disease. Pain control can be managed by some patients with the use of paracetamol, and some patients may benefit from the use of non-steroidal anti-inflammatory drugs (NSAIDs), either orally or topically applied. Local heat or cold applied to the affected region may help to ease the pain.

The patient may need to be referred to a physiotherapist who can advise about exercise regimens, and an occupational therapist who can help with adaptations to the home if they are needed. Referral to an orthopaedic surgeon may be required if joint replacement is an issue. If the patient is overweight or obese, weight reduction is recommended as this can reduce weight on the joint, decrease other symptoms and prevent progression of osteoarthritis in the affected joint.

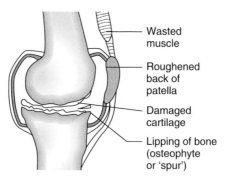

Figure 16.7 A knee joint with osteoarthritis.

Osteoporosis

In the elderly, osteoporosis is a major cause of death. The impact of fractures because of osteoporosis can have an enormous effect on the quality of a person's life. Osteoporosis is a metabolic disease resulting in loss of bone mass, particularly in postmenopausal women (Conaghan and Sharma, 2009). The skeleton is affected, bone breakdown occurs faster than bone is built, and the bones become weak and break.

Osteoporosis means porous bones and is defined as a reduction in bone density, along with degenerate microarchitecture, leading to increased skeletal fragility and threat of fracture after minimal trauma. Everyone loses bone as they age, and the amount varies from person to person. Some people lose much more bone than others and their bones become fragile and break more easily.

Risk factors

Everyone is at risk of developing osteoporosis as they age, but there are some factors that make some people more at risk. Risk factors that are associated with the development of osteoporosis are associated with an interaction of multiple factors in a genetically susceptible person:

- advancing age – risk of osteoporosis and fractures increases with age
- sex hormone deficiency
- low body mass index (underweight)
- medications (such as steroids)
- chronic disease, e.g. chronic liver disease, inflammatory bowel or coeliac disease
- previous fracture
- early menopause
- family history of maternal hip fracture
- immobility
- environmental hazards, such as an unsafe carpets and rugs in the home
- smoking
- alcohol abuse.

The person who suffers with osteoporosis may experience immobility and this can bring with it an increase in dependence on others; for some people the result may be death. There is personal distress as a result and this is also accompanied with financial expense.

Diagnosis

Diagnosis is usually made after the patient has suffered a fracture, but sometimes diagnosis of osteoporosis can be overlooked. Diagnosis can also be made by carrying out a number of investigations as well as taking an in-depth health and medical history, coupled with physical examination. X-ray cannot diagnose osteoporosis; it can, however, reveal fractures of the vertebra that have occurred as a result of osteoporosis. Special scans called dual energy X-ray absorptionmetry (DEXA) can be used to measure the density of the bone (bone mineral density); this can confirm diagnosis as well as quantifying the risk of fracture that may be due to osteoporotic changes. Blood tests are required to assess a variety of biochemical substances, e.g.:

- serum calcium, albumin, phosphate
- serum creatinine

- serum thyroid-stimulating hormone
- alkaline phosphatase and liver transaminases.

Care and management

Increasing awareness and encouraging activities to reduce risk can prevent the personal and financial hardships from occurring. Pain is a key feature of osteoporosis – immediately when a bone fractures or in the long term in association with hip, wrist or vertebral fractures; the pain of osteoporotic fractures can be both acute and chronic. There are some over-the-counter analgesics that may help some patients and the pharmacist may be able to provide advice; there are some patients who may, however, need stronger analgesia. Acute pain can be incapacitating and the healthcare professional may need to engage the help of other healthcare professionals, e.g. those working in pain services; strong analgesics may be required, e.g. opiates.

Lifestyle advice is also a part of the care and management of the person with osteoporosis:

- regular weight-bearing exercise
- adequate nutrition (eating foods that are rich in calcium and vitamin D)
- avoidance of smoking
- avoidance of excessive alcohol intake.

486

There is a range of pharmacological interventions that can be used to improve bone mass (Table 16.4).

Alternative methods of pain relief include:

- Transcutaneous electrical nerve stimulation (TENS) – electrical signals are used to block or reduce pain impulses from getting to the brain.
- Complementary therapies, e.g. aromatherapy, homeopathy and acupuncture, may help to relieve pain as well as increasing well-being.

As well as the physical aspects, the healthcare professional must also consider the psychological aspects associated with osteoporosis. Pain can result in lack of sleep, as well as having the potential to make the patient depressed. Psychological assessment and interventions may be required, as well as consideration of the use of antidepressants.

Table 16.4   Pharmacological agents that may be used in the treatment for osteoporosis.

Drug	Action
Biphosphonates	Decreases bone loss and fracture rate
Strontium ranelate	Increases bone formation and decreases resorption of bone
Selective oestrogen receptor modulator (SERM)	Inhibit bone resorption
Hormone replacement therapy (HRT)	Postpones postmenopausal bone loss and decreases fractures

Adapted from Davies *et al.* (2006).

Measures must be taken to reduce the risk of falls and the damage that can be caused by falls (i.e. fractures). Falls are one of the biggest risk factors for fractures and there is an increase in the tendency to fall as the patient ages.

Gout

Gout, also known as crystal-induced arthritis, is an inflammatory disease (Tortora and Derrickson, 2011) of the joints as the result of the deposition of crystals of the sodium salt of uric acid; it is the most common cause of inflammatory joint disease in men aged 40 years and over. The patient experiences intermittent episodes of joint pain due to the uric crystals. Uric acid is the waste product formed from the breakdown of food and protein in the blood and tissues; the crystals, formed after supersaturation of the tissues, are needlelike and can cause inflammation and painful swelling of the joints. There are three joints that are commonly (but not exclusively) affected:

- the first metatarso-phalangeal joint
- the mid-tarsal joints
- the knee.

Gout is more common in men than women,, affecting men aged between 30 and 60 years; in women it tends to occur later in life between 50 and 80 years ((Belavic, 2010; Watkins, 2010). There are a number of predisposing factors that put a person more at risk of contracting gout:

487

- family history
- obesity
- excessive alcohol intake
- high purine diet (purines are found in many foods, e.g. meat, game and seafood)
- acute infection
- use of diuretics
- ketosis
- surgery
- leukaemia
- cytotoxic drugs
- hypertension
- renal failure.

Diagnosis

The person may experience intermittent episodes of acute joint pain; this is a characteristic sign, often beginning during the night, and can be brought about by trauma or another illness; it reaches a peak within a few hours. The pain may be so great that the patient is unable to tolerate the weight of bed clothes. As well as painful swollen joints, the skin over the affected area may be red and shiny, it may also peel; there may be pyrexia and fever; and the patient may have loss of appetite and malaise. More than one joint can be affected (this is termed polyarticular); particularly in the elderly person, and the joint may feel hot to touch.

Diagnosis is confirmed by in-depth history taking, examination and investigation; investigations are not carried out until the acute phase is over. Blood tests are required and may show an elevated white blood cell count and an increase in blood urate. In some instances, the fluid in the joint (the synovial fluid) may be aspirated (removed through a needle and syringe) and analysed;

analysis of the synovial fluid will exclude the possibility of septic arthritis. Renal function tests may also be needed to rule out renal disease. X-rays will be unhelpful as they will usually only reveal soft tissue swelling.

Care and management

Treatment is threefold:

- pain management
- lifestyle modification
- lowering of urate levels.

Pain relief is a central aspect of the care and management of the person with gout. NSAIDs such as diclofenac or indomethacin may help, with the caution that such medications may cause gastrointestinal disturbances (e.g. gastric haemorrhage); if these occur, alternative medications must be given. The patient should rest, the affected limb should be elevated, and the application of an ice pack may be helpful; a bed cradle should be used to take the weight of the bed clothes off the patient's joints. The injection of steroid preparations into the joint is also effective.

As a health educator the healthcare professional should encourage the patient to reduce weight if overweight or obese, and alcohol should be reduced as well as those foods that are high in purine (e.g. sardines, liver and red meats) – lifestyle modification is needed. If the patient is receiving aspirin (salicylate) or diuretic medications, these should be reviewed with a view to stopping them if possible.

There are some medications, e.g. allopurinol, that lower the level of uric acid. They do not control pain and once started, have to be taken for a lifetime; therefore, the decision to commence this type of medication must be carefully explained to the patient using a language that they understand in order for them to arrive at an informed decision.

Case study

James Segal is a 62-year-old man who presents at his general practitioner's surgery complaining of pain and swelling over his left great toe at the metatarsal phalangeal joint. When Mr Segal's foot is examined by the practice nurse, Stella Brent, she finds the great toe is erythematous, warm, swollen and tender to touch. He has had at least three other episodes of this type of pain, lasting for about 2 or 3 days, but he tells Nurse Brent that the pain is now worse and he has had it for 6 days. During the examination, Nurse Brent also notices a small rounded, subcutaneous nodule, which is tender and rubbery to the touch. The patient has a history of type 2 diabetes mellitus controlled by diet and of hypertension (controlled with hydrochlorothiazide). A tentative diagnosis of gout is made.

Take some time to reflect on this case and then consider the following.

1. What examinations do you think the nurse will request in order to make a definitive diagnosis?
2. Why might these be required and what might they reveal?
3. What treatment might be required in order to help Mr Segal with his condition?
4. Are there any health promotion activities the nurse might wish to discuss with Mr Segal?

Chapter 16

Myasthenia gravis

This condition is a chronic autoimmune neurological disease. According to McCance *et al.* (2010), myasthenia gravis is a complicated condition that is not fully understood. The condition fluctuates in severity as well distribution throughout the body and the person can experience relapses and remissions. In some patients, the condition resolves spontaneously, but in others it persists for life. There are three myasthenias:

● myasthenia gravis
● congenital myasthenias
● the Lambert–Eaton myasthenic syndrome.

This section will briefly consider myasthenia gravis. The disease is a progressive neuromuscular disease of the lower motor neurons characterised by muscle weakness and fatigue. Chapter 10 discusses the central nervous system and associated disorders in more detail. Christensen and Kockrow (2011) note that the condition can occur at any age, but it is more common in those aged between 10 and 65 years. The peak age of onset in women is 20–30 years. In younger people, more women are affected than men, but in the older age group the distribution between the genders is equal.

Electrical activity in the muscles

For skeletal muscle to contract, it needs to receive electrical nerve impulses from the fibres of motor neurons – these are nerve cells. The electrical impulses originate in the central nervous system (the brain or spinal cord). They travel to a nerve cell close to the muscle via the nervous system where chemical messengers (also called neurotransmitters) are released into the gap between the nerve cell and muscle cell. A neuromuscular junction is formed where the end of the nerve cell is in close contact with the muscle cell membrane; this structure is similar to a synapse. Acetylcholine is the neurotransmitter that is released into the neuromuscular junction.

Acetylcholine only has short distance to travel across the nerve cell to the muscle membrane. When it reaches the muscle membrane, it attaches itself to receptors, generating electrical impulses in the muscle. Calcium is released into the muscle cell when the impulses occur and this usually results in muscle contraction.

In myasthenia gravis, the action of acetylcholine is not fully effective. The body's immune system produces autoantibodies that attack the muscle cells (receptors) at the neuromuscular junction and neurons are unable to stimulate the muscle cells adequately (Richardson, 2006). The result of this ineffective activity is weak and ineffective muscular contraction. Muscle weakness, particularly in the face, throat and eyes, and progressing to all four limbs and the muscles of the respiratory tract, occurs. Classification by severity is (McCance *et al.*, 2010):

● Grade I – ocular disease
● Grade II – generalized mild weakness
● Grade IIa – mild weakness
● Grade IIb – moderate weakness
● Grade III – severe generalized weakness
● Grade IV – myasthenic 'crisis' with respiratory failure.

It can affect all races, but there are some patients who may be more at risk of developing myasthenia gravis than others. Those who have a tendency to inherit autoimmune diseases, such as diabetes mellitus and thyroid disease, are at an increased risk. Risk also increases if the person has a relative with an autoimmune disease. Myasthenia gravis is not an inherited disease and does not occur in families.

Case study

Annie Morgan is a university physiotherapy student who swam for the university team. In her last race she swam abysmally and felt miserable as she had let her team mates down. She had been experiencing blurred vision lately, but puts off doing anything about it as she considered it the result of work, her lenses and the chlorine in the pool. She was experiencing aching in her fingers and hands as she needed to type up more assignments for her course. As she walked up the stairs to leave the gym, she was gasping for breath, finding it a challenge. Her friend Sheena noticed this and had noticed that Annie was becoming increasingly short of breath over the last month or so.

When Annie arrived home she went straight to bed telling Sheena she was exhausted. Sheena had to wake Annie and Annie commented on how hard it was to keep her eyes open these days again, putting this down to the enormous amount of course work she had. Sheena prepared the meal (Annie was again sleeping) and when they sat to eat Annie was finding it difficult to grasp the cutlery. Sheena suggested that Annie should see her GP and they agreed that after the weekend she would go and see him. Annie slept for long periods over the weekend. When Monday arrived, Annie said she was feeling so much better and she might cancel the appointment. She said it was amazing what rest can do. Sheena convinced Annie she needed to see the GP just to check things out.

Annie and Sheena went to see the GP who asked about the problems. Annie explained about her eyes, the tiredness, her shortness of breath, her difficulty grasping things like keys and cutlery, and the tiredness she felt in her hands and fingers when typing. An appointment was made for Annie to see the neurologist at her local hospital.

Take some time to reflect on this case and then consider the following.

1.   What do you think the diagnosis might be? Might there be any other possible diagnoses (is there a differential diagnosis)?
2.   How would explain what myasthenia gravis is to Annie and Sheena?
3.   What tests and investigations might the neurologist request in order to make the diagnosis?
4.   What is the Tensilon test?

Diagnosis

Patient history and examination will help to reveal a diagnosis. The patient may experience abnormal muscle fatigability and muscle weakness. The most common manifestations are ptosis and diplopia. There may also be an accompanying dysarthria, dysphagia, ocular palsy, and facial and limb weaknesses. Respiratory involvement will lead to breathlessness; in the acute stage respiratory distress can occur and this may lead to respiratory arrest followed by cardiac arrest.

There are a number of tests that can be used to confirm or refute the diagnosis. The most common test used to confirm diagnosis is the Tensilon test (Hickey, 2009). Tensilon (edrophonium) is an anticholinesterase and is injected intravenously; those patients who show an improvement in muscular strength after the test have tested positive for the disease. This anticholinesterase increases the effective amount of acetylcholine at the neuromuscular junction in those patients with myasthenia gravis. The response is measured over 1 minute and lasts no longer than 5 minutes; it is vital that resuscitation equipment is at hand when performing this test.

Blood tests may also be needed, e.g. testing for the antibodies to acetylcholine receptors. These antibodies, according to Clarke (2005), are found in no other condition. An electromyogram (EMG) is a test that involves measuring the electrical activity within the muscle after a fine needle is inserted into the muscle; however, not all centres offer such a facility. There are some patients with myasthenia gravis who also have an enlarged thymus gland (this may be due to a tumour) and a chest X-ray may need to be performed.

Care and management

No single treatment works for all patients; it is advocated that an individualised care package be designed once a diagnosis has been made. The condition can be life-threatening, but with appropriate treatment, advice and support the majority of patients can become symptom free. Careful explanation regarding the condition must be provided and the patient should be advised to avoid activities that may put them in danger if they suddenly become weak, e.g. swimming alone. The healthcare professional should communicate clearly with the patient, encouraging concordance with medications and to avoid activities such as stress-inducing activities that may exacerbate the condition. As some patients with myasthenia gravis suffer with respiratory difficulties, they should be advised to have annual influenza immunisations. A co-ordinated, multidisciplinary approach to care should be adopted as there are several different healthcare professionals who may need to intervene and provide care for the patient, e.g. physiotherapist, occupational therapist and dietician. The diagnosis of a long-term potentially life-threatening disease can instil fear and anxiety in patients and they may as a result experience depression; careful assessment of the patient's psychological state is required and where appropriate referral to the most suitable healthcare professional, e.g. a psychologist and/or counsellor.

Medications such as oral anticholinesterase can be prescribed, e.g. pyridostigmine; this prolongs the action of acetylcholine by inhibiting the production of cholinesterases. Immunosuppressive medications, e.g. corticosteroids, may be of value as they have an immunosuppressive effect. If there is thymus involvement, then thymectomy may improve prognosis. Plasmapheresis, can also have some impact in some patients as this procedure attempts to remove the destructive antibodies. Another option is the injection of intravenous immunoglobulin; this, it is thought, reduces the function or production of antibodies (Clarke, 2005). Plasmapheresis and intravenous immunoglobulins produce a rapid improvement in symptoms but this only last for approximately 6 weeks.

Conclusion

Every activity of living is associated with mobility and the degree of mobility/immobility will alter as the patient traverses the lifespan. The ability to move about freely allows us to meet our basic needs, e.g. eating, drinking and elimination, as well as being able to carry out leisure and work-related activities that will enable us to maintain our social contact and enhance our self-esteem.

491

Some patients may become totally dependent on others for their care; some may become transiently dependent on others and will then return to carrying out their activities of daily living in an independent manner. All body systems can be affected by the hazardous effects of immobility; the longer the patient is immobilised the greater the consequences (McCance et al., 2010). There are many potential complications associated with bed rest that can cause discomfort (physically and psychosocially); therefore, the healthcare professional has to assume an active role in the prevention or minimisation of the potential problems. The key elements of the healthcare professional's role are predominantly threefold – to comfort, educate and prevent.

It is not possible in a chapter of this size to address in depth all concerns associated with the musculoskeletal system and the reader is advised to read more detailed texts in order to inform clinical practice with the aim of improving their clinical skills.

Test your knowledge

- Describe the role and function of the healthcare professional in relation to the care of the person who has a musculoskeletal problem.

- Discuss the environmental, physical, psychological, politico-economic and sociocultural factors that need to be taken into account when caring for a person with a musculoskeletal problem.

- Describe the ways in which the musculoskeletal system is able to perform and fulfil several different roles.

- Provide a range of health promotion activities that would reduce the risk of osteoarthritis.

- Identify the muscles of the body where it would be safe administer an intramuscular injection. Give the reasons for your responses.

Activities

Here are some activities and exercises to help test your learning. For the answers to these exercises, as well as further self-testing activities, visit our website at www.wiley.com/go/fundamentalsofappliedpathophysiology

Fill in the blanks

Some of the _____ that make up _____ are lost as part of normal _____. From about the age of 35, you gradually lose bone _____. For some people this can lead to _____, a condition in which bones become _____ and _____ easily. These _____ are called _____ fractures. These fractures are most common in bones of the _____, _____ and _____ , but affect other bones in the _____ and _____. Women who have gone through the _____ are at increased _____ of osteoporosis because their _____ no longer produce _____, which protects against bone _____. Osteoporosis can affect men, younger women and children.

Choose from:
Ovaries; Fragile; Ageing; Fractures; Oestrogen; Arms; Pathological; Osteoporosis; Break; Bone; Density; Loss; Spine; Menopause; Wrists; Matter; Hips; Risk; Pelvis

Label the diagram

Using the list of words supplied, label the diagram that is depicting the muscles.

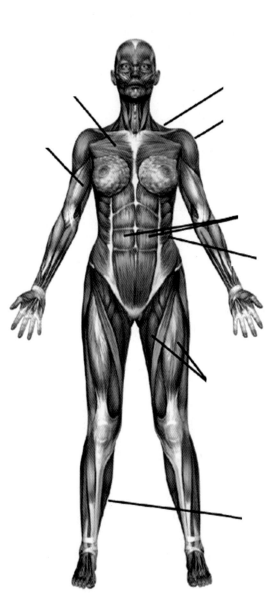

Abdominals; Quadriceps; Biceps; Trapezius; Deltoids; Pectorals; Obliques; Soleus.

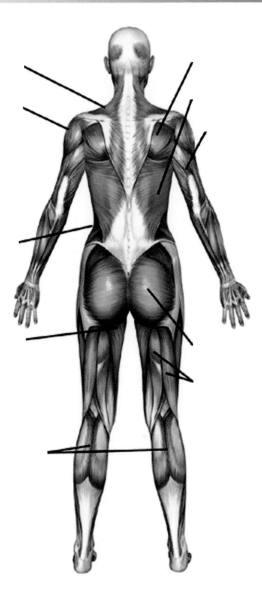

Trapezius; Gluteus Maximus; Calves; Hamstrings; Adductors; Triceps; Rhomboid; Deltoids; Obliques; Latissimus dorsi.

Word search

I	E	H	T	E	C	A	P	O	S	T	U	R	E
M	U	N	N	C	A	O	N	O	I	X	E	L	F
U	U	O	P	T	T	L	N	S	S	N	E	I	A
S	B	I	S	L	S	A	R	T	O	R	I	U	S
C	C	T	C	L	A	A	A	E	R	K	T	D	A
L	E	C	G	L	A	T	L	O	O	A	N	O	D
E	S	U	A	U	A	S	E	B	P	C	C	O	D
S	R	D	O	R	R	C	R	L	O	L	R	T	U
N	S	B	E	B	T	R	T	A	E	E	O	T	C
T	R	A	P	E	Z	I	U	S	T	K	T	D	T
S	N	A	A	E	I	S	L	T	S	A	S	S	I
S	I	T	I	R	H	T	R	A	O	E	T	S	O
N	Z	B	T	U	I	E	I	T	G	L	E	E	N
C	A	S	S	I	E	N	O	D	N	E	T	U	M

Abduction	Flexion	Pain
Adduction	Metatarsals	Posture
Bone	Muscle	Sartorius
Calcium	Osteoarthritis	Skeletal
Cartilage	Osteoblast	Tendon
Contract	Osteoporosis	Trapezius

Further resources

National Institute for Health and Clinical Excellence (NICE)

http://www.nice.org.uk/

NICE provides guidance, sets quality standards and manages a national database to improve people's health and prevent and treat ill health. There are many excellent resources on this website that can help guide and inform practice.

The Myasthenia Gravis Association

https://www.mga-charity.org/
The Myasthenia Gravis Association provides a contact point that puts sufferers and their families in touch with each other so that they do not feel isolated in dealing with this rare disease. The Association also puts members in touch with other appropriate agencies for any specific problems they are facing, e.g. problems with benefits.

Arthritis Care

http://www.arthritiscare.org.uk/
Arthritis care supports people with arthritis. This is the largest arthritis charity. The website provides a range of information for people with arthritis and healthcare professionals.

National Osteoporosis Society

http://www.nos.org.uk/
The National Osteoporosis Society is the only UK-wide charity dedicated to improving the diagnosis, prevention and treatment of osteoporosis. The website is easy to navigate and offers a wealth of useful information for people with osteoporosis and their families, and for those who care for people with osteoporosis.

497

Muscular Dystrophy Campaign

http://www.muscular-dystrophy.org/
The Muscular Dystrophy Campaign provides free and expert information to anyone affected by muscle disease. There is a telephone and email information service provision offering support and signposting to anyone with questions about muscle disease. The Muscular Dystrophy Campaign funds world class research aiming to find effective treatments and cures.

Brittle Bone Society

http://www.brittlebone.org/
The Brittle Bone Society provides practical and emotional support for people affected by the rare bone condition osteogenesis imperfecta. It also provides short-term loan of specialist wheelchairs and other equipment when required, And acts as a signpost to organisations that may be able to help with queries, such as benefits and welfare issues.

Glossary of terms

Actin:	a microfilament protein.
Anticholinesterase:	an agent that blocks nerve impulses by inhibiting the activity of an enzyme called cholinesterase.

Cartilage:	a type of connective tissue that contains collagen and elastic fibres. This strong tough material on the bone ends helps to distribute the load within the joint; the slippery surface allows smooth movement between the bones. Cartilage can withstand both tension and compression.
Cholinesterase:	an enzyme that breaks down acetylcholine to stop its action.
Claudication:	ischaemia of the muscles, causing lameness and pain on by walking, particularly in the calf muscles.
Crepitus:	a crinkling, cracking or grating feeling or sound in the joints.
Cytokine:	a hormone-like protein that regulates the intensity and duration of immune responses.
Diplopia:	a condition where a single object is perceived as two objects.
Dyarthria:	a disturbance of speech and language.
Dysphagia:	difficulty in swallowing.
Effusion:	a collection of fluid.
Haematoma:	a localised collection of blood due to a break in the wall of a blood vessel that is often clotted.
Haemopoiesis:	the formation and development of blood cells.
Immunosuppressive:	pertaining to immunosuppression – prevention or interference with the development of an immunological response.
Lesion:	a wound or injury; refers to a change in the tissues.
Ligament:	a tough fibrous band that holds two bones together in a joint.
Macrophage:	a phagocyte produced from monocytes that engulfs and digests cellular debris, microbes and foreign matter.
Menisectomy:	the removal of the meniscus (ligament within the knee).
Opiate:	a powerful analgesic agent derived from opium that stimulates opiate receptors within the central nervous system.
Ossification:	the formation of bone.
Osteoblast:	a cells that arises from fibroblasts; a bone-forming cell.
Osteoclasts:	a cell that breaks down bone tissue and thus releases the calcium used to create bones.
Osteophyte:	an overgrowth of new bone around the side of osteoarthritic joints; also known as spurs growth.
Osteoporosis:	a condition characterised by reduced bone density and an increased risk of fractures.
Plasmapheresis:	**the** removal of whole blood from the body and separation of cellular elements.

Proximal:	nearest to the trunk or point of origin.
Ptosis:	drooping of the upper eye lid.
Septic arthritis:	a pus-forming bacterial infection of a joint space.
Synapse:	the junction where two neurons meet or where a neuron meets tissue.
Uric acid:	the end product of the purine nucleotide (nucleoprotein) metabolism.

References

Belavic, J.M. (2010). Febuxostat provides new gout treatment options. *Nurse Practitioner.* 35(3): 9–10.

Bulstrode, C.J.K. and Swales, C. (2010). *The Musculoskeletal System at a Glance.* Oxford: Wiley Blackwell.

Chartered Institute of Personnel and Development (2009). *Absence Management: Annual Survey 2009.* London: Chartered Institute of Personnel and Development.

Christensen, B.L. and Kockrow, E.O. (2011). *Adult Health Nursing,* 6th edn. St Louis: Mosby.

Clarke, C.R.A. (2005). Neurological disease. In: Kumar, P. and Clark, M. (eds). *Clinical Medicine,* 6th edn. Edinburgh: WB Saunders, pp. 1173–1271.

Conaghan, P.G. and Sharma, L. (2009). *Fast Facts: Osteoarthritis.* Abingdon: Health Press.

Davies, R., Everitt, H. and Simon, C. (2006). *Musculoskeletal Problems.* Oxford: Oxford University Press.

Davis, G. (2006). The musculoskeletal system: Physiology, conditions and common drug therapies. *Nurse Prescribing.* 4(10): 406–411.

Department of Health (2010) *Improving the Health and Well-being of People with Long Term Conditions.* London: Department of Health.

Docherty, B. (2007). Skeletal system. Part two – Bone growth and healing. *Nursing Times.* 103(6): 28–29.

Hickey, J.V. (2009). *The Clinical Practice of Neurological and Neurosurgical Nursing,* 6th edn. Philadelphia: Lippincott.

Brown, A. and Mclennan, A. (2007). Moving and handling. In: Jamieson, E.M., McCall, J.M., Whyte, L.A. and McCall, J.M. (eds). *Clinical Nursing Practices,* 5th edn. Edinburgh: Churchill Livingstone.

Langstaff, D. (2000). Fracture healing and principles of fracture management. In: Langstaff, D. and Christie, J. (eds). *Trauma Care: A Team Approach.* Oxford: Heinemann.

McCance, K.L., Huether, S.E., Brashers, V.L. and Rote, N.S. (2010). *Pathophysiology: The Biologic Basis for Disease in Adults and Children,* 6th edn. St. Louis: Mosby.

McRae, R. (2006). *Pocket Book of Orthopaedics and Fractures,* 2nd edn. Edinburgh: Churchill Livingstone.

Perez, E. (2011). Mobility and biomechanics. In: Daniels, R., Grendell, R.N. and Wilkins, F.R. (eds). *Nursing Fundamentals: Caring and Clinical Decision Making,* 2nd edn. New York: Delmar, pp. 1308–1391.

Richardson, M. (2006). Muscle physiology. Part 4: Movement and muscle problems. *Nursing Times.* 102(50): 26–27.

Spray, M.E. (2011). Care of the patient with a musculoskeletal disorder. In: Christensen, B.L. and Kockrow, E.O. (eds) *Adult Health Nursing,* 6th edn. St. Louis: Mosby, pp 1345–1410.

Tortora, G.J. and Derrickson, B. (2011). *Principles of Anatomy and Physiology. Organization, Support and Movement, and Control Systems of the Human Body,* Vol 1, 13th edn. New Jersey: Wiley.

Tortora, G.J. and Grabowski, S.R. (2006). *Principles of Anatomy and Physiology,* 11th edn. New Jersey: Wiley.

Watkins, J. (2010) A case of gout. *Practice Nurse.* 21(4): 210–211.

17

Fluid and electrolyte balance and associated disorders

Ian Peate

Visiting Professor of Nursing, School of Nursing, Midwifery and Healthcare, Faculty of Health and Human Sciences, University of West London, Brentford, Middlesex, UK; Independent Consultant and Editor-in-Chief British Journal of Nursing

Contents

Fundamentals of Applied Pathophysiology: An Essential Guide for Nursing and Healthcare Students, Second Edition. Edited by Muralitharan Nair and Ian Peate.
© 2013 John Wiley & Sons, Ltd. Published 2013 by John Wiley & Sons, Ltd.

Key words

- Diffusion
- Hypovolaemia
- Intracellular
- Oedema
- Electrolytes
- Hypervolaemia
- Osmosis
- Extracellular
- Interstitial fluid
- Osmotic pressure

Test your prior knowledge

- In the human body, where are the extracellular compartments?
- Where is most of the fluid volume found – in the intracellular or extracellular compartments?
- Define the function of body fluids and electrolytes.
- Define the terms hypotonic, hypertonic and isotonic solutions.
- What are the signs and symptoms of dehydration?

Learning outcomes

On completion of this section the reader will be able to:

- Identify the fluid compartments of the body.
- List the major electrolytes of the extracellular and intracellular compartments of the body.
- Define the term osmosis.
- Define the term diffusion.

Don't forget to visit to the companion website for this book (www.wiley.com/go/ fundamentalsofappliedpathophysiology) where you can find self-assessment tests to check your progress, as well as lots of activities to practice your learning.

Introduction

Fluid and electrolytes are essential for body function and to maintain homeostasis. Fluid and electrolytes are not static in the body. There is constant movement of fluid and electrolytes between the intracellular and extracellular compartments. The movement of fluid and electrolytes ensures that the cells have a constant supply of electrolytes such as sodium, chloride, potassium, magnesium, phosphate, bicarbonate and calcium for cellular function (see Chapter 1 for a description of cellular functions). Changes in the movement of fluid and electrolytes between compartments occur as a result of disease. This chapter considers fluid and electrolyte balance and some diseases resulting from fluid and electrolyte imbalance.

Body fluid compartments

Fluid forms approximately 60% of the body weight in an adult male, 50% in an adult female and 70% in an infant (McCance *et al.*, 2010). The percentage of fluid distribution varies with age and gender. Women have less body fluid compared to men as women have more body fat and men have more muscle mass (McCance *et al.*, 2010). Fat cells contain less water than muscle cells.

The two principal body fluid compartments are intracellular and extracellular. The intracellular compartment is the space inside a cell and the fluid inside the cell is called intracellular fluid (ICF). The extracellular compartment is found outside the cell and the fluid outside the cell is called extracellular fluid (ECF). However, the extracellular compartment is further divided into the interstitial compartment and the intravascular compartment (Figure 17.1). Two-thirds of body fluid is found inside the cell and one-third outside the cell. Eighty per cent of the ECF is found in the interstitial compartment and 20% in the intravascular compartment as plasma (Figure 17.2).

Composition of body fluid

The body fluid is composed of water and dissolved substances such as electrolytes (sodium, potassium and chloride), gases (oxygen and carbon dioxide), nutrients, enzymes and hormones. The total body water constitutes 60% of the total body weight and water plays an important part in cellular function. Water is essential for the body as it:

- acts as a lubricant
- transports nutrients, gases such as oxygen, hormones and enzymes to the cells, and waste products of metabolism, e.g. carbon dioxide, urea and uric acid, from the cells for excretion
- helps in the regulation of body temperature
- provides an optimum medium for the cells to function
- provides a medium for chemical reactions
- breaks down food particles in the digestive system.

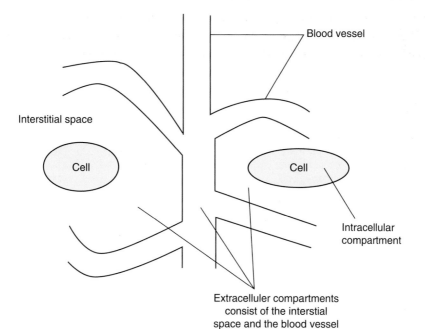

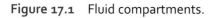

Blood vessel

Interstitial space

Cell

Cell

Intracellular
compartment

Extracelluler compartments
consist of the interstial
space and the blood vessel

Figure 17.1   Fluid compartments.

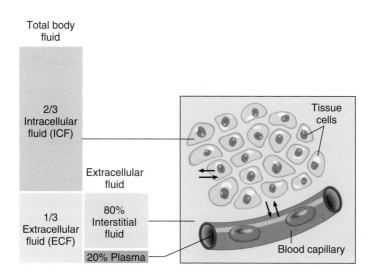

Total body
fluid

2/3
Intracellular
fluid (ICF)

Extracellular
fluid

1/3
Extracellular
fluid (ECF)

80%
Interstitial
fluid

20% Plasma

Tissue
cells

Blood capillary

Figure 17.2   Fluid distribution.

Table 17.1   Fluid intake and output.

Intake (mL)		Output (mL)	
Drinking	1500–2000	Urine	1500–2000
Water from food	700–1000	Faeces	100
Cellular metabolism	300–400 mL	Expiration	600–800
		Skin	300–600
Total balance	2500–3400		2500–3400

Adapted from McCance *et al.* (2010).

Body fluid balance

The term fluid balance indicates that the body's required amount of water is present and distributed proportionally among the compartments. Generally, water intake equals water loss and the body fluid remains constant. However, fluid intake varies with individuals; but the body regulates fluid volume within a narrow range. Most of the water essential for body function is obtained from drinking water, some from the food consumed and some from cellular metabolism. The kidneys play a vital role in fluid balance as water is excreted in the urine; some water is lost in respiration, skin and in faeces. See Table 17.1 for fluid intake and output.

The body regulates body fluid volume via the thirst receptors. When there is an excess of water loss through excessive sweating or by not drinking, then the body fluid balance is disrupted, which can result in dehydration. Dehydration stimulates the thirst reflex in three ways:

- The blood osmotic pressure increases, resulting in the stimulation of the osmoreceptors of the hypothalamus.
- Circulating blood volume decreases, which initiates the renin–angiotensin system, resulting in the stimulation of the thirst centre in the hypothalamus.
- As a result of dehydration, the mucosal lining of the mouth is dry and the production of saliva decreases, which stimulates the thirst centre in the hypothalamus.

Osmosis

Osmosis is a process by which water moves from an area of high volume to an area of low volume through a selective permeable membrane. The movement of water depends on the number of solutes dissolved in the solution and not their molecular weights (Thibodeau and Patton, 2010). Therefore, the number of dissolved particles determines the concentration of the solution, which is expressed as the osmolality of the solution. The selective permeable membrane will allow water molecules to move across, but is not permeable to solutes such as sodium, potassium and other substances. Water accounts for the osmotic pressure in the tissues and cells of the body. Water movement between the intracellular and the extracellular compartments occurs through osmosis.

At times the term tonicity is used instead of osmolality. Thus, solutions can be regarded as hypertonic, hypotonic or isotonic. The term hypertonic solution indicates that the solution has high amount of solutes dissolved in it, e.g. 5% dextrose. A hypotonic solution is one that has a low concentration of solutes dissolved in it, e.g. 0.45% normal saline. An isotonic solution has the same osmolality as body fluids, e.g. 0.9% normal saline (Stanfield, 2011).

Electrolytes

Fluid balance is linked to electrolyte balance. Electrolytes are chemical compounds that dissociate in water to form charged particles called ions. They include potassium (K), sodium (Na), chloride (Cl), magnesium (Mg) and phosphate (HPO_4). Electrolytes are either positively or negatively charged. Positively charged ions are called cations (e.g. Na^+ and K^+) and negatively charged ions are called anions (e.g. Cl^- and HCO_3^-). Remember that an anion and a cation will combine to form a compound, e.g. potassium (K^+) and chloride (Cl^-) will combine to form potassium chloride (KCl). The composition of electrolytes differs between the intracellular and the extracellular compartments (Figure 17.3).

Functions

Electrolytes have numerous functions in the body:

- regulation of fluid balance
- regulation of acid–base balance
- essential in neuromuscular excitability
- essential for neuronal function
- essential for enzyme reaction.

505

Table 17.2 summarises of the principal electrolytes and their functions.

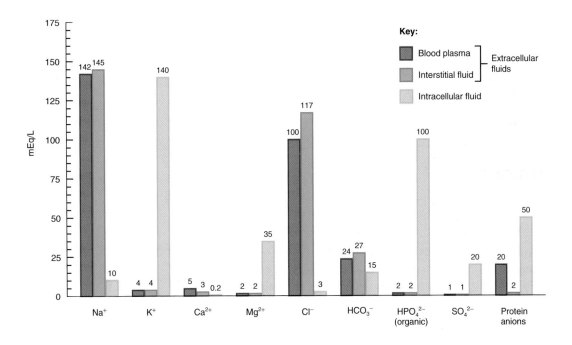

Figure 17.3   Electrolytes of intracellular and extracellular compartments.

Table 17.2   Principal electrolytes and their functions.

Electrolytes	Normal values in extracellular fluid (mmol/L)	Function	Main distribution
Sodium (Na^+)	135–145	Important cation in generation of action potentials. Plays an important role in fluid and electrolyte balance	Main cation of the extracellular fluid
Potassium (K^+)	3.5–5	Important cation in establishing resting membrane potential. Regulates pH balance. Maintains intracellular fluid volume	Main cation of the intracellular fluid
Calcium (Ca^{2+})	2.1–2.6	Important clotting factor. Plays a part in neurotransmitter release in neurons. Maintains muscle tone and excitability of nervous and muscle tissue	Mainly found in the extracellular fluid
Magnesium (Mg^{2+})	0.5–1.0	Helps to maintain normal nerve and muscle function; maintains regular heart rate, regulates blood glucose and blood pressure. Essential for protein synthesis	Mainly distributed in the intracellular fluid
Chloride (Cl^-)	98–117	Maintains a balance of anions in different fluid compartments	Main anion of the extracellular fluid
Hydrocarbons (HCO_3^-)	24–31	Main buffer of hydrogen ions in plasma. Maintains a balance between cations and anions of intracellular and extracellular fluids	Mainly distributed in the extracellular fluid
Phosphate – organic (HPO_4^{2-})	0.8–1.1	Essential for the digestion of proteins, carbohydrates and fats and absorption of calcium. Essential for bone formation	Mainly found in the intracellular fluid
Sulphate (SO_4^{2-})	0.5	Involved in detoxification of phenols, alcohols and amines	Mainly found in the intracellular fluid

Diffusion

Diffusion is a process by which solutes move from an area of high concentration to an area of low concentration. Diffusion is further subdivided into simple and facilitated diffusion. Liquid-soluble molecules and gases move by a process of simple diffusion through a concentration gradient (Figure 17.4). Larger molecules such as glucose and amino acids are transported across a cell membrane by a carrier protein and concentration gradient (Figure 17.5).

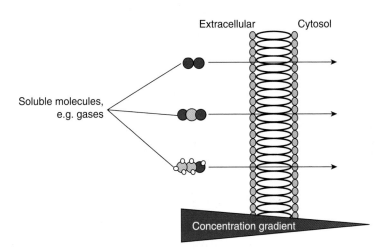

Figure 17.4 Simple diffusion.

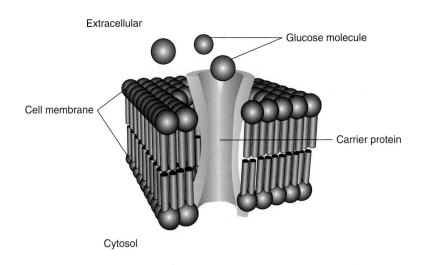

Figure 17.5 Carrier protein (facilitated diffusion).

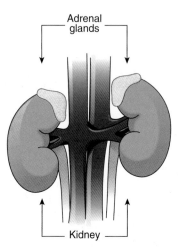

Figure 17.6   Adrenal glands.

Hormones that regulate fluid and electrolytes

The two principal hormones that regulate fluid and electrolyte balance are antidiuretic hormone (ADH) and aldosterone (Thibodeau and Patton, 2010). Antidiuretic hormone regulates fluid balance in the body. This hormone is produced in the hypothalamus by neurons called osmore-ceptors and the hormone is stored by the posterior pituitary gland. Osmoreceptors are sensitive to plasma osmolality and a decrease in blood volume. The target organs for ADH are the kidneys. ADH acts on the distal convoluted tubule and the collecting ducts (see Chapter 8) and make them more permeable to water, thus increasing reabsorption of water.

Aldosterone is a steroid hormone produced by the cortex of the adrenal glands, which are situated at the top of each kidney (Figure 17.6). The adrenal gland is divided into the cortex and the medulla (Figure 17.7). Aldosterone regulates electrolyte and fluid balance by sodium and water retention.

Oedema

Oedema is the abnormal accumulation of fluid, mainly water in the body (Kumar and Clark, 2009) in the interstitial space. It is a problem of fluid distribution and does not indicate fluid excess (McCance et al., 2010). The term is derived from the Greek word meaning swollen condition. The accumulation of fluid may be localised as in thrombophlebitis or generalised as in heart failure affecting all tissues. Localised oedema is normally temporary and resolves without intervention. Generalised oedema is regarded as an abnormal condition that requires treatment.

Oedema can either be pitting or non-pitting. If an indentation develops after gently pressing the swollen lower limb with a finger, this is termed pitting oedema. The causes of oedema include:

- heart failure
- obesity resulting in increased fluid pressure and salt retention

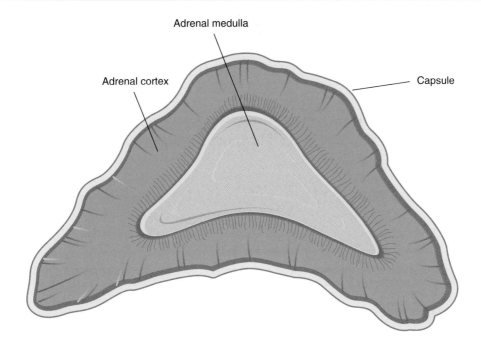

Adrenal medulla

Adrenal cortex

Capsule

Figure 17.7   Cross-section of the adrenal gland.

- drugs such as calcium antagonists, e.g. verapamil and nifedipine, and prolonged steroid therapy
- renal conditions such as nephrotic syndrome
- venous stasis resulting from immobility
- varicose veins
- liver cirrhosis causing hypoalbuminaemia.

Pulmonary oedema

Pulmonary oedema is a condition where there is accumulation of fluid in the lungs, resulting in impaired gas (oxygen and carbon dioxide) exchange and pulmonary function. Pulmonary oedema can result from:

- congestive heart failure
- fluid overload as a result of renal failure
- myocardial infarction with left ventricular failure
- chest injury as a result of a road traffic accident
- upper airway obstruction
- severe chest infection.

Peripheral oedema

Peripheral oedema is a condition where there is localised soft tissue swelling as a result fluid accumulation in the interstitial space. Fluid accumulates in parts of the body affected by gravity, e.g. the lower limbs in a mobile patient or around the sacral region in a patient who is immobile and on bed rest. Peripheral oedema can result from:

- immobility
- obesity
- heart failure
- pregnancy as a result of fluid retention and venous stasis
- liver diseases such as cirrhosis of the liver
- prolonged steroid therapy.

Disorders associated with fluid and electrolyte imbalance

Learning outcomes

On completion of this section the reader will be able to:

- Describe the importance of maintaining a fluid balance chart.

- Discuss the significance of adequate hydration and the benefits of this for the health and well-being of the patient.

- Outline the management and interventions related to the patient who is nauseous and may be vomiting.

- Outline the management and interventions related to the patient who has pulmonary and/ or peripheral oedema.

Maintaining fluid balance charts

Fluid balance, according to Daniels and Nicoll (2012), is a state where the amount of fluid taken into the body equals the amount of fluid that leaves the body. Maintenance of fluid balance is an important activity and is essential for optimal health. If a patient has too much fluid and there is an imbalance, this can cause health problems; likewise if the patient has too little fluid, this too can cause problems. There are some pathophysiological conditions that can result in fluid over-loading, e.g. kidney disease and some types of heart disease; when this occurs the person finds it difficult to rid the body of excess water and can experience oedema, i.e. there is too much fluid in the tissues of the body (care of the patient with oedema is discussed later).

For those patients who are experiencing problems associated with fluid balance, the monitoring of fluid balance becomes important. The healthcare professional uses a chart called a fluid balance chart in order to monitor the patient's input and output (Figure 17.8). Sometimes these charts are known as fluid intake and output charts or intake and output flow charts. Each time the patient takes in fluids or fluids leave the body, the healthcare professional has a responsibility to record this on the fluid balance chart. The amounts are calculated at the end of a 24-hour period – usually

Ward:				Date:			
Surname:				Hospital Number:			
Forename:							
Date of Birth:							

	Fluid intake				**Fluid output**		
Time	**Oral**	**Intravenous**	**Other (specify)**	**Urine**	**Vomit**	**Other (specify)**	
01.00							
02.00							
03.00							
04.00							
05.00							
06.00							
07.00							
08.00							
09.00							
10.00							
11.00							
12.00							
13.00							
14.00							
15.00							
16.00							
17.00							
18.00							
19.00							
20.00							
21.00							
22.00							
23.00							
24.00							
Total							

Figure 17.8   A fluid balance chart.

this is from 12 midnight to 12 midnight the next night. A comparison is made between the amount of fluid taken in and the amount of fluid the patient passes out; this is the patient's fluid balance.

Reid *et al.* (2004) suggest that fluid balance charts that are family-friendly (user-friendly) should be provided. These fluid balance charts encourage patients and their families to fill them in themselves; this can help to promote independence.

Measuring fluid balance

Intake

All of the fluid that a patient drinks and also those foods that are liquid, milk on cereals and ice cream are considered fluid intake. There are other fluids that are considered a part of fluid intake, e.g. enteral feeds and intravenous fluids. All fluid intake must be measured and documented on the patient's fluid balance chart. The healthcare professional needs to know how much various receptacles, such as cups and glasses, hold in order to chart intake effectively.

The amount of enteral feed, gastrostomy and nasogastric feeding and intravenous fluid (including blood and or blood products) being infused must also be monitored, measured and documented. There are some patients who require fluid via the subcutaneous or rectal route and the same is required here; the fluid intake must be recorded.

Output

The following are deemed fluid output, and these (just like intake) must be monitored, measured and documented on the fluid balance chart:

- urine (in seriously ill patients with a urinary catheter *in situ* this may need to be measured and recorded hourly)
- vomit
- aspirate from a nasogastric tube
- diarrhoea
- effluent from a stoma
- exudate from a wound and wound drain.

There may be some instances when it is impossible to measure output accurately, e.g. where the patient has diarrhoea or a wound has excessive exudate. In these instances the healthcare professional may need to weigh incontinence pads or dressings to determine the amount of fluid being lost via this route.

A positive fluid balance exists when the patient's intake exceeds their output and a negative balance occurs when output exceeds intake. Brooker (2007) points out that a record of the daily balance over several days should be carried out so that an assessment of trend can occur.

Maintaining hydration

Florence Nightingale stated that the very first requirement in a hospital is that it should do the sick no harm; this statement was made back in 1854. Having enough to eat and drink is one of the most basic of human needs (Royal College of Nursing and National Patient Safety Agency, 2007). Most people are able to maintain an adequate level of hydration – they are prompted by thirst or hunger to seek fluids or food; however, those who are ill and dependent are unable to do this and they may be at risk of becoming dehydrated. Dehydration is a common fluid and electrolyte imbalance in older people (Daniels and Nicoll, 2012).

This section considers the healthcare professional's responses that need to be made to ensure that patients are adequately hydrated. It draws on previous sections of the chapter in respect to fluid and electrolyte balance. Green and Simpson (2007) define hydration as the state of fluid balance of the body. Rapid weight loss as a result of dehydration can be the consequence of a lack of fluid intake or hyponatraemia (sodium depletion) with an accompanying loss of water.

Benefits of good hydration

Water is vital to health and should be seen as an essential nutrient. As people age their body's needs and health concerns change as a result of an increasing susceptibility to pathophysiological disease. There are many benefits associated with good hydration. The implications of poor hydration from a pathophysiological perspective can have many ramifications and some of these are discussed here.

Those patients who are poorly hydrated have the potential to develop pressure sores (decubitus ulcers); the more an individual becomes dehydrated, the more at risk they become. Dehydration results in a reduction in padding over bony prominences. Fluid intake to correct poor hydration can increase oxygen levels with the possibility of enhancing ulcer healing. Poor outcomes of care and the person's quality of life are directly linked to dehydration (Courtney et al., 2009).

One of the most frequent causes of chronic constipation is inadequate fluid intake. Those patients who are inadequately hydrated can, by drinking more water, increase stool frequency and enhance the beneficial effects of daily dietary fibre intake (LeMone et al., 2011).

It is important in the prevention of urinary tract infection to ensure that the patient maintains adequate hydration. Water helps to maintain a healthy urinary tract and promotes renal function. Consumption of water at regular intervals can help by diluting bile and stimulating gallbladder emptying, which in turn has the potential to reduce and prevent gallstone formation.

In relation to heart disease, hydration reduces the risk of coronary heart disease as adequate hydration decreases blood viscosity, thereby protecting against clot formation. Extracellular volume depletion as result of dehydration is the result of a net loss of total-body sodium with a reduction in intravascular volume (Mentes, 2006).

Dehydration can worsen diabetic control, and water is an essential aspect of dietary management of diabetes mellitus. In those patients who have poorly controlled diabetes, there can be an increase in urinary output and this in turn can result in dehydration; good hydration levels can slow down the development of diabetic ketoacidosis, helping to maintain healthy blood sugar levels (Thibodeau and Patton, 2010).

Dehydration is a risk factor that is associated with falls in older people (LeMone et al., 2011). Dehydration can cause disorientation, dizziness, headache and tiredness, increasing the risk of fainting and falling. Adequate hydration in the older population can be part of an effective falls prevention strategy.

Failure to ensure that the patient is adequately hydrated can lead to a number of pathophysiological changes that can put the health and well-being of the individual at risk. It is therefore vital that this aspect of care is given the priority it deserves. People should be able to access food and drink any time according to their needs and preferences (Department of Health, 2010).

There may be instances where the patient requires an intravenous infusion to replace fluid loss or to hydrate them. An alternative to intravenous fluid replacement (particularly in the frail elderly person) is hypodermoclysis (Arinzon et al., 2004). Hypodermoclysis involves the insertion of a small cannula (a butterfly cannula) into the subcutaneous tissues (often this is in the abdomen). Subcutaneous infusions can be carried out in the home setting if service users, relatives or carers feel confident and can be assessed by the district nurse to demonstrate safe techniques in caring for infusion and cannula sites. The cannula is secured using an occlusive type of dressing and the prescribed infusion begins. The rate and duration of fluid to be transfused is determined by prescription, and the care and management of the patient is in accordance with local policy. It is vital that all fluids (input and output) are recorded on the fluid balance chart.

Nausea and vomiting

There are many reasons why a person may feel nauseous and/or vomit. Johnson et al. (2006) point out that most patients will experience nausea and/or vomiting during a disease process; this may be as a result of the disease pathology or the consequence of treatment. Nausea and vomiting may indicate pathophysiological changes that are occurring within the body. Both nausea and vomiting can be particularly upsetting for the patient as well as for their family; they can also impact on the person's ability to perform the activities of daily living.

Nausea

Crumbie (2007) described nausea as an unpleasant sensation that produces a feeling of discomfort in the region of the stomach with a feeling of a need to vomit. Nausea can be short-lived or long-lasting. A person may experience nausea alone, with no vomiting, or they may vomit without any feeling of nausea beforehand. Some people experience nausea and then go on to vomit. Nausea, therefore, does not always lead to vomiting.

Nausea is a symptom of many conditions; it can be due to physical or psychological issues. It is not an illness and not all of the causes are necessarily related to the stomach, e.g. those patients who are receiving chemotherapy may experience nausea. Nausea can be caused by adverse drug reactions; nausea is also a common symptom of pregnancy. Usually, the presence of nausea means that there may be an underlying pathological condition occurring in the body. The following can also cause nausea:

- diabetes mellitus
- influenza
- gastroenteritis
- renal failure
- adrenal insufficiency
- peptic ulcer
- vertigo.

Treatment of nausea will depend on its cause. Avoidance of foods in the short-term may help to reduce the feelings associated with nausea. Removing or avoiding strong smells such as perfume or aftershave can also help to alleviate nausea. Some people experience nausea when they are, for example, travelling in a car, and stopping the car and sitting still can help alleviate the feelings of nausea that are caused by perceived movement and actual movement.

The healthcare professional may advise the patient to eat small meals throughout the day as opposed to three large meals, and encourage the patient to eat slowly, avoiding foods that are hard to digest. If it is the smell of food that is provoking the nausea, then foods should be eaten cold or at room temperature, avoiding the smell of cooked food or food that is cooking.

An anti-emetic (e.g. metochlopromide), a medicine that is given to prevent or stop nausea and vomiting, may also be administrated. There are also a number of mechanical aids that are used to help prevent nausea (and vomiting). These devices work by applying continuous pressure on specific acupressure points located on the wrist and can be used by children and adults.

Vomiting

Vomiting is a complex physiological activity. It can be defined as the forceful expulsion of gastric contents through the mouth and/or nose.

Excessive vomiting can have a profound effect on a person's fluid and electrolyte balance (Brooker, 2007). The vomiting centre (sometimes also known as the emetic centre) situated in the medulla oblongata of the brain is responsible for the initiation of vomiting. Both physical and psychological impulses can excite the vomiting centre, causing the patient to vomit. Some causes of excitement of the vomiting centre include:

- fear/anxiety
- odours
- pain
- unpleasant sights
- side effects of some drugs
- radiotherapy
- hypercalcaemia.

The sensitivity of the vomiting centre varies in different people and as such the healthcare professional should treat each person on an individual basis.

It is important to determine, if possible, the cause of vomiting; removal of the causative factor, if possible, should be the first line of treatment. Caring for the patient who is vomiting will include the following:

- Ask the patient if they have any tried and tested methods of dealing with vomiting and if appropriate implement these.
- Ensure the patient is cared for in an upright (unless contraindicated) position.
- Care for the patient in the lateral position if they are unconscious and unable to protect their own airway.
- Administer prescribed anti-emetic medication.
- Ensure privacy (e.g. curtains are drawn and doors closed).
- Provide easy access to a vomit bowl and tissues (ensure a receptacle is available to dispose safely of used tissues).
- Remove the dirty vomit bowl and replace with a clean one as soon as possible.
- Offer the patient physical comfort by being with them and holding the vomit bowl or mopping their brow.
- Observe, measure, record and report vomitus.
- Provide the patient with the opportunity to use a mouthwash.
- Provide the patient with the opportunity to 'freshen up' after they have finished vomiting.
- Change any soiled clothing/bedding.
- Try to avoid strong odours such as food, perfumes and aftershaves that may induce nausea and vomiting.

If the extent of vomiting or retching has been excessive, the patient may complain of exhaustion or headache, and muscle soreness can also occur. An explanation of why the person may feel like this, as well as the administration of a prescribed analgesic, can help to provide comfort.

Excessive vomiting and anorexia as a result of this will impinge on a person's hydration status, leading to dehydration and loss of weight. Attention must be paid to the effects of excessive vomiting as extreme gastric secretion can lead to electrolyte imbalance and an ensuing acid–base (i.e. acidosis) discrepancy. The management of this will depend on the extent of vomiting and the patient's overall condition.

Case study

Tomaz Kwiatkowski is an 86-year-old retired carpenter who lives in warden-controlled accommodation. He was admitted to the accident and emergency department via a GP locum referral. His oldest son, Tomas, was due to arrive in the next hour or so. Mr Kwiatkowski gave a

Continued

confusing account of a 4-day history of severe generalised abdominal pain accompanied by a grossly distended abdomen. Mr Kwiatkowski had not opened his bowels for the last 3 days, he felt nauseous and had vomited twice already today and three times yesterday; he was anorexic. Previously he had opened his bowels on a daily basis. He had no mobility problems but, over the last few days, he had been so tired and unwell that he had not been able to get up. He had had an uneventful transurethral resection of the prostate gland 11 years ago. He was hypotensive with a pulse of 120 beats per minute and a temperature of 37.2 °C. Mr Kwiatkowski was in pain and reluctant to move, his tongue was dry and coated. He appeared anxious.

Take some time to reflect on this case and then consider the following.

1. With regards to the care of Mr Kwiatkowski, what are his immediate needs?
2. What other indicators could suggest that he is dehydrated and what would be the safest, most effective method of correcting his dehydration?
3. How can you help meet Mr Kwiatkowski's needs? Your answer should include addressing his psychosocial and emotional needs.

Caring for the patient with oedema

The abnormal collection of fluid in the interstitial spaces is known as oedema (Kumar and Clark, 2009). This section provides an overview of the care required for the patient with oedema in order to maintain a safe environment and provide comfort. The causes of pulmonary and peripheral oedema have been discussed above.

Pulmonary oedema

Many patients who are diagnosed with pulmonary oedema will be acutely ill and they (and their families) may be highly anxious and afraid. The healthcare professional must provide care that takes both the physical and psychological aspects of the condition into account for both the patient and family.

The first line of treatment should be to determine the cause of pulmonary oedema and to take steps to eliminate or reduce this; attempts should be made to reverse the specific cause(s). For example, if the cause is left-sided heart failure, then measures should be taken to improve the pumping action of the left side of the heart.

Signs and symptoms

The signs and symptoms can include some or all of the following:

- dyspnoea/orthopnoea
- wheeze
- tachycardia and tachypnoea
- hypotension
- cardiogenic shock
- sweating

- pallor/cyanosis
- nausea
- anxiety
- dry or productive cough (if productive pink frothy sputum).

Investigations

It is important to remember that pulmonary oedema can result in mild to severe dyspnoea; therefore, when obtaining a history from the patient in order to make a diagnosis this must be borne in mind; questioning of the patient should be kept to an absolute minimum. The healthcare professional should ask questions that are only absolutely necessary and framed in such a way that the patient need only nod or shake their head in order to make a response. After a detailed history has been undertaken from the primary source (the patient) or secondary sources (i.e. other healthcare professionals, the patient's spouse, family or friends), then the following investigations may be required:

- chest X-ray
- blood gas analysis
- estimation of cardiac enzymes
- liver function tests
- estimation of urea and electrolytes
- electrocardiograph.

Care and management

Treatment of the specific cause of pulmonary oedema should continue and the patient's airway must also be managed if dyspnoea becomes so severe that this is in danger; in the acute phase the patient may need to be resuscitated. The key aim should be to improve oxygenation, and this can be done by the administration of prescribed oxygen therapy via a facemask. As pulmonary oedema indicates that there is an abnormal collection of fluid in the interstitial spaces, it is imperative that there is strict control of fluid balance and in some cases a urinary catheter may need to be inserted to provide close monitoring of urinary output. Here is an overview of the management of the patient with pulmonary oedema; this is not a comprehensive list and care will be dictated by the patient's condition and response to therapeutic interventions, and as such the patient requires close monitoring and the provision of skilled care.

- Reassurance, psychological and physical support and explanations (for the patient and family) with regards to care interventions.
- Provide the patient with a nurse call bell; leave this in close proximity.
- Provide easy access to a sputum pot and tissues (ensure a receptacle is available to dispose safely of used tissues).
- Care for the patient in an upright position (unless this is contraindicated), supported by pillows.
- Administer prescribed humidified oxygen via a face mask.
- Administer prescribed medication, e.g. diuretics (i.e. furosemide) and with caution diamorphine, to alleviate anxiety, pain and distress.
- Strict monitoring of fluid balance (may include hourly urine measurements if a urinary catheter is *in situ*).

- Fluid restriction if indicated.
- Monitor, measure and report oxygen saturation, blood pressure, respiratory rate, depth and rhythm; monitoring of pulse frequency, dictated by the patient's condition.
- Assistance with all activities of daily living as appropriate.

Peripheral oedema

Whilst pulmonary oedema, as its name suggests, causes problems associated with breathing as a result of excessive fluid in the lungs, peripheral oedema presents as a collection of excessive fluid within the tissues that pools in the dependent regions, e.g. the legs, ankles, feet and sacral region (Riley, 2007); sacral oedema tends to occur more in those patients who are bed bound. The pooling of fluid can be associated with lack of mobility, the consequence of gravitational pull, as well as the physiological factors that are related to oedema formation as described earlier.

Pitting oedema is the more serious type of oedema. The area of skin, e.g. around the ankles, when lightly pressed remains indented (a pit forms); this is a more serious type of oedema than the type that does not pit. Riley (2007) suggests that peripheral oedema does not appear or become visible until the body has retained 4 L of fluid. If, for example, a patient retains 5.5 L of fluid, this is equivalent to 5.5 kg of weight; hence a way of determining if the patient is retaining fluid, is to record daily weight, along with meticulous fluid balance monitoring.

Case study

Anne Patton is a 47-year-old woman who was admitted to the ward after being referred by the oncology nurse consultant. Ms Patton presented with severe lymphoedema (this was classed as stage III lymphoedema) to the right leg. She tells the physiotherapist who is carrying out an assessment of her needs that her oedema began 9 years ago after she received treatment for cervical cancer. She says she feels ashamed and embarrassed about the 'state she had got herself into'. The oedema had advanced so much that it is impacting on her ability to mobilise independently and safely, as well as having a detrimental effect on her self-esteem. Ms Patton rarely leaves her home. Her husband had become 'distant' and her children and grandchildren have stopped coming around to see her. Her treatment 9 years ago was extensive and necessitated a partial hysterectomy along with radiation therapy. She had metastasis to her spine, causing her much pain; this was also treated with radiation and a range of analgesics. She has been hospitalised twice since for the treatment of cellulitis with oral and intravenous antibiotic therapy. Recently, she has experienced lymph fluid leakage from the pores of her skin, so much so that it has damaged the soft furnishings in her home and she feels this is causing her home to smell.

Take some time to reflect on this case and then consider the following.

1. Explain the pathophysiological factors associated with Ms Patton's lower limb oedema.
2. It is clear Ms Paton is distressed. How can the healthcare team, working in an integrated way, help Ms Patton from a psychosocial perspective?
3. What might the proposed treatment consist of to help reduce the oedema and the detrimental effects it is having on Ms Patton's health and well-being?

Skin that has become oedematous predisposes the patient to the development of pressure sores (decubitus ulcers) and infection, particularly when the skin over the oedematous area has broken down. This risk can become more evident when healthcare professionals who handle patients with oedema have long or sharp fingernails, watches, pens, badges and scissors that can potentially catch the patient's skin and cause more trauma; hence the importance of short nails and the covering of items of equipment in the healthcare professional's pockets. It is important that the patient's fingernails are also kept short to prevent them from inadvertently causing damage to their skin. The principles of care for the patient who has peripheral oedema include:

- a clear explanation of the condition to the patient and, if appropriate, their family
- assessment of skin condition in association with local policy for skin assessment
- careful washing and patting dry (not rubbing) of the oedematous skin
- fluid balance monitoring
- daily weight measurement
- administration of prescribed diuretics (e.g. furosemide)
- elevation of oedematous ankles when sitting out of bed to aid drainage of the pooled fluid
- assistance with those activities of daily living that the patient is unable to carry out independently.

Conclusion

519

Understanding the complex concepts and processes of fluid and electrolyte balance is vital if safe and effective care is to be provided to patients who may sometimes, as a result of fluid and electrolyte imbalance, be critically ill. The healthcare professional has a pivotal role to play when helping people who are experiencing pathophysiological changes associated with fluid and electrolyte imbalance.

This chapter has explained how the dynamics of fluid balance can have a profound effect on an individual's health and well-being. The subtle changes associated with fluid balance have to be recognised quickly by the healthcare professional in order to avert harm; this can be done in many ways using all the senses as well as implementing the fundamentals of science.

It is not possible in a chapter of this size to address in depth all concerns associated with fluid and electrolyte balance and the associated disorders. The reader is advised to access more detailed texts and other forms of information related to fluid and electrolytes with the key aim of providing care that is safe, effective and founded on a sound evidence base.

Test your knowledge

- List the functions of water.
- Explain how fluid and electrolytes move between compartments.
- List the major electrolytes and their functions.
- How would you encourage an older person to increase their fluid intake in order to prevent them from becoming dehydrated?
- Outline the care of a person who is feeling nauseous and vomiting.
- Describe how you would monitor a bed-bound person's fluid intake.

Activities

Here are some activities and exercises to help test your learning. For the answers to these exercises, as well as further self-testing activities, visit our website at www.wiley.com/go/fundamentalsofappliedpathophysiology

Fill in the blanks

The _____ and _____ of dehydration vary depending on the degree of dehydration. Dehydration occurs when fluid _____ exceeds fluid _____. Those people who are at _____ risk of dehydration are the very _____ or the _____. The person experiences _____ and _____, the blood pressure _____ and pulse _____. The person may _____ in severe dehydration as a result of _____ shock. There are many cause of dehydration, e.g. _____, _____, vomiting and _____. The person may need to be hospitalised and fluid _____ via the _____ route. A fluid _____ chart is essential and all fluid is _____. Appropriate _____ is needed if all _____ of the body are to perform _____.

Choose from:
Hydration; Burns; Output; Signs; Elderly; Cells; Collapse; Thirst; Intake; Balance; Recorded; Effectively; Falls; Increases; Symptoms; Greater; Discomfort; Hypovolaemic; Young; Diarrhoea; Intravenous; Haemorrhage; Replaced

Label the diagram

Using the list of words supplied, label the diagram.

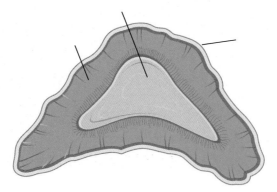

Adrenal cortex; Adrenal medulla; Capsule

Word search

C	Y	N	E	I	I	E	C	L	S	A	H	A	L	I	A	C
L	H	I	A	L	T	O	I	H	S	C	C	P	N	O	E	O
H	Y	N	O	I	T	A	R	D	Y	H	E	R	I	N	O	T
G	P	M	C	H	L	O	R	I	D	E	R	L	E	O	H	A
N	O	O	P	A	E	A	H	A	D	L	T	L	L	I	R	A
I	T	A	M	H	D	I	C	P	O	I	A	S	E	S	R	S
T	O	E	U	M	O	N	E	H	O	O	C	H	C	U	A	C
I	N	O	I	S	N	E	T	O	P	Y	H	M	T	F	I	U
M	I	A	S	Y	T	C	D	R	C	D	Y	C	R	N	D	O
O	C	S	S	E	N	N	A	E	I	I	C	S	O	O	Y	O
V	C	Y	A	N	O	S	I	S	M	T	A	T	L	C	C	O
N	D	I	T	N	R	N	O	I	T	A	R	D	Y	H	E	D
I	O	H	O	D	N	T	D	S	H	E	D	R	T	D	Y	Y
L	I	S	P	I	O	Y	A	E	P	U	I	N	E	A	A	E
C	N	E	P	N	H	E	C	Y	E	C	A	M	S	N	A	N
S	O	D	I	U	M	L	H	O	N	H	A	S	P	I	A	U
O	R	C	A	L	C	I	U	M	Y	C	I	C	D	O	N	L

521

Electrolytes	Isotonic	Diaphoresis
Sodium	Vomiting	Diarrhoea
Potassium	Hydration	Renal
Chloride	Dehydration	Hypotension
Calcium	Cells	Tachycardia
Hypotonic	Oedema	Cyanosis
Hypertonic	Lymphoedema	Confusion

Further resources

National Institute for Health and Clinical Excellence (NICE)

http://www.nice.org.uk/
NICE provides guidance, sets quality standards and manages a national database to improve people's health and prevent and treat ill health. There are many excellent resources on this website that can help guide and inform practice.

Lymphoedema Support Network

http://www.lymphoedema.org/
The Lymphoedema Support Network is the only national patient-led organisation offering information and support to people with this condition and has a unique understanding of the patients' experience. It provides a high standard of information as well as promoting self-help.

Water UK

http://www.water.org.uk/
This website includes a section called Water for Health and it describes The Water for Health initiative that was launched to guide and inform health professionals and health authorities, to stimulate interest and research in hydration, and to help move water up the public health agenda. This is a user friendly, helpful site.

Department of Health – Heat Wave Plan

http://www.dh.gov.uk/prod_consum_dh/groups/dh_digitalassets/documents/digitalasset/dh_127235.pdf
This document provides the heat wave plan for England and has some helpful hints and tips about ways in which dehydration can be prevented and people protected. The plan has been issued as a part of raising both public and professional awareness. The Plan's purpose is to enhance resilience in the event of a heat wave. It is an important component of overall emergency planning.

Age UK

http://www.ageuk.org.uk/
This national website is packed with information for the general public and healthcare professionals concerning the older population. It includes a section called professional resources; this contains links to (amongst other things) policy and research.

British Lung Foundation

http://www.lunguk.org/
The British Lung Foundation is the only national charity associated with lung disease. There are video clips on this site and a range of other resources that would be of interest to healthcare

professional and members of the public. There is a really useful section (there are many) about how to live with a lung condition. This is a very practical and user friendly website that is easy to navigate.

Glossary of terms

Amine:	organic compound that contains nitrogen.
Anion:	negatively charged ion.
Anti-emetic:	a drug that reduces nausea and vomiting.
Cation:	positively charged ion.
Dehydration:	excessive fluid loss from the body.
Detoxification:	removal of toxic substances from the body.
Electrolyte:	a chemical element or compound that includes sodium, potassium, calcium, chloride and bicarbonate.
Extracellular:	outside the cell.
Hypertonic:	solution that has large amounts of solutes dissolved in it.
Hypodermoclysis:	Insertion of a small cannula into the subcutaneous tissues.
Hypotonic:	a solution that has a low concentration of solutes.
Interstitial space:	space between cells.
Intracellular:	inside the cell.
Isotonic:	a solution that has the same osmolality as the body fluids.
Metabolism:	the collective name for all the physical and chemical processes occurring within a cell/living organism, but often referring only to reactions involving enzymes..
Nausea:	an unpleasant sensation that produces a feeling of discomfort in the region of the stomach with a feeling of a need to vomit.
Oedema:	the abnormal accumulation of fluid in the interstitial spaces. It may be localised (following an injury = swelling) or it may be generalised (as in heart failure).
Osmolality:	osmotic concentration of a solution.

Osmosis: the passive movement of water through a selectively permeable
                    membrane from an area of high concentration of a chemical to an area
                    of low concentration.

Osmotic pressure: the pressure that must be exerted on a solution to prevent the passage
                    of water into it across a semipermeable membrane from a region of
                    higher concentration of solute to a region of lower concentration of
                    solute.

Plasma: fluid component of the blood.

Stoma: any opening; a mouth. Usually used to refer to a surgically-created
                    opening.

Tonicity: another term for osmolality.

Vomiting: a disagreeable experience that occurs when the stomach contents are
                    reflexly expelled through the mouth or nose.

524 References

Arinzon, Z., Feldman, J., Feldman, Z. Gepstein, B. and Berner, Y. (2004). Hypodermoclysis (subcutaneous infusion): Effective mode of treatment of dehydration in long-term care patients. *Archives of Gerontology and Geriatrics.* 38(2): 167–173.

Brooker, C. (2007). Promoting hydration and nutrition. In: Brooker, C. and Waugh, A. (eds). *Foundations of Nursing Practice: Fundamentals of Holistic Care.* London: Mosby, pp. 531–568.

Courtney, M., O'Reilly, M., Edwards, H. and Hassall, S. (2009). The relationship between clinical outcomes and quality life for residents of aged care facilities. *Australian Journal of Advanced Nursing.* 26(4): 49–57.

Crumbie, A. (2007). Caring for the patient with a disorder of the gastrointestinal system. In: Watson, M. and Crumbie, A. (eds). *Watson's Clinical Nursing and Related Sciences*, 7th edn. Edinburgh: Bailliere Tindall, pp. 427–495.

Daniels R. and Nicoll, L. (2012) *Contemporary Medical-Surgical Nursing*. New York: Delmar.

Department of Health (2010) *Essence of Care* London Department of Health http://www.dh.gov.uk/prod_consum_dh/groups/dh_digitalassets/@dh/@en/@ps/documents/digitalasset/dh_119978.pdf [accessed 11 September 2012].

Green, S.M. and Simpson, P.M. (2007). Eating and drinking. In: Hogston, R. and Marjoram, B.A. (eds). *Foundations of Nursing Practice: Leading the Way*, 3rd edn. Basingstoke: Palgrave, pp. 121–153.

Johnson, A., Harrison, K., Currow, D., Luhr-Taylor, M. and Johnson, R. (2006). Palliative care and health breakdown. In: Chang, E., Daly, J. and Elliott, D. (eds). *Pathophysiology Applied to Nursing Practice*. Sydney: Mosby, pp. 449–471.

Kumar, P. and Clark, M. (2009). *Clinical Medicine*, 7th edn. Edinburgh: Elsevier.

LeMone, P., Burke, K. and Bauldoff, G. (2011). *Medical – Surgical Nursing; Critical Thinking in Client Care*, 4rd edn. New Jersey: Pearson.

McCance, K.L., Huether, S.E., Brashers, V.L. and Rote, N.S. (2010). *Pathophysiology: The Biologic Basis for Disease in Adults and Children*, 6th edn. St. Louis: Mosby.

Mentes, J. (2006). Oral hydration in older adults. *American Journal of Nursing.* 106(4): 40–49.

Reid, J., Robb, E. and Stone, D. (2004). Improving the monitoring and assessment of fluid balance. *Nursing Times.* 100(20): 36–39.

Riley, J. (2007). Breathing and circulation. In: Brooker, C. and Waugh, A. (eds). *Foundations of Nursing Practice: Fundamentals of Holistic Care*. London: Mosby, pp. 463–500.

Royal College of Nursing and National Patient Safety Association (2007). *Water for Health: Hydration Best Practice Tool kit for Hospitals and Healthcare*. London: RCN/NPSA. http://www.rcn.org.uk/newsevents/campaigns/nutritionnow/tools_and_resources/hydration [accessed 11 September 2012].

Stanfield, C.L. (2011). *Principles of Human Physiology*, 5th edn. New Jersey: Pearson.

Thibodeau, G.A. and Patton, K.T. (2010). *The Human Body in Health and Disease*, 5th edn. St. Louis: Elsevier Mosby.

18

The skin and associated disorders

Ian Peate

Visiting Professor of Nursing, School of Nursing, Midwifery and Healthcare, Faculty of Health and Human Sciences, University of West London, Brentford, Middlesex, UK; Independent Consultant and Editor-in-Chief British Journal of Nursing

Contents

Fundamentals of Applied Pathophysiology: An Essential Guide for Nursing and Healthcare Students, Second Edition. Edited by Muralitharan Nair and Ian Peate.
© 2013 John Wiley & Sons, Ltd. Published 2013 by John Wiley & Sons, Ltd.

Key words

- Dermis
- Dermatology
- Health promotion
- Epidermis
- Self-esteem
- Chemotherapy
- Integumentary system
- Cancer
- Radiotherapy

Test your prior knowledge

- Name the layers of the skin.
- What are the appendages of the skin?
- Describe the role of the skin in health.
- What aesthetic properties does the skin have?
- How might the healthcare professional help to prevent skin cancer?

Learning outcomes

On completion of this section the reader will be able to:

- Discuss the anatomy and physiology of the skin.
- Describe the various functions of the skin.
- Discuss the appendages.
- Outline the management of some skin conditions.
- Describe the role of the healthcare professional as health educator.

Don't forget to visit to the companion website for this book (www.wiley.com/go/ fundamentalsofappliedpathophysiology) where you can find self-assessment tests to check your progress, as well as lots of activities to practise your learning.

Introduction

Skin diseases affect 20–30% of the population at any one time, seriously interfering with activity in 10%. (Lawton, 2001). They can affect a person's ability to carry out activities of daily living and also have an impact on their sense of well-being. Healthcare professionals observe the patient's skin on a daily basis whilst carrying out care activities; it is vital therefore that they have an understanding of the function of the skin in order to recognise problems that may occur. There are many areas of practice where the healthcare professional will come into contact with people who suffer with problems of the skin and they are ideally placed to offer these people support with respect to some of these conditions.

Some skin conditions have the potential to cause stigma, such as eczema and psoriasis; the healthcare professional, as advocate, can dispel any misunderstanding regarding contagion and enhance the individual's social well-being. Appearance and image are often associated with success and achievement, and the blemish-free individual portrayed in the media (in most Western societies) is the image to which many strive; this is not always possible for those with skin conditions. Society places much emphasis on physical appearance and for those who have skin problems this can become increasingly challenging. People with skin problems may experience difficulties in other aspects of their lives, e.g. from a sexual relationship perspective, and also concerning issues surrounding self-esteem and self-concept – altered body image can have a profound effect on the individual, their partner and their family.

Patients may report feeling ostracised, stigmatised and isolated. It is unusual for skin diseases to kill, but the psychological morbidity they cause is massive and often largely unrecognised or ignored by healthcare professionals. Every disease brings with it a psychological as well as a physical burden, but the visual nature of skin diseases means that those people with skin disease are more susceptible to embarrassment and as a result of this loss of self-esteem.

Mitchell and Kennedy (2006) note that skin disease is not just a cosmetic nuisance, emphasising that it can have a profound impact on a person's life; they suggest that it can help to think of the five 'Ds' in association with dermatology:

- **D**isfigurement
- **D**iscomfort
- **D**isability
- **D**epression
- **D**eath.

Page (2006) summarises some of the problems that patients with skin conditions may experience (Table 18.1).

Dermatology is the study of the skin and its diseases; dermatologists are specialist practitioners who diagnose and treat diseases of the skin, nails and hair. The healthcare professional can help enhance the quality of life for the person who has a skin problem.

This chapter introduces the reader to the structure and function of the skin. The skin (including its appendages), the only visible and largest organ of the body, is also known as the integumentary system. An overview of the anatomy and physiology of the skin is provided; the function of the

Table 18.1   Problems that patients with skin conditions may experience.

Emotional problems	Low self-esteem Feeling unclean Problems with relationships Feeling stared at Being regarded as infectious or contagious
Clothing restrictions	Avoiding wearing short sleeves Avoiding the wearing of dark clothing due to skin shedding Avoiding the wearing of summer clothing which exposes the skin Clothing can become stained or ruined when using greasy oily skin preparations
Social restrictions	Skin becomes itchy in hot places where people congregate Avoiding swimming or sports facilities Avoiding communal changing rooms
Financial implications	Routine prescriptions are expensive but essential No allowances are made to replace clothing or bedding No allowances are made for fuel bills due to extra laundering and bathing

Adapted from Page (2006).

skin is also discussed, and a number of skin conditions are considered along with the management of a patient with a skin disorder. A brief discussion is also provided of the skin appendages – hair follicles, eccrine and apocrine glands, and nails. This chapter considers preventative strategies that the healthcare professional may wish to introduce to prevent conditions such as skin cancer.

The anatomy and physiology of the skin

The skin in humans (as in most other mammals) consists of two layers: the outer layer – the epidermis; and an underlying layer made of fibrous tissue – the dermis. Below the dermis is subcutaneous fat. At a cellular level the skin is composed of a number of types of cells; these cells and their functioning are essential to maintaining health and the promotion of well-being (Figure 18.1).

The skin is estimated to weigh between 2.5 and 4 kg in an adult and is thickest at the palms and soles (approximately 1 mm thick) and at the eyelids it is at its thinnest (approximately 0.1 mm thick). There are over one million nerve endings in the skin and it covers a surface area of $2\,m^2$.

The skin has a number of vital functions:

- protection from harmful external factors (such as microbes, ultraviolet light and chemicals)
- internal homeostasis (a balanced internal environment)
- shock absorber
- thermoregulation
- insulation

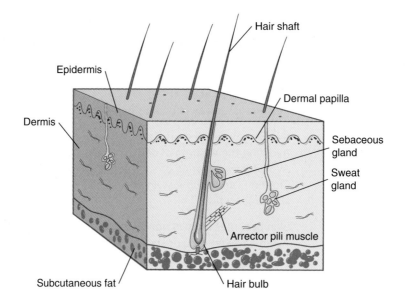

Figure 18.1   The structure of the skin.

- sensation
- lubrication
- protection and grip
- calorie reserve
- synthesis of vitamin D
- body odour
- psychosocial

The epidermis

The epidermis is the outer layer of the skin and is composed primarily of keratinocytes (approximately 95% of cells), including other specialised cells, e.g. melanocytes, Langerhans cells and Merkel cells. Table 18.2 outlines the functions of these cells.

The epidermis is composed of stratified epithelium and it has no blood vessels. The cellular nourishment (including oxygenation) and the removal of waste products occur through diffusion from the vascular network in the superficial dermis.

The prime functions of the epidermis are to provide a physical and biological barrier to the environment – the penetration of irritants is prevented by the epidermis, as is the loss of water, and the management of internal homeostasis. There are three key factors associated with the various layers of the epidermis:

- division and migration of epidermal cells to the skin surface on a regular basis
- keratinisation of the epidermal cells
- rubbing away of the epidermal cells (desquamation).

Table 18.2   The functions of melanocytes, Langerhans and Merkel cells.

Cells	Functions
Melanocytes	These cells are located in the basal layer of the epidermis. The melanocytes produce the pigment melanin; melanin is found in the eyes, hair and skin. Melanin is responsible for providing protection and the absorption of ultraviolet rays. Melanin is the primary determinant of human skin colour
Langerhans cells	Langerhans cells are one part of the body's immune system, they activate the immune response and in particular the T-helper cells. They play an important role in contact allergies
Merkel cells	These cells are found in small numbers in the basal layer. They play a role in sensation, are associated with sensory nerve endings and are found in specific areas such as the palms, soles and genitalia. Their exact function is unclear

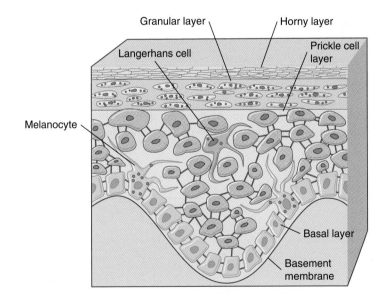

Figure 18.2   The layers of the epidermis.

The layers of the epidermis are shown in Figure 18.2. The basal layer (also called the stratum basale) is located close to the cells that are nearest to the dermis at the dermo-epidermal junction; it is at this point that cell division takes place. Cells migrate upwards from the dermo-epidermal junction and over a period of approximately 12–18 days they keratinise prior to being shed.

The next layer is the prickle cell layer (stratum spinosum), and this protects against shearing forces or trauma to the skin; the cells in this layer move upwards above the basal layer.

Fine granules are formed from within the granular layer (stratum granulosum). These granules are the precursor of keratin, which eventually replaces the cytoplasm of the cells.

The clear cell layer (stratum lucidium) is only present in areas where the skin is thick, e.g. the soles and palms. The cells in this layer have large amounts of keratin; they are flattened and closely packed. When injury or trauma occurs, the production of these cells is increased and calluses or corns are formed.

The horny layer (stratum corneum) is the uppermost part of the epidermis and is made up of thin, flat and non-nucleated cells. These are dead cells and are shed from the skin.

The dermis

The dermis is chiefly composed of a network of connective tissue (mainly collagen) underlying the epidermis of the skin, which acts as the anchor that joins the dermis and epidermis (Figure 18.3). The connective tissue gives strength and elasticity, as well as providing a supportive mesh-work for the specialised structures throughout the dermis. This layer of the skin is much thicker than the epidermis; the key function is to support and sustain the epidermis. The dermis provides a protective pad for the deeper structures, protecting them from trauma, and it also nourishes the epidermis and has a vital role to play in wound healing.

The dermis has a number of specialised cells, e.g. mast cells and fibroblasts, as well as:

- blood vessels
- lymphatics
- nerves
- sweat glands.

Just as the epidermis has layers, so too does the dermis; the dermis has two layers. The first layer, the superficial papillary dermis, is made up primarily of loose connective tissue that contains

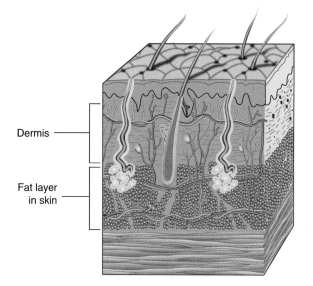

Figure 18.3   The structure of the dermis.

blood vessels in the form of capillaries; elastic fibres and collagen are also components. The depth of the superficial papillary dermis depends on age and anatomical location.

The second layer is called the reticular dermis. This layer is thicker than the superficial papillary dermis, dense connective tissue and larger blood vessels are interlaced with elastic fibres (providing pliability) and thick bundles of collagen are present. There are also mast cells and fibroblasts as well as nerve endings and lymphatic vessels. These structures are surrounded by a viscous gel that bathes the structures, allowing nutrients, hormones and waste products to pass through the dermis. The viscous gel helps to provide bulk, allowing the dermis to act as a buffer.

Blood supply

Thermoregulation is primarily controlled by a complex network of blood vessels within the dermis. Lying close to the epidermal border is the superficial plexus, which is made up of a number of interconnecting arterioles; these vessels wrap themselves around the structures in the dermis and through this interconnecting network, oxygen and nutrients are supplied to the cells. At the border with the subcutaneous layer (the dermis) is the deep plexus. These vessels, in comparison to those in the superficial plexus, are more substantial; they connect vertically to the superficial plexus.

Lymph vessels

The lymph vessels play an important role in draining excess tissue fluid and plasma proteins from the dermis; this results in internal homeostasis – ensuring that there is the correct volume and composition of tissue fluids. Lymph also searches for foreign matter such as bacteria and antigenic substances.

533

Nerves

Free sensory nerve endings (the Merkel cells) are found in the basal layer of the epidermis and the dermis, and detect pain, irritation and temperature. The skin is supplied with approximately one million nerve fibres; sensory perception is an important protective mechanism of these cells. Specialist receptors responding to pressure and vibration (Pacinian corpuscles) and touch/ sensitivity (Meissner's corpuscles) are also found in the dermis. Autonomic nerves supply the blood vessels and sweat glands and the Arrector pili muscles.

The subcutis

The subcutis is a subcutaneous layer that lies below the dermis. The layer, composed mainly of fat (adipose tissue), provides the skin with support and acts as a shock absorber (Figure 18.3). The subcutis is also responsible for insulating the body and storage of nutrients; the subcutis is interlaced with blood vessels and nerves.

The appendages

There are three important components of the skin known as the appendages of the epidermis:

- the sweat glands
- hair follicles and sebaceous glands
- nails.

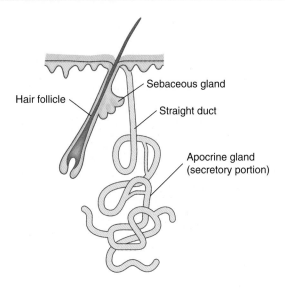

Figure 18.4   Sweat gland.

Sweat glands

Sweat glands are coiled tubes of epithelial tissue; they open out to pores on the skin surface (Figure 18.4). Each gland has its own nerve and blood supplies. The glands secrete a slightly acidic fluid containing water and salts (excess excretory products). Keratin maintains its suppleness because of the action of sweat. There are two types of sweat glands – eccrine and apocrine. The production of secretions by the eccrine glands in response to, for example, heat or fear, is controlled by the sympathetic nervous system. These glands are found all over the body; however, they are more numerous at some sites, e.g. the forehead, axillae, soles and palms.

The apocrine glands are also coiled; they are not as numerous as the eccrine glands and are found in more localised sites – the pubic and axillary regions, the nipples and perineum – and are not functional until puberty; it is understood that they secrete pheromones released into the external environment. A viscous material is excreted that causes body odour when acted upon by the surface bacteria.

Hair follicles and sebaceous glands

Hair is found on all surfaces of the body except the palms, soles and lips; its amount, distribution, colour and texture vary depending on its location, and the sex, age and ethnic group of the individual. It contributes to an individual's unique appearance. Hair colour is determined by the melanocytes that are within the hair bulb and hair growth is influenced by genetic and hormonal factors.

Hair is a keratin structure of the epidermis; each hair is a thread of keratin and is formed from cells at the base of a single follicle. It has several functions:

● sexual
● social

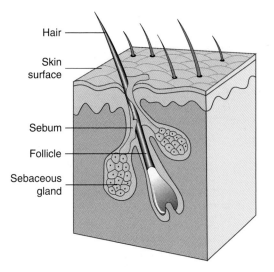

Hair
Skin surface
Sebum
Follicle
Sebaceous gland

Figure 18.5   The pilosebaceous unit.

- thermoregulation
- protection.

The key role of hair is to prevent heat loss. The whole skin surface is provided with hair follicles; each pore is an opening to a follicle and they are situated deep in the dermis above the dermis. Attached to each gland is a small collection of smooth muscle called the Arrector pili; these muscles contract and become erect in response to cold, fear and emotion. The contraction of the muscle can be seen on the skin in the form of 'goose bumps'. When heat leaves the body through the skin, it becomes trapped in the air between the hairs.

The hair follicles are accompanied by sebaceous glands, and sebum (a liquid substance) is secreted by these glands, providing moisturization to the skin as well as ensuring that the skin and hair are waterproof. Sebum is a slightly acidic substance that has antibacterial and antifungal properties (Waugh and Grant, 2010). The distribution of the sebaceous glands varies; they are most prominent on the scalp, face, upper torso and anogenital region, and during puberty these glands are at their most active – sebum production is influenced by sex hormone levels. Figure 18.5 demonstrates what is known as a pilosebaceous unit; the pilosebaceous unit is composed of the follicle, the hair shaft, the sebaceous gland and the Arrector pili.

Nails

The final appendage is the nails; these too are made of keratin and they have a tough texture because the keratin is formed in concentrated amounts; they can be described as horn-like. There are no nerve endings in nail. They act as protectors; fingernails and toenails afford some protection to the digits. Nails also make it easier to grab or grasp things, acting as a counterforce to the fingertips which have many nerve endings to allow an individual to receive a lot of information about the objects we touch.

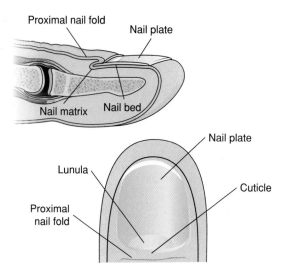

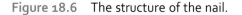

Figure 18.6   The structure of the nail.

The rate of nail growth varies; on average, nails grow at a rate of 0.1 cm per day (1 cm per 100 days). Fingernails require 4–6 months to regrow completely; toenails take longer to grow, between 12 and 18 months to regrow completely. The rate of growth depends upon factors such as the age of the person, the time of year, the amount of exercise undertaken and hereditary factors (Haneke, 2006). Nail growth can be impeded by trauma and inflammation; changes in the integrity of the nails can be the result of injury or infection and in some instances is evidence of systemic diseases, e.g. chronic cardiopulmonary disease (Timby and Smith, 2010). Figure 18.6 demonstrates the structure of the nail.

Learning outcomes

On completion of this section the reader will be able to:

- Describe some of the pathophysiological changes that may occur to the skin.

- Highlight the role and function of the healthcare professional when caring for those who may suffer with a skin condition.

Disorders of the skin

There is an old saying – a picture is worth a thousand words; this saying is particularly true when caring for people with skin, hair and nail disorders. It is important that you understand what some of the most common skin lesions look like. The reader may benefit from consulting a colour skin atlas to enhance their skills of observation (Wolff *et al.*, 2005). When discussing skin conditions, the term lesion describes a small area of disease, whereas a rash or eruption describes a widespread area of skin.

Box 18.1   Some components of the history.

- Any known allergies
- Onset, initial site continuous or intermittent, how long
- Associated symptoms such as itch, burning, redness, oozing, scaling, blisters
- Actions that might make the condition worse, e.g. exposure to heat or cold, any stress including activities
- Family history, e.g. genetic predisposition, anyone at work/school with a similar condition
- Associated systemic symptoms, e.g. asthma
- Current prescribed medications, including any medications that are being applied to the skin as well as any oral preparations. How often are they taken and effect
- Current over-the-counter medications, including any medications that are being applied to the skin as well as any oral preparations. How often are they taken and effect
- Social history, including details about occupation, hobbies, amount of exercise, housing, smoking, alcohol intake and use of recreational drugs
- Impact of the disorder on them as an individual, their self-esteem, self-image, ability to manage on a daily basis and any coping mechanisms used
- Impact of the disorder on others they live or work with

Adapted from Buxton and Morris-Jones (2009).

Many skin lesions can be diagnosed on sight; however, there is still the need to adopt a systematic approach to diagnosis and this will entail a detailed health and medical history as well as a physical examination. To confirm diagnosis, other investigations may also be needed. Page (2006) provides details of what a full history should entail (Box 18.1). The healthcare professional needs to use effective and sensitive communication skills to help reveal the diagnosis and also the person's description and understanding of the disorder, as well as their perception and the perceptions of others of living with it.

Wolff *et al.* (2005) report that the type, frequency and prevalence of skin disorders is closely associated with and depends on an individual's social, economic, geographical and cultural circumstances. There are a number of factors that can predispose a person to skin disorders; both extrinsic and intrinsic (Table 18.3).

Skin disorders can be minor or life-threatening, with people sometimes seeking their own remedies to some of the problems they encounter. There are, however, a number of conditions that require more intensive interventions; these interventions can take place in the patient's own home, in the primary care setting or there may be a need for the person to be admitted to hospital.

Skin cancer

Sunlight is the main cause of skin cancer and the incidence of this cancer has increased steadily over the years (National Institute of Health and Clinical Excellence, 2010) In the UK, skin cancer is the second most common form of cancer (Foss and Farine, 2007). There are three forms of skin cancer:

Table 18.3   Some intrinsic and extrinsic factors that can predispose a person to skin disease.

Extrinsic	Intrinsic
Extremes of heat	Genetic/hereditary factors
Allergens	Internal disease
Chemicals	Medications
Irritants	Infections
Trauma	Psychological factors
Friction	
Infections	
Sunshine	
Sun lamps	

Adapted from Hunter *et al.* (2002).

- malignant melanoma
- basal cell carcinoma (BCC)
- squamous cell carcinoma (SCC).

Malignant melanoma

This is the most dangerous form of skin cancer and it accounts for 10% of all cases of skin cancer (Wolff *et al.*, 2005). The cells of the body that become cancerous in malignant melanoma are the melanocytes. Melanoma usually develops in a naevus (also known as a mole); it can metastasise rapidly via the circulatory and lymphatic systems.

This type of skin cancer spreads rapidly and because of the speed with which it spreads, it is the most dangerous type. These cancers are more common in young people and are closely related to sunburn and overexposure (Foss and Farine, 2007).

Risk factors

- exposure to sun
- use of sunbeds
- being female (evidence to suggest that hormones play a part if risk is inconclusive)
- age
- presence of moles
- being fair skinned
- history of sunburn, having been sunburned at least once and risk rises if this occurred as a child
- geographical factors (where the person was born)
- family history.

There is one key risk factor for melanoma, i.e. sun or sunbeds (ultraviolet light). There are, however, some people who are more at risk than others. More women than men get melanoma; it is the seventh most common cancer in women. The disease is rare in those who are aged under 14 years; after age 15 years, the incidence steadily rises and the highest incidence is in those aged 80 years and over. Risk increases the more moles a person has.

Those who are fair skinned are more at risk than those who are dark skinned; however, dark skinned people can and do get malignant melanoma. Those who are fair and have a tendency to freckle in the sun are more at risk as are those who do not tan at all; these people are usually those who peel before getting a tan. People with melanoma are twice as likely to have been badly sunburned at least once in their lives; sunburn as a child is even more damaging than sunburn as an adult, because during childhood the skin is at its most vulnerable. Risk is also associated with geography and where the person was born. Those who are fair skinned and were born in hot country, e.g. Australia, have an increased risk of melanoma for life, in contrast to those who went to live there as a teenager or those with similar skin colour who live in cooler climates. The skin would have been exposed to the effects of the sun whilst the person was young, when the skin was at its most delicate. A family history, i.e. a family member who has had melanoma, places a person at risk.

Signs and symptoms

There are a number of warning signs that may indicate malignant melanoma (Page, 2006):

- new or existing moles getting bigger
- changes in the shape of a mole; if there is a change in the edge of the mole, it becomes irregular in shape around the edges
- changes in the colour of a mole – it gets darker or becomes patchy or multi-shaded
- a mole becomes itchy or painful
- a mole starts to bleed or becomes crusty
- any surrounding or underlying inflammation.

Diagnosis

A patient's history as well as full physical examination is required. The healthcare professional should examine and observe the whole of the body. Hutchinson's freckle (also known as lentigo maligna) is a premalignant melanoma condition (Mitchell and Kennedy, 2006). Hutchinson's freckle can be seen on the face or other areas of the body that are exposed to the sun; in some patients, the condition will have been slowly enlarging for a number of years.

Dermatoscopy may be performed in order to examine the lesion. This is a painless test that has the ability to magnify the area up to ten times.

The only method used to confirm diagnosis of a malignant melanoma is to take a biopsy of the lesion and subject it to histological testing (histology). Usually, the specimen is obtained under a local anaesthetic but this will depend on the part of the body where the lesion is. The lesion is measured and usually photographed in order to make comparisons at a later stage.

Urgent referral must be made if the lesion is suspected to be cancerous. A seven-point scale is advocated by the National Institute for Health and Clinical Excellence (NICE, 2006) to help make the decision to refer to a specialist (Table 18.4). Within the scale, there are three major features and four minor ones. Two points are given for any of the major features and one for the minor features; if the mole (the lesion) scores three points or above, then urgent referral is required.

Table 18.4   Assessing changes in moles (lesions).

Characteristic	Points
Change in size*	2
Change in colour (e.g. getting darker, becoming patchy or multi-shaded)*	2
Change in shape*	2
7 mm or more across in any direction	1
Inflammation	1
Oozing or bleeding	1
Change in sensation (e.g. itching or pain)	1

*Major feature.
Adapted from NICE (2006).

However, NICE (2006) suggests that if there is any cause for concern, regardless of the score, then the person should be referred to a specialist.

Care and management

Precancerous moles can be treated by excision under local anaesthetic; early malignant melanomas can also be treated in this way. The longer a suspicious mole is left, the more difficult it can be to treat and the poorer the prognosis. If the mole is removed, the patient will have sutures in place and they will need to stay *in situ* for up to a week; the patient returns to the centre where the lesion was removed and usually receives the results of the histology. If the histology reveals that the lesion was non-cancerous, then no further treatment is needed; however, if there is evidence of cancerous cells, more tests will be required.

One of the proposed tests will determine how deep the melanoma is – this is called staging. The deeper the cancerous cells, the more likely it is that the cancer has spread within the body (Thompson *et al.*, 2005). The following tests may also be required:

- blood tests
- chest X-ray
- ultrasound scan
- bone scan
- CT scan.

Wide local excisions may be required depending on the individual's unique circumstances, e.g. how much of the mole (lesion) was left behind and how deep the melanoma has grown into the tissues. In some circumstances, if a large area of skin has been excised, this may require skin grafting.

Lymph node removal, if there is lymph involvement, may be needed and treatment can also include chemotherapy; another type of treatment that may be offered is interferon treatment.

Chemotherapy and interferon (biological therapy) is also known as adjuvant treatment. Radiotherapy, the use of high-energy radiation, to kill cancer cells can also be used; again this will depend on the individual needs and circumstances. Sharpe (2006) suggests that there is no improvement regarding survival when adjuvant therapy is used; however, disease-free intervals may be prolonged.

Often patients are anxious and concerned about the results of test and the decisions they will have to make. The healthcare professional has a duty to provide the patient with physical and psychological support before, during and after all interventions; this will include providing information in a manner that the patient understands and is able to assimilate, so that they can make an informed decision.

Regular follow-up is needed and the frequency at which this is required will depend on the individual circumstances. The aim of follow-up is to see how the patient is coping and to determine if they need any further physical or psychological support, if there is recurrence around the scar, if there is any spread to the lymph nodes or other parts of the body or if there are any new melanomas.

Basal cell carcinoma and squamous cell carcinoma

BCC is a skin cancer of the epidermis. BCC is slow to develop and commonly occurs on the face. SCC occurs to the outermost layers of the skin. Often it appears as a scaly or crusty patch of skin bigger than 1 cm (but it may be smaller); it does not heal. Both these types of cancer are called non-melanoma skin cancers and are the most common type of cancer in the UK (NICE, 2006). Usually, they appear on body parts that are exposed:

- face
- neck
- ears
- forearms
- fingers
- hands.

These types of skin cancer are more common in the older population (NICE, 2010). Prognosis for those with this type of cancer is very good.

The main treatment for BCC and SCC is surgery (NICE, 2010). The type of surgery is classed as minor surgery and involves the use of a local anaesthetic to remove the cancer. Radiotherapy may be used to treat large areas of skin cancer or if the cancer is in a difficult place to operate on or if the patient is unable, due to ill health or incapacity, to have surgery performed safely (Sharpe, 2006). Chemotherapy is another option, but for BCC and SCC this is rarely used. Creams that contain chemotherapeutic medications may, however, be used, particularly when the cancer is limited to the top layer of the skin.

In all cases of skin cancer, malignant or non-malignant, and for all patients, the healthcare professional should be prepared to provide health promotion advice. Healthcare professionals in any situation can encourage regular checking of the skin; they are ideally placed to provide information concerning skin self-examination. Effective treatment depends on early detection of skin cancer and a prompt diagnosis (NICE, 2006).

Case study

Roland Cunliffe is a 62-year-old married man with two children. He has been aware of a lesion on his skin on his upper chest for about the last 4 years. Initially the lesion appeared to be a harmless red spot; since then it has grown gradually. Recently, it has started to crust a little. He has been prescribed a number of creams but none of these has helped.

Mr Cunliffe could not recall any particular skin problems in the past; however, he did remember his mother having something removed from her face a good few years ago. He is skin type II and he has a holiday home in Spain, spending 2 weeks each year there.

When examined there was a red, mainly flat lesion on his upper chest measuring 1.75 cm in diameter. Closer inspection using a good light source and magnifying glass showed a very delicate raised whipcord edge. Further examination revealed two similar lesions on his back. No further lesions were identified on his face or limbs. A basal cell carcinoma was suspected.

Take some time to reflect on this case and then consider the following.

1. What tests need to be undertaken to allow a diagnosis to be made?
2. How will you explain these tests to Mr Cunliffe so that he can make an informed decision?
3. What modes of treatment may be needed?

Health promotion advice – skin cancer

When the opportunity arises, the healthcare professional should be proactive in providing health promotion advice concerning the damaging effects of the sun and the avoidance of skin cancer to those who may need it, e.g. those working outdoors and younger members of the population.

Not everyone's skin offers the same protection in the sun and because of this, it is important to know about skin types (Table 18.5). Those with skin types I–IV need to take most care in the sun, particularly those who have skin types I and II. Those who have skin types V and VI generally only need to protect their skin when the sun is particularly strong or they go out in the sun for a long period of time. Box 18.2 provides some advice the healthcare professional can give to patients concerning sun protection. Skin cancer is a significant and increasing health problem for the nation; prevention according to Sharpe (2006) is a long-term issue and will require major attitude and behavioural changes of the population.

New legislation is now in force to protect people aged under 18 years from the harmful effects of sunbeds (ultraviolet tanning equipment). The Sunbeds (Regulation) Act 2010, which is enforced by local councils, requires sunbed operators to ensure that no person under the age of 18 uses a sunbed on their premises.

There is much evidence to suggest that sunbeds can lead to malignant melanoma. The International Agency for Research on Cancer (IARC, 2007), an expert body that examines the evidence on causes of cancer, have re-classified sunbeds as a Group 1 carcinogen. This classification is the highest cancer risk category and is reserved for things where the evidence is strongest. IARC has demonstrated that, on average, people who start using sunbeds under the age of 35 years increase their risk of malignant melanoma by 75%.

Table 18.5   Skin types.

Type	Characteristics
Type I	Pale skin, burns very easily and tans rarely. Generally these people have light coloured or red hair and freckles
Type II	These people usually burn but may gradually tan. Often they have light hair, blue or brown eyes. Some may have dark hair but still have fair skin
Type III	Generally tan quite easily, but with long exposure to the sun burn. Usually, they have dark hair with brown or green eyes
Type IV	Tan very easily, but with long exposure to the sun will burn. Often they have olive skin, brown eyes and dark hair
Type V	Naturally brown skin with dark hair and brown eyes. These people burn only with prolonged exposure to the sun and their skin further darkens easily
Type VI	Have black skin with dark brown eyes and black hair. These people burn only with extreme exposure to the sun and their skin further darkens easily

Adapted from British Association of Dermatologists (2007).

Box 18.2   Some points related to sun protection.

- Select a waterproof sunscreen, one with an adequate sun protection factor (SPF). An SPF of 15 multiplies the period of time it takes to burn by 15. An SPF of at least 15 should be used by everyone. Those who have paler skin should use a higher SPF rating. The sunscreen should screen out both ultraviolet A (UVA) and ultraviolet B (UVB) rays. A lip balm with a high SPF should also be applied to the lips
- The sunscreen should be rubbed in well and applied approximately 15–30 minutes before going out into the sun. Every 2 hours throughout the day the sunscreen should be reapplied and also after swimming
- Avoid excessive exposure to the sun. Light-coloured loose fitting clothing should be worn as this will help the person feel cooler. Garments should be closely woven as lightweight clothing provides little protection to UV light which will pass through it. A wide brimmed hat protects the head and neck
- The sun should be avoided between 1100 hours and 1500 hours, particularly in those countries that are close to the equator
- Sunglasses should be worn as prolonged exposure can cause damage to the lens of the eye, resulting in an opaqueness (cataract). Sunglasses that conform to British standards are advocated
- The skin's sensitivity is increased when cosmetics are worn in the sun; therefore they should be avoided
- UV light can be reflected by water, snow and buildings; therefore, it is important to apply sunscreen when sitting in the shade. Cloud is no barrier to UV light, and it is still possible to burn on a cloudy day as UV light can penetrate cloud

Adapted from Foss and Farine (2007).

Eczema

According to Mitchell and Kennedy (2006), the word eczema comes from the Greek word meaning to boil over. The terms eczema and dermatitis are used synonymously; they can be described as acute or chronic (Waugh and Grant, 2010) and the severity can vary. The condition can affect all age groups. There is no specific diagnostic test for eczema and the diagnosis is based on clinical assessment (NICE, 2007). With the correct treatment, the inflammation can be reduced; however, there is currently no cure for eczema.

As with most skin conditions that are visible, eczema can have a profound effect on an individual's self-esteem. The patient may also experience disturbed sleep as a result of the clinical manifestations. For younger patients, there may be a significant impact on their behaviour and development as a result of disturbed sleep, lowered self-esteem and social isolation (ostracism). Frequent visits to the doctor, the need to apply messy topical applications and the use of special clothing can add to the burden of the disease. Eczema can have a profound effect not only on the patient but also on their family.

The pathophysiology of atopic eczema is a complex interaction of susceptible genes, environmental triggers, defects in the skin barrier and immunological responses (Akdis *et al.*, 2006). Raised serum immunoglobulin E (IgE) levels are seen in atopic eczema, but the exact role of IgE in the disease is unclear (Flohr *et al.*, 2004).

Wolff *et al.* (2005) describe the characteristics of both acute and chronic eczema. Acute eczema is characterised by:

- pruritus
- erythema
- vesiculation

and chronic eczema by:

- pruritus
- xerosis
- lichenification
- hyperkeratosis
- fissure formation (rare).

Endogenous eczema

Atopic eczema

This condition is described as a chronic relapsing inflammatory skin condition; the patient tends to scratch and itch at a red rash that is often found in skin creases, such as the elbows and behind the knees. Mitchell and Kennedy (2006) note that other features include:

- crusting
- scaling
- cracking
- swelling of the skin.

The cause of atopic eczema is unknown. The condition is also associated with other diseases such as hay fever and asthma. Adults make up nearly one-third of community cases of atopic eczema.

544

Pathophysiological changes are the result of complex interactions between:

- the skin barrier
- genetic responses
- environmental issues
- pharmacological factors
- immunological causes.

Microscopically, atopic eczema appears as excessive fluid between the cells in the epidermis (this is known as spongiosis); when the condition worsens, the fluid erupts into the epidermis and forms vesicles – small collections of fluid, and vesiculation occurs (Mitchell and Kennedy, 2006). In atopic eczema, a hypersensitivity response occurs in reaction to an antigen and antibody effect; however, Wolff *et al.* (2005) suggest that the antigen–antibody response is still not fully understood. A genetic predisposition and a combination of allergic and non-allergic factors appear to be influencing features.

Discoid eczema

Also called nummular eczema, the aetiology of this type of eczema is unknown. It appears to peak twice a year in autumn and winter (Wolff *et al.*, 2005) and is more common in middle-aged and older people; it usually lasts for only a few weeks (Page, 2006). Characteristically, the disease appears as coin-shaped plaques with small papules and vesicles on an erythematous base, more common on the lower legs.

545

Seborrhoeic eczema

The main areas affected are the hairy areas of the body, and the patient may complain of itching and have a red scaly rash (Mitchell and Kennedy, 2006). The disease is more common in men and may be associated with patients who are immunosuppressed, e.g. those with human immunodeficiency virus (HIV). This type of eczema can become complicated as a result of fungal infection.

Varicose eczema

This type of eczema commonly affects the lower limbs and can occur with or in the presence of varicose ulcer (Page, 2006). The aetiology is associated with chronic venous stasis; often the area involved becomes red and itchy and the patient may also have varicose veins and oedema (Gawkrodger, 2003).

Diagnosis

It has already been stated that diagnosis is made on clinical examination; referral to a dermatologist may be required. Other diagnostic tests include:

- blood tests
- patch test
- allergy tests.

Exogenous eczema

In industrial settings, exogenous eczema is common (Mitchell and Kennedy, 2006). It is usual for this type of eczema to erupt at the point of contact and the way in which the patient presents will depend on the irritant. The immune system overreacts to a substance that would otherwise be harmless.

There are many irritants that can cause allergic contact dermatitis, e.g. the wearing of earrings or jewellery that contains nickel may cause allergic contact dermatitis and hypersensitivity will occur; perfumes and cosmetics can also cause contact dermatitis. Dermatitis may be triggered by the wearing of disposable gloves; if this is the case the user should be advised to use hypoaller-genic, commercially supplied, disposable gloves. In such cases the person may have to consider a change in occupation. Occupations that are considered high risk include:

- hairdressing
- catering
- healthcare
- printing
- engineering
- agriculture
- horticulture
- construction
- cleaning.

Care and management

The care and management of the various types of eczema are similar. In atopic eczema, one of the main complications is infection (bacterial and fungal) as a result of a break in the skin. When the skin is infected, it contains pustules that are green or yellow in colour, with large blisters; the patient may feel unwell and have a raised temperature. The role of the healthcare professional is to prevent infection in this instance and this can be done by educating the patient in how the infection may be caused and spread by scratching.

The healthcare professional should explore with the patient what it is that causes or makes the eczema worse; the answers to these questions can provide information that will lead to the testing of the patient for certain things with a patch test. If an allergen or irritant is identified, then this should, if possible, be avoided. The following outlines the general approach to the management of atopic eczema; however, it should be noted that approaches to care should be tailored to meet individual needs.

- Remove, if possible, the irritant or allergen that causes the antibody–antigen reaction.
- Offer support to the patient and their family to empower, educate and motivate. The overall aim should be to raise self-esteem and self-awareness and as such to prevent stigma.
- If the eczema, for example, is varicose eczema, then the patient may be advised to wear support hosiery or if appropriate and possible, surgical intervention may be required.
- Creams, ointments and oils can be used to act as emollients to reduce the drying and itching effects of the disease.
- Aqueous cream may be used as a substitute for soap. Soaps can have the effect of further drying the skin. Perfumed products should be avoided.
- If infection occurs, then antibiotics or antifungal medication may need to be prescribed. These medications are often given systematically but may be applied topically.
- In some instances, topical steroid preparations can be used to reduce inflammation, but these should be used with caution and should not be used for longer than is necessary.

- Topical preparations containing both antibiotics and steroids are available, but again these should only be used for the short-term.
- Antihistamines may be prescribed.

Examples of other issues that will need to be considered are:

- Encourage rest as sleeping may be difficult for some patients.
- Dietary advice may be needed if the allergen is a food product; a multidisciplinary approach is advocated with referral to a dietician.
- Complementary therapies may help some patients. Complementary therapies are complementary and not a substitute for conventional medicine; however, the healthcare professional must respect the patient's wishes.
- At all times when applying medications, wear gloves not only to combat the risk of cross-infection but also to avoid absorbing the patient's medicines.

Case study

Martin Halpin is a 25-year-old retail assistant in a large DIY store. He is shortly to be interviewed for a promotion. He has had eczema for over 10 years; this comes and goes but is particularly bad during periods of stress. The eczema is usually symmetrical. Mr Halpin's skin itches uncontrollably and this can have an impact on his sleep. Mr Halpin has used steroid cream which his doctor prescribed which helped the itching but it was less effective when the situation became severe and the itching became worse. Mr Halpin is an asthmatic and uses an inhaler when his breathing troubles him and this is often as a result of dust and during the winter.

Currently he is experiencing itching at his elbow and in the elbow crease, and behind the knees. He feels very tired and is hot and irritable. Red thick areas with erythema located at the back of knees and elbows are present on examination.

Take some time to reflect on this case and then consider the following.

1. What are the factors that might cause a flare up of eczema?
2. Are there any ways in which you can help promote comfort?
3. How might you help Mr Halpin with this condition?
4. Are there any complications that may arise? What are they?

Psoriasis

There are several forms of psoriasis; this skin disorder is a non-infectious, inflammatory disorder that can appear as a red, raised demarcation of skin patches with silvery whitish scales (Mitchell and Kennedy, 2006); the condition can vary from mild to severe. The aetiology is unknown.

The patient may also experience an itch. If itching occurs the scales are easily shed. It occurs most frequently on the back, elbows, knees and scalp. This skin condition has the potential to cause the patient to feel ashamed and dirty.

Pathophysiologically, the cells of the basal layers of the epidermis reproduce and the more rapid upward progression of these cells through the epidermis results in an incomplete maturation of the upper layer (Waugh and Grant, 2010); there is an overproduction of skin cells. Sometimes psoriasis is associated with arthritis and this is called psoriatic arthropathy. The rash associated with psoriasis can occur when the patient is experiencing an episode of arthritis.

Thirty-five per cent of the patients with this condition have a family history (Mitchell and Kennedy, 2006); Page (2006) points out that there are other precipitating/aggravating factors:

- infection (streptococcal throat infection)
- some medications, e.g. antimalarials, antidepressants, beta-blockers
- sunlight (can help or hinder)
- hormones – psoriasis can get better or worse during pregnancy or menstruation
- psychological stress, e.g. bereavement, divorce or sitting examinations
- trauma, e.g. burns, the site of an injury or a surgical scar.

Naldini and Gambini (2007) suggest that the diagnosis of psoriasis is made on clinical presentation. Skin biopsy, skin swab, throat swab and blood tests as well as clinical examination will be required to confirm diagnosis (Page, 2006). Treatment will include psychological support for the patient and the family.

There are a range of topical therapies that are available to manage psoriasis. The healthcare professional has a role to play in motivating and encouraging the patient to apply the therapies meticulously, adhering to the treatment regimen. The following is a list of some of the topical therapies. It must be noted that whatever treatment is chosen, this is not a cure for the disease and no single treatment will suit everyone and individual assessment is required (Mitchell and Kennedy, 2006):

- Emollients with the aim of lubricating the skin and easing scaling, as well as providing patient comfort.
- Coal tar ointments – these preparations have an antipruritic and anti-inflammatory effect (they may stain clothing).
- Dithranol – this is used to suppress cell proliferation.
- Vitamin D analogues such as calcipotriol, tacalcitol and calcitriol; these are used amongst other things to inhibit cell proliferation.
- Phototherapy can be used to inhibit cell division in some forms of psoriasis.
- Methotrexate – this is often used in the treatment of cancer; it causes inhibition of cell division.
- Retinoids – these influence the activity of the epidermis.
- Topical steroids – used only for a short period.

Conclusion

The skin, also called the integumentary system, is the largest organ in the body and has several important functions. This chapter has provided an overview of the skin and has discussed a number of pathological changes that can result in disease or illness. Some of the more common skin conditions have been discussed with an emphasis on skin cancer. The reader is advised to consult other texts to fully appreciate the scope and potential the healthcare professional has in helping people with skin conditions; this chapter has merely touched on the topic. The healthcare professional has a vital role to play in assisting the individual with problems associated with the skin; however, this can only be achieved with insight and understanding.

As well as the physiological disturbances resulting in problems of skin, there are also important psychological ramifications that must be given much consideration. The healthcare professional has a role to play in empowering and motivating the patient in order to adhere to prescribed treatment regimens that can often be messy and potentially damage clothing and bedding. Many patients with skin conditions and their families voice concerns about social isolation and ostracism; education and explanation may help to reduce these feelings; the healthcare professional is ideally placed to do this, acting as a key resource.

Test your knowledge

- Describe the care of the patient with atopic eczema.

- Outline the role and function of the healthcare professional when providing advice to a patient or group of patients concerning skin cancer avoidance.

- Describe the pathophysiological changes that occur during wound healing.

- Discuss the potential psychosocial impact a disfiguring skin condition can have on the person.

- List the complications that may be associated with a full thickness burn.

Activities

Here are some activities and exercises to help test your learning. For the answers to these exercises, as well as further self-testing activities, visit our website at www.wiley.com/go/fundamentalsofappliedpathophysiology

Fill in the blanks

Skin forms the _____ organ of the body and performs many vital roles as both a _____ and as a _____ where it has regulating influence between the _____ world and the controlled _____ within the body. _____ body temperature (core temperature) is _____ through several processes, including _____ production and the rate of _____ flowing through the _____ of blood _____ within the skin. Skin and the fat layer _____ it also act as good _____. _____ of sweat from the skin greatly _____ the rate at which _____ can be lost from the body. The physical _____ of the skin prevents _____ of harmful chemicals and invading _____ such as _____ and _____. It also acts as a _____ absorber for the more sensitive tissues and organs underneath.

Choose from:
Viruses; Heat; Internal; Outside; Entry; Environment; Regulator; Controlled; Strength; Bacteria; Organisms; Barrier; Shock; Sweat; Network; Largest; Insulators; Blood; Increases; Evaporation; Beneath; Vessels

Label the diagram

From the list of words supplied, label the diagram.

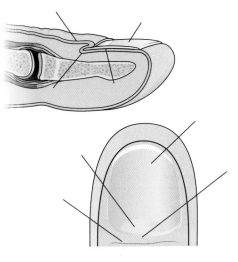

Lunula; Nail matrix; Hyponychium (nail bed); Nail body (plate); Eponychium (cuticle); Proximal nail fold

Word search

P	O	S	S	I	I	I	A	A	E	S	I	S	E	R
S	S	O	E	E	S	M	P	B	C	L	I	A	A	O
M	E	E	T	L	E	N	P	S	S	M	A	O	E	I
B	E	A	Y	Z	C	M	E	N	R	M	A	A	E	L
S	U	B	C	U	T	A	N	E	O	U	S	N	P	O
I	I	E	O	A	L	C	D	N	L	I	I	A	A	C
S	H	S	N	V	M	U	A	I	M	C	S	A	P	A
Y	U	N	A	E	I	L	G	R	S	M	I	E	U	O
L	I	O	L	I	E	E	E	C	C	E	A	S	L	R
O	N	R	E	M	R	D	E	O	R	I	E	S	E	E
H	I	T	M	C	I	O	R	P	A	S	N	L	R	V
C	C	S	Y	P	A	S	S	A	E	S	L	O	C	M
Y	A	U	E	O	C	B	C	P	C	N	S	S	M	S
N	P	U	S	T	U	L	E	M	A	E	A	D	U	A
O	G	U	N	A	L	E	I	S	T	R	A	T	U	M

Psoriasis	Eczema	Macule
Onycholysis	Lesion	Papule
Dermis	Sebaceous	Vesicle
Epidermis	Apocrine	Pustule
Appendage	Pacini	Stratum
Melanoma	Meissner	Subcutaneous
Carcinoma	Lanugo	Melanocytes

Further resources

National Institute for Health and Clinical Excellence

http://www.nice.org.uk/

The National Institute for Health and Clinical Excellence (NICE) provides guidance, sets quality standards and manages a national database to improve people's health and prevent and treat ill health. There are many excellent resources on this website that can help guide and inform practice.

Cancer Research UK

http://aboutus.cancerresearchuk.org/

Cancer Research UK is the world's leading charity dedicated to beating cancer through research. This website offers much useful information for the public and healthcare professionals.

British Association of Dermatologists

http://www.bad.org.uk/

This website provides information sheets about skin diseases, as well as general information about the skin, current issues in skin disease, and changes to dermatology services in the UK and those areas experiencing problems with providing access to care for their patient population.

UK National Eczema Society

http://www.eczema.org/

The National Eczema Society has two key aims: first, to provide people with independent and practical advice about treating and managing eczema; second, to raise awareness of the needs of those with eczema among healthcare professionals, teachers and the government. A very useful, practical site.

The Psoriasis Association

http://www.psoriasis-association.org.uk/

The Psoriasis Association is the leading national membership organisation for people affected by psoriasis – patients, families, carers and healthcare professionals. This site provides easy to understand information concerning psoriasis as well as offering information concerning research related to the condition.

Changing Faces

http://www.changingfaces.org.uk/

Changing Faces is the leading UK charity that supports and represents people who have disfigurements to the face, hand or body from any cause. Changing Faces helps people to face the challenges of living with a disfigurement and equips them with the appropriate tools to build self-confidence and self-esteem. Its work involves providing support for children, young people, adults and their families, working with schools and employers to ensure a culture of inclusion and with health and social care professionals to provide better psychological care for people with disfigurement, and campaigning for better policies and practices that are inclusive of people with disfigurements and for social change by working with the media, government and opinion leaders.

Glossary of terms

Adjuvant:	an agent that modifies the effects of another agent.
Antibiotic:	a drug used to kill bacteria.
Antifungal:	a drug used to treat fungal infections.
Chemotherapy:	the use of chemical substances to treat diseases, primarily to treat cancer.
Dermatitis:	inflammation of the skin.
Dermatoscopy:	a magnifier with a light allowing illumination of the lesion.
Erythema:	a superficial redness of the skin.
Extrinsic:	originates externally.
Fissure:	a groove or tear.
Histology:	the study of a tissue's microscopic anatomy.
Hyperkeratosis:	excess keratins are produced resulting in thickening of the skin.
Integumentary:	the external covering of the body – the skin.
Intrinsic:	originates internally.
Keratin:	a tough insoluble protein.
Keratinise:	to convert into keratin.
Lichenification:	thickening of the skin as a result of chronic scratching.
Naevus:	a pigmented lesion of the skin.
Pheromone:	a chemical that triggers an innate behavioural response in another.
Prognosis:	a prediction about how a person's disease will progress.
Pruritus:	itchy sensation on the skin.
Radiotherapy:	the medical use of radiation to treat cancer.

Relapsing (relapse):   when the person is again affected by a condition that has occurred in the past.

Sebum: an oily substance made of fat and the debris of fat-producing cells.

Suture: stitch.

Topical: a medication applied to the body surface.

Vesiculation: collection of fluid in the skin.

Viscous: relating to the thickness of a fluid.

Xerosis: dry skin.

References

Akdis, C.A., Akdis, M., Bieber, T. *et al*. (2006) Diagnosis and treatment of atopic dermatitis in children and adults: European Academy of Allergology and Clinical Immunology/American Academy of Allergy, Asthma and Immunology/PRACTALL Consensus Report. *Allergy.* 61: 969–987.

British Association of Dermatologists (2007). *Know Your Skin Type.* Available at http://www.bad.org.uk/site/715/default.aspx [accessed 11 September 2012].

Buxton, P.K. and Morris-Jones, R. (2009) *ABC of Dermatology*, 5th edn. London: British Medical Association.

Flohr, C., Johansson, S.G., Wahlgren, C.F. and Williams, H. (2004). How atopic is atopic dermatitis? Journal of Allergy and Clinical *Immunology* 114(1): 150–158.

Foss, M. and Farine, T. (2007). *Science in Nursing and Health Care*, 2nd edn. Harlow: Pearson.

Gawkrodger, D.J. (2003). *Dermatology: An Illustrated Colour Text*, 3rd edn. Edinburgh: Churchill Livingstone.

International Agency for Research on Cancer (2007). The association of use of sunbeds with cutaneous malignant melanoma and other skin cancers: A systematic review. *International Journal of Cancer* 120(11): 116–122.

Haneke, E. (2006). Surgical anatomy of the nail apparatus. *Dermatology Clinic.* 24(3): 291–296.

Hunter, J., Savin, J. and Dahl, M. (2002). *Clinical Dermatology*, 3rd edn. Oxford: Blackwell Scientific.

Lawton, S. (2001). Assessing the patient with a skin condition. *Journal of Tissue Viability.* 11(3): 113–115.

Mitchell, T. and Kennedy, C. (2006). *Common Skin Disorders*. Edinburgh: Churchill Livingstone.

Naldini, L. and Gambini, D. (2007) The clinical spectrum of psoriasis. *Clinics in Dermatology.* 25: 510–518.

National Institute for Health and Clinical Excellence (2006). *Improving Outcomes for People with Skin Tumours Including Melanoma: The Manual.* London: NICE.

National Institute for Health and Clinical Excellence (2007). *NICE Clinical Guideline 57. Management of Atopic Eczema in Children from Birth up to the Age of 12 years.* London: NICE.

National Institute for Health and Clinical Excellence (2010). *Improving Outcomes for People with Skin Tumours including Melanoma (update): The Management of Low-risk Basal Cell Carcinomas in the Community.* London: NICE.

Page, B.E. (2006). Skin disorders. In: Alexander, M.F., Fawcett, J.N. and Runciman, P.J. (eds). *Nursing Practice, Hospital and Home: The Adult*, 3rd edn. Edinburgh: Churchill Livingstone, pp. 525–552.

Sharpe, G. (2006). Skin cancer: Prevalence, prevention and treatment. *Clinical Medicine.* 6: 333–334.

Thompson, J.F., Scolyer, R.A. and Kefford, R.A. (2005). Cutaneous melanoma. *Lancet.* 365: 687–701.

Timby, B.K. and Smith, N.E. (2010). *Introductory Medical Surgical Nursing*, 11th edn. Philadelphia: Lippincott.

Waugh, A. and Grant, A. (2010). *Ross and Wilson Anatomy and Physiology in Health and Illness*, 11th edn. Edinburgh: Churchill Livingstone.

Wolff, K., Allen-Johnson, R. and Suurmond, S. (2005). *Fitzpatrick's Color Atlas and Synopsis of Clinical Dermatology*, 5th edn. New York: McGraw-Hill.

19

The ear, nose and throat, and eyes, and associated disorders

Carl Clare

Senior Lecturer, Department of Adult Nursing and Primary Care, School of Health and Social Work, University of Hertfordshire, Hatfield, Hertfordshire, UK

Contents

Fundamentals of Applied Pathophysiology: An Essential Guide for Nursing and Healthcare Students, Second Edition. Edited by Muralitharan Nair and Ian Peate.
© 2013 John Wiley & Sons, Ltd. Published 2013 by John Wiley & Sons, Ltd.

Key words

- Pinna

- Tympanic membrane

- Eustachian tube

- Cochlea

- Septum

- Turbinates

- Epiglottis

- Larynx

- Iris

- Retina

- Sclera

- Humour

557

Test your prior knowledge

- Which part of the ear contains the sensory organ for balance?

- Which structure is completely removed from the throat during a laryngectomy?

- Which part of the eye is affected by a cataract?

- How many sections is the ear divided into?

Learning outcomes

On completion of this section the reader will be able to:

- Describe the functions of each of the three sections of the ear.

- Explain the functions of the nose in respiration.

- Describe the functions of the true vocal cords and the false vocal cords.

- Describe the roles of the two types of photoreceptors of the eye.

Don't forget to visit to the companion website for this book (www.wiley.com/go/ fundamentalsofappliedpathophysiology) where you can find self-assessment tests to check your progress, as well as lots of activities to practise your learning.

Introduction

Disorders of the structures of the head and neck range from the relatively minor to some of the most challenging you may be asked to care for. The special senses of the ear, nose and eye are something that are often taken for granted, but conditions that affect these senses can have an immense effect on the daily activities of a person. The aim of this chapter is to introduce the reader to the physiology and associated disorders of the special senses and, in line with the speciality of ear, nose and throat (ENT) care, the physiology and disorders of the throat will also be reviewed.

Physiology of the ear, nose and throat

Ear

The ear is divided into three sections (Figure 19.1):

- external
- middle
- inner.

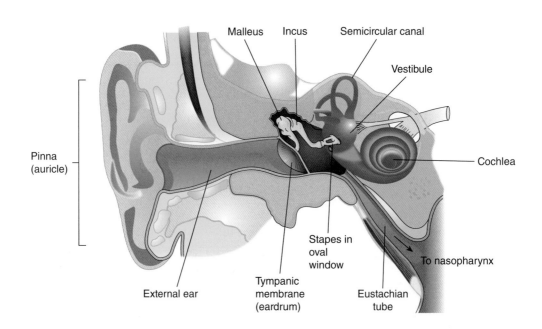

Figure 19.1   The ear.

Each of these three sections is integral to the process of hearing and the inner ear is also essential to the maintenance of the sense of balance.

External ear

The external ear consists of the pinna, the external ear canal and the tympanic membrane.

- Pinna – a skin covered flap of elastic cartilage shaped somewhat like the end of a horn and surrounding the end of the external auditory canal.
- External ear canal – a slightly 'S'-shaped tube lined with skin, fine hairs, sebaceous (oil) glands and ceruminous (wax) glands. The purpose of the oils and the wax is to lubricate the ear canal, kill bacteria and, in conjunction with the hairs, keep the canal free of debris (Lewis *et al.*, 2010).
- Tympanic membrane – composed of epithelial cells, connective tissue and mucous membrane. It acts as a partition between the external and middle ears and is responsible for the transmission of sound from the external to the middle ear.

Middle ear

The middle ear is an air space lined with mucous membrane; it is connected to the nasopharynx by the eustachian tube, thus allowing for the equalisation of air pressure between the middle ear and the throat (and therefore atmospheric air). This equalisation of pressure ensures free movement of the tympanic membrane in response to sound waves conducted along the external ear canal.

Within the middle ear are three bones (the ossicles or ossicular chain):

- hammer (malleus)
- anvil (incus)
- stirrup (stapes).

These interlink and are connected with the tympanic membrane. Vibrations of the tympanic membrane are conducted along the bones to the oval window; these vibrations are then transmitted via the oval window into the fluid of the inner ear. Movement in this fluid leads to stimulation of the hearing receptors.

Inner ear

The inner ear is also known as the labyrinth due to the complicated series of canals it contains (Tortora and Derrickson, 2011a). The inner ear is composed of two main, fluid-filled parts:

- Bony labyrinth – a series of cavities within the temporal bone that contains the main organs of balance (the semicircular canals and the vestibule) and the main organ of hearing (the cochlea).
- Membranous labyrinth – a series of sacs and tubes that is contained within the bony labyrinth. Movement of the fluid within the membranous labyrinth contained within the cochlea stimulates the hearing receptors, leading to the generation of nerve impulses that are transmitted to the hearing centres of the brain (Guyton and Hall, 2010).

Nose

The nose is the first part of the respiratory tract and also contains the receptors for the sense of smell. The functions of the nose are threefold:

- warming, moistening and filtering inhaled air
- detecting olfactory stimuli
- resonance chamber that modifies the quality of speech.

The nose can be divided into external and internal sections:

- External nose – a framework of bone and cartilage covered by muscle and skin and lined with a mucous membrane. This framework is attached to the frontal and maxillary bones of the skull. The external nose is divided into two airways (nares or nostrils) of roughly equal size by the septum, which forms part of the framework of bone and cartilage.
- Internal nose – a large chamber lined with ciliated mucous membrane and containing coarse hairs that filter out large particles from inhaled air. Finer particles that enter the nose become trapped in the sticky mucus created by the membrane and are then transported to the nasopharynx by the ciliary system. The internal nose is divided into two by a continuation of the septum. Each side contains three shelves formed by projections of bone known as the turbinates (Figure 19.2); these increase the surface area that inhaled air must pass over (Guyton and Hall, 2010). The internal nose has an extremely rich vascular supply, which in conjunction with the turbinates maximises the humidification and warming of the air passing through. The internal nose also contains openings (ostia) from the sinus cavities (contained within the bones of the skull).

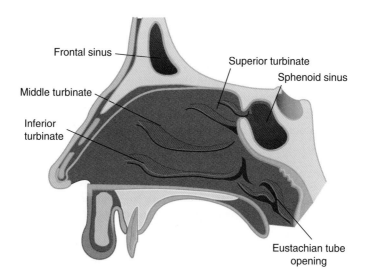

Frontal sinus

Superior turbinate

Sphenoid sinus

Middle turbinate

Inferior turbinate

Eustachian tube opening

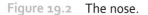

Figure 19.2   The nose.

Throat

The throat consists of the oropharynx and the hypopharynx (Figure 19.3).

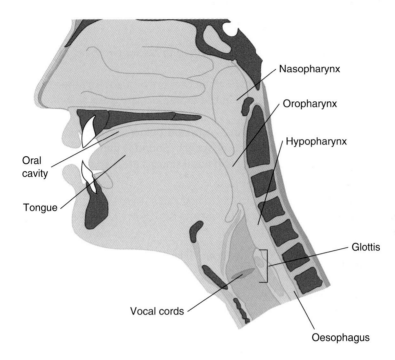

Nasopharynx

Oropharynx

Hypopharynx

Oral cavity

Tongue

Glottis

Vocal cords

Oesophagus

Figure 19.3   The throat.

Oropharynx

Tonsils

The tonsils are five collections of lymphatic nodules mostly located in a ring around the junction of the oral cavity and the oropharynx (Tortora and Derrickson, 2011b):

- two palatine tonsils located at the back of the oral cavity
- two lingual tonsils located at the base of the tongue
- a single pharyngeal tonsil (adenoid) located at the junction of the nasal cavity and the nasopharynx.

The role of the tonsils is to participate in the fight against inhaled or ingested foreign substances.

Hypopharynx

Larynx

The larynx is a short tube that connects the lower hypopharynx with the trachea. It is composed of a mucous membrane covering several pieces of cartilage including:

- thyroid cartilage (Adam's apple)
- epiglottis – a large piece of cartilage that covers the opening of the glottis during swallowing, thus protecting the airway
- cricoid cartilage – a ring of cartilage that forms the inferior wall of the larynx and connects to the first cartilage ring of the trachea.

The mucous membrane of the larynx is formed to create two pairs of folds:

- Ventricular folds (false vocal cords) – when they are brought together, they enable the holding of the breath against the pressure in the thoracic cavity, such as when lifting a heavy object (Tortora and Derrickson, 2011b).
- Vocal cords (folds; true vocal cords) – situated below the ventricular folds, the vocal cords are fundamental to the generation of speech. Sound is generated by the vibration of these cords, but the mouth, nasal cavity and nasal sinuses are also required to create recognisable speech (Guyton and Hall, 2010).

Physiology of the eye

The eyeball (globe) is made up of three layers (Figure 19.4):

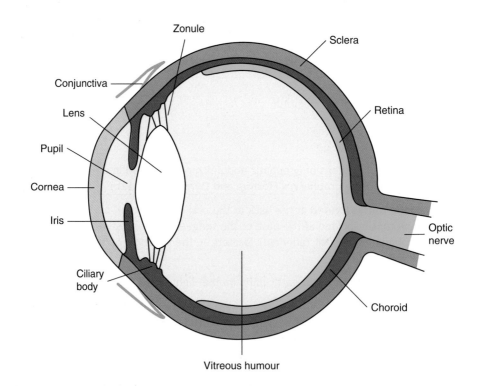

Figure 19.4   The eye.

- a tough outer layer – fibrous tunic
- a middle layer – vascular tunic
- the retina – sensory tunic.

Fibrous tunic

This layer is composed of the cornea and the sclera, and contains no blood vessels. The cornea is a curved, transparent coat which helps focus light onto the retina. The sclera (the 'white' of the eye) covers the entire eyeball, except where the cornea is present; it gives shape and protection to the eyeball. The anterior sclera (but not the cornea) is covered by the conjunctiva, which produces a lubricating mucus that prevents the eye from drying out (Marieb and Hoehn, 2010).

Vascular tunic

The vascular tunic (uvea) is composed of the iris, the ciliary body and the choroid.

- Choroid – a highly vascular membrane; its blood vessels supply nutrition to all the tunics of the eye (Marieb and Hoehn, 2010).
- Ciliary body – at the front of the eye the choroid becomes the ciliary body – a thickened ring of smooth muscle that circles the lens and has an important role in controlling the shape of the lens. The choroid is connected to the lens by a suspensory ligament (zonule).
- Iris – coloured part of the eye lying between the cornea and the lens; it contains a hole (the pupil) through which light can enter the eye. The size of the pupil is controlled by the contraction and relaxation of two separate layers of muscle fibres contained within the iris.

Sensory tunic

The retina has two layers; however, only the neural layer is directly involved with vision (Marieb and Hoehn, 2010). Within this neural layer are the photoreceptors:

- rods for peripheral and dim light vision
- cones for bright light and colour vision.

Impulses generated as a result of stimulation of these photoreceptors are transmitted to the visual cortex via the optic nerve.

Internal structure

Internally, the eye is divided into two chambers by a barrier formed by the lens and the zonule:

- Anterior segment – in front of the lens and zonule. This chamber is filled with aqueous humour, which is constantly formed and drained. Aqueous humour provides the lens and the cornea with nutrients and oxygen.
- Posterior segment – filled with a gel-like substance called vitreous humour. The thick vitreous humour supports the back of the lens, holds the retina against the choroid and contributes to intraocular pressure, thus helping to maintain the shape of the eye (Jenkins *et al.*, 2010).

563

Lens

The lens is the main apparatus for focusing light onto the retina. The thickness of the lens is varied by the contraction and relaxation of the ciliary muscles, depending on whether the eye is focusing on near or far objects.

Movement of the eye

Movement of the eye is controlled by the extrinsic eye muscles; neuromuscular co-ordination ensures the simultaneous movement of both eyes (Lewis *et al.*, 2010).

Disorders of the ear, nose and throat, and eye

Learning outcomes

On completion of this section the reader will be able to:

- Describe the care of a patient following ear surgery.

- Describe the care of a patient following nasal surgery.

- Explain the difference between a tracheostomy and a laryngectomy.

- Discuss the two types of glaucoma.

Disorders of the ear, nose and throat

Ear

Ear wax

Impaction of ear wax in the external ear canal is a common complaint often related to a patient's attempts to remove ear wax with fingers or cotton buds. Impaction of ear wax reduces the ability of sound to travel the length of the external ear canal and the responsiveness of the tympanic membrane to sound waves, leading to a temporary reduction in the ability to hear. This is especially common in older patients who have a tendency to produce more and drier wax (Clegg *et al.*, 2010).

One method for the removal of ear wax is the syringing of the external ear canal, often preceded by the use of a cerumenolytic (substance that actively helps to break down wax) or a wax softener (Clegg *et al.*, 2010).

Otitis externa

This is diffuse inflammation of the external ear canal, often associated with regular swimming ('swimmer's ear') (Kaushik *et al.*, 2010). The condition is characterised by pain, itching and a discharge from the ear canal. The discharge is usually watery at the beginning but becomes purulent as the condition progresses.

The spread of infection can lead to pyrexia and systemic symptoms such as malaise. The infection is usually caused by a mixture of micro-organisms and swabs should be sent for microbiological culture and sensitivity.

The care of this condition includes:

- Careful removal of any debris from the external ear canal.
- The administration of topical antibiotics and a steroid preparation (Kaushik *et al.*, 2010).
- If the infection has become systemic (entered the bloodstream) or extensive. the patient may require oral antibiotics, analgesia and bed rest.
- The patient should be discouraged from scratching the affected ear and advised to prevent water from entering the ear canal (Pankhania *et al.*, 2011).

Tympanic membrane rupture

Rupture of the tympanic membrane due to improper ear syringing technique, blows to the side of the head or blast injuries are often self-healing as long as infection is not present.

Patients should be advised to avoid:

- the entry of water into the ear
- introducing foreign objects such as cotton buds.

Persistent deafness may indicate damage or displacement of the ossicular chain and may require surgical intervention.

565

Otitis media

Acute otitis media is a condition that is often associated with upper respiratory tract infections and sinusitis (Benninger, 2008). The infection tracks up into the middle ear via the eustachian tube, leading to infection and the collection of pus. The infection and the pressure resulting from the collection of pus may lead to a range of potential symptoms including (Gopen, 2010):

- pain
- pyrexia
- malaise
- headache
- nausea and vomiting
- tinnitus
- reduction in hearing.

Treatment includes:

- antibiotics
- pain relief
- antipyretics
- nasal decongestants may reduce inflammation of the eustachian tube and allow drainage of the middle ear into the nasopharynx (Canaday and Salata, 2008)

- application of warmth to the affected ear in order to reduce pain
- avoidance of water entering the ear canal.

Untreated or repeated episodes of acute otitis media may lead to chronic infection of the middle ear, which may eventually spread to the mastoid process of the temporal bone of the skull (mastoiditis) (Kumar and Wiet, 2010). Tympanic membrane rupture is common and destruction of the bones of the ossicular chain is also possible (Kumar and Wiet, 2010). Symptoms include:

- purulent discharge
- pain – may be associated with redness and swelling of the bone behind the pinna (mastoid process)
- pyrexia
- hearing loss
- nausea and vomiting
- vertigo.

Treatment for the chronic complications of otitis media is usually surgical and depends on the structures that are affected:

- myringoplasty – repair of the tympanic membrane, often using grafted tissue
- ossiculoplasty – reconstruction of the ossicular chain
- tympanoplasty – myringoplasty and ossiculoplasty performed at the same time
- mastoidectomy – removal of infected tissue from the middle ear and mastoid bone; often performed with a tympanoplasty.

The care of patients following surgery of the ear is detailed in Box 19.1.

Box 19.1   Care of the patient following ear surgery.

- Recovery period – position the patient flat on the opposite side to the operation side with no pillows
- Advise the patient to avoid sudden movements of the head
- Administer analgesia as prescribed
- Pillows are introduced for comfort when the patient feels able to tolerate them; most patients are able to tolerate sitting up after 24 hours
- Following operations on the inner ear, observe for signs of neurological damage (neurological observations at least 4 hourly for the first 24 hours)
- Facial nerve damage may occur at the time of the operation or subsequently due to inflammation or oedema. The patient should be asked to show their teeth or smile to assess for facial palsy
- Patient should avoid coughing, sneezing and blowing their nose, or straining during bowel movements for 7–10 days as this will lead to an increased pressure in the ear via the eustachian tube. If coughing or sneezing is unavoidable, then the patient is advised to keep the mouth open to reduce the pressure on the middle ear (Lewis et al., 2010). Laxatives may be provided to avoid straining during bowel movements
- Most patients can be discharged after 2–3 days, but should be advised to avoid water entry into the ear, crowded places (where respiratory infections may be contracted) and changes in air pressure (such as flying or high altitudes) until advised by the surgeon (Lewis et al., 2010)

Otosclerosis

Otosclerosis is the formation of new bone around the footplate of the stapes. It is often hereditary (Schrauwen, 2010) and is associated with a gradual deterioration in hearing. The treatment is surgical (e.g. stapedectomy or stapedotomy) and involves the removal of part of the stapes and insertion of a prosthesis (Bajaj *et al.*, 2010).

Ménière's disease

Ménière's disease is a disorder of the inner ear characterised by episodes of:

- vertigo
- nausea and vomiting
- tinnitus
- varying hearing loss
- aural fullness (a feeling of 'stuffiness' in the ear)
- 'drop attacks' – a feeling of being pulled to the ground; alternatively some patients feel as though they are whirling through space.

The duration of an episode may be hours or days. The care of a patient experiencing an acute episode of Ménière's disease includes:

- reassurance and counselling
- a quiet, darkened, environment
- comfortable position (often semi-recumbent)
- avoidance of sudden head movements
- fluorescent and flickering lights, and watching television should be avoided as they can exacerbate symptoms
- vomit bowls should be provided
- all drugs should be administered parenterally
- the bedside call bell should be put in the patient's reach and the patient advised not to mobilise without assistance.

Treatment of the disease requires lifestyle changes and long-term medication (e.g. diuretics or steroids). Patients who experience a reduced quality of life (frequent incapacitating attacks and/or loss of employment) may require surgery (Sajjadi and Paparella, 2008).

Nose

Epistaxis (nose bleed)

Epistaxis is often associated with trauma to the nose or upper respiratory tract infections. Control is achieved by applying pressure to the upper part of the nose by pinching it between the finger and the thumb whilst the patient sits with their head tilted forward to avoid blood draining into the throat and being swallowed. Nasal packing may be required and in some cases this may be modified by the use of a Foley catheter or postnasal pack to provide a firm base against which to pack the nose (Schlosser, 2009). Further care for difficult-to-control bleeds may include:

- frequent observations (blood pressure and pulse half hourly)
- assessment of blood loss and blood transfusion if hypovolaemia is suspected
- cold compresses applied to the nose and back of the neck to reduce blood flow to the nose
- antihypertensive drugs for hypertensive patients
- cauterisation or surgical ligation of blood vessels (Manes, 2010).

Deviated nasal septum

This is a condition that may be congenital or acquired (due to trauma); the patient may present with nasal obstruction. Treatment is normally surgical:

- submucous resection (SMR) – removal and resection of the parts of the septum causing the deviation
- septoplasty – septum is completely freed and the removal of areas around its margin may allow it to be repositioned in the midline.

The care of patients following surgery of the nose is detailed in Box 19.2.

Nasal polyps

These are soft fleshy swellings inside the nose and are the end product of prolonged oedema of the nasal mucosa caused by prolonged infection or allergy. The patient may present with nasal obstruction, nasal discharge and headaches. The treatment for severe cases is the surgical removal of the polypi (ethmoidectomy) and treatment of the underlying cause (DeMarcantonio and Han, 2011), although some cases may be managed medically.

Sinusitis

Following a viral infection of the nose, the natural resistance of the mucosa is reduced and a secondary bacterial infection occurs, which rapidly spreads into the sinuses. The swelling of the

---

Box 19.2   Care of the patient following nasal surgery.

- In the immediate postoperative period, patients will normally have a nasal pack in place. This is removed 24–48 hours after the operation
- Monitoring of the patients' airway is essential in the immediate postoperative period due to the risk of blood or nasal packing entering the respiratory tract
- When the patient is fully conscious, their head should be raised above the level of the heart and they should be encouraged to sleep with at least three pillows. This reduces bleeding and swelling. Ice packs may also be used to reduce swelling if allowed by the surgeon
- Administer analgesia and antibiotics as prescribed
- Patient should avoid sneezing, blowing their nose and straining during bowel movements for 10–14 days as this may lead to bleeding. If sneezing is unavoidable, then the patient is advised to keep the mouth open to reduce the pressure on the nose. Laxatives may be provided to avoid straining during bowel movements
- After the removal of nasal packs, steam inhalations or a saline spray will help to keep the nasal mucosa moist and loosen any crusts

mucosa may close off the ostia of the sinuses; thus, the infected mucus is unable to escape. The symptoms include:

- pain
- nasal obstruction
- malaise
- pyrexia
- localised tenderness

If untreated there is the possibility of complications such as:

- spread of infection to the eyes
- intracranial infection or abscess formation
- osteomyelitis (infection of the bone).

The treatment of sinusitis includes:

- nasal decongestants to reduce the mucosal swelling and allow drainage
- antibiotics
- pain relief
- antral lavage – introduction of a trocar and cannula into the maxillary (antral) sinus to allow the cavity to be flushed with normal saline (Masood *et al.*, 2007)
- abscesses require surgical intervention.

The care of patients includes:

- a warm, well-ventilated environment
- fluid intake of at least 3 L a day
- good oral hygiene
- use of a humidifier (Walsh, 2007)
- bed rest may be required for 24–48 hours
- whilst recovering, the patient should avoid extremes of temperature, crowded environments and smoking.

Throat

Tonsillitis and quinsy

Tonsillitis is a condition characterised by inflammation of the tonsils, leading to the patient presenting with:

- bilateral sore throat
- dysphagia
- pyrexia
- malaise.

Treatment is usually:

- antibiotics
- encourage a fluid intake of 1–3 L per day
- pain relief
- good oral hygiene
- recurrent bouts of tonsillitis may require surgical removal of the tonsils (tonsillectomy).

A peritonsillar abscess (quinsy) may develop and patients may present with:

- an inflamed tonsil with swelling due to the collection of pus
- worsening dysphagia often with an associated inability to swallow saliva
- worsening pain on one side of the throat
- trismus – an inability to open the mouth due to spasm of the jaw muscles.

This is considered a much more serious condition and needle aspiration (with antibiotic cover) is recommended (McKerrow and Bradley, 2007); occasionally surgical incision and drainage is still performed.

Tracheostomy

Tracheotomy is the surgical procedure of making an incision in the anterior tracheal wall for the purpose of creating an airway; a tracheostomy is the opening (stoma) that is created by the tracheotomy (Lewis *et al.*, 2010). Tracheostomies are created for several reasons:

- relief of upper airways obstruction
- protection of the lungs from the aspiration of food or regurgitation of the stomach contents
- respiratory insufficiency
- long-term ventilation
- following a laryngectomy.

Most tracheostomies are temporary and a plastic or metal tube is inserted into the stoma to maintain the patency of the airway (Figure 19.5). Following a laryngectomy, the trachea is brought to the surface of the neck and a permanent stoma is formed (Feber, 2006).

Potential complications following tracheostomy include:

- tube dislodgement – avoided by correctly securing the tube with tapes and sutures
- tube obstruction – due to the build-up of secretions or the formation of a mucous plug which is then coughed into the tube
- surgical emphysema – the escape of air into the soft tissue of the neck, characterised by a 'crackling' sensation when palpated
- pneumonia
- tracheo-oesophageal fistula – created by excessive or prolonged inflation of a cuffed tracheostomy tube leading to necrosis of the tracheal wall and the development of a hole (fistula) between the trachea and the oesophagus; the fistula allows the entry of food and fluids into the lungs.

The care of a patient following the creation of a tracheostomy includes:

- Position the patient upright to reduce oedema formation.
- Frequent observations – blood pressure, pulse, respirations and oxygen saturations should be noted every 15 minutes for the first 2 hours, then reducing to half hourly for 2 hours and then hourly for 24 hours.
- A low pressure cuffed tracheostomy tube (Box 19.3) should be placed in the operating theatre and should be left inflated for the first 24 hours to reduce the chance of bleeding. To reduce

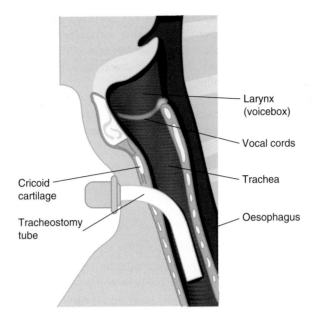

Figure 19.5   Temporary tracheostomy.

Box 19.3   Cuffed and uncuffed tracheostomy tubes.

Cuffed tracheostomy tubes have an inflatable cuff towards their distal end; this is used to create an airtight seal in the trachea. They are generally used in patients who require a tracheostomy for ventilation (e.g. in intensive care) or for patients who are at risk of aspirating food or body fluids (e.g. immediately post-tracheostomy formation, there is a risk of bleeding from the operative site). Cuffed tracheostomy tubes have a low pressure cuff and therefore there is no requirement to deflate the cuff regularly so long as the pressure is checked with a pressure gauge.

Uncuffed tracheostomy tubes (as in Figure 19.5) are much more common. However, in the acute setting it is recommended that a cuffed tracheostomy tube of the correct size is kept by the bedside for use in an emergency situation (such as resuscitation).

the chance of pressure necrosis, the cuff pressure should be checked every 8 hours. The correct cuff pressure is maintained by the use of a pressure gauge (Lewis *et al.*, 2010).
- Suctioning – this is dependent on patient requirements (patients will produce secretions at different rates). The type and quantity of the suctioned mucus should be monitored and recorded (Lewis *et al.*, 2010).
- Humidification – as the air entering the patient's lungs is no longer warmed and humidified by the upper airway, the provision of humidification is essential to prevent the formation of crusts which may block the tracheostomy tube (Fairhurst-Winstanley, 2007).

- Dressings should be kept clean and dry as wet dressings encourage the growth of bacteria and may lead to wound infections or, if inhaled, respiratory infections (Feber, 2006).
- The tracheostomy tube is first changed after 48 hours – this is a procedure that should only be carried out by two members of the multi-disciplinary team at least one of whom should be experienced in this procedure.

Longer term care of the patient with a tracheostomy is geared towards enabling the patient to perform their own care (including tube care, tube changes, suctioning and dressing changes).

Laryngectomy

Case study

John Davis is a 47-year-old man who is being cared for on the ward having undergone a laryngectomy for cancer. He currently has a tracheostomy tube in place and is beginning to mobilize around the ward. He is frequently visited by his wife and 13-year-old daughter, although his daughter does not seem keen to stay at the bedside and is often to be found in the day room whilst her mother stay's at her father's bedside. Mr Davis was a police officer and will not be returning to work as he has been advised to retire on health grounds. He is depressed and anxious about the future but finds it hard to communicate and thus he can become quite frustrated.

Take time to reflect on this case study and then consider the following.

1. What are Mr Davis's immediate care needs on a daily basis?
2. What should be done to prepare Mr Davis for his eventual discharge?
3. It is too early for Mr Davis to begin using artificial speech, so what can be done to help him communicate in the short term?
4. Mr Davis and his family have psychological needs. What are these and how could the family be aided in overcoming and adapting to the new situation?

Laryngectomy is the removal of the entire structure of the larynx (Figure 19.6) and is the standard treatment for advanced laryngeal cancer (Scottish Intercollegiate Guidelines Network, 2006).

During a laryngectomy the trachea is brought to the surface of the neck and a permanent tracheostomy is formed through which the patient breathes; therefore, there is no connection between the mouth, nose and lungs. Immediately postoperatively the stoma will be protected by a tracheostomy tube and the care of the patient is similar to that of a patient with a temporary tracheostomy. The greater trauma to the trachea raises the risk of bleeding and oedema formation, and it is therefore common practice for oxygen saturations to be monitored with pulse oximetry continuously for 24 hours and then overnight for 2–3 days. Once the risk of bleeding and oedema formation has reduced, about 5–10 days postoperatively, the tracheostomy tube is removed and replaced with a silicone stoma button or stud to prevent the closure of the stoma as scar tissue forms (Feber, 2006). Patients are normally discharged 14 days postoperatively.

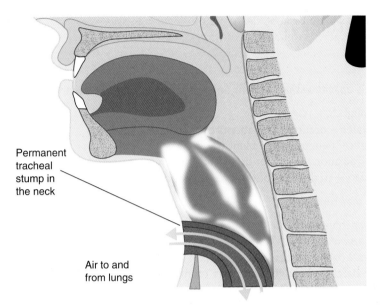

Permanent
tracheal
stump in
the neck

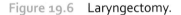

Air to and
from lungs

Figure 19.6   Laryngectomy.

573

The loss of the normal humidification and warming mechanisms of the mouth and nose will lead to the drying of the mucous lining of the lower respiratory tract and a significant increase in water loss via exhaled air. This leads to changes in respiratory mechanisms and a significantly increased risk of respiratory infections (Feber, 2006). The loss of moisture will lead to the creation of thick secretions and crust formation, which may completely block the stoma and thus threaten life. Humidification is essential for a laryngectomy patient and once the patient is discharged, they must use a passive heat and moisture exchanger (HME) worn over the stoma; these are usually made of foam that traps the heat and moisture in expired air, which are then transferred into the inspired air.

The loss of the patient's voice following laryngectomy can have significant psychological effects and several communication methods are available (Kazi et al., 2010):

- Voice prostheses (speaking valve) – a valve placed between the trachea and the oesophagus which diverts expired air into the oesophagus when the tracheostomy is manually blocked; thus air passes into the mouth.
- Electrolarynx – a battery-powered device held against the mouth that creates speech with the use of sound waves.
- Artificial larynx – similar to an electrolarynx except that the device is held to the neck rather than the mouth.
- Oesophageal speech – this involves the patient swallowing air, trapping it in the oesophagus and releasing it to create sound.

It is important that laryngectomy patients wear a medical alert bracelet identifying them as a 'neck breather' in the event of an emergency situation.

Disorders of the eye

Cataracts

A cataract is opacity within the lens and has several causes (Allen and Vasavada, 2006):

- congenital
- age related – occurring in patients over the age of 60 years
- traumatic – penetrating or blunt trauma
- toxic – radiation therapy or drugs such as topical steroids
- secondary – to diseases of the eye or systemic disease such as diabetes mellitus.

Patients may report:

- decrease in vision
- 'misty vision'
- abnormal colour perception
- glare – dazzling by bright lights due to abnormal light refraction.

The treatment of cataracts is surgical and requires the removal of the diseased lens and replacement with a prosthetic lens (Riaz *et al.*, 2006). The procedure is normally carried out under local anaesthetic and the patient is given sedation. Postoperatively, the patient can be discharged when the effects of sedation have worn off (Lewis *et al.*, 2010). Postoperative self-care advice may include:

- administration of antibiotic and steroid eye drops as prescribed
- cover the eye with an eye patch and protective shield for 24 hours, then only at night
- avoid situations that increase intraocular pressure (stooping, coughing or lifting)
- a reduction in visual acuity in the immediate postoperative period is not unusual – it may take up to 2 weeks for vision to improve
- once full healing has occurred (approximately 6–8 weeks), a prescription for glasses will be required as the prosthetic lens is not able to correct for near vision (e.g. reading).

Macular degeneration

Case study

Joyce Kirkpatrick is a 72-year-old widow who has previously been fit and active. Recently, she has noticed that her eyesight is deteriorating and she finds that she is unable to focus on objects that are in front of her and has to turn her head in order to 'catch them in the corner of my eye'. A recent visit to the optician led to a referral to the ophthalmologist at the local hospital who informed Mrs Kirkpatrick that she has macular degeneration in both eyes. The left eye has mostly dry macular degeneration but the right eye has both wet and dry macular degeneration. The ophthalmologist has advised Joyce that there is little that can be done for the left eye at present but she can help to prevent worsening. The ophthalmologist has also advised Mrs Kirkpatrick that a treatment is available for the wet macular degeneration which involves injecting a drug into the eye, but it is still quite new and expensive so permission to use the treatment will need to be sought from the local health authority.

Take some time to reflect on this case and then consider the following.

1. What is the treatment the ophthalmologist referring to for the treatment of the wet macular degeneration?
2. What can Mrs Kirkpatrick do to help prevent the worsening of her macular degeneration?
3. What support groups are available to help Mrs Kirkpatrick with her condition?
4. Mrs Kirkpatrick lives alone and would like to continue living in her house. What changes to the home could be made to maintain her safety and independence?

Macular degeneration is characterised by a gradual loss of central vision, but peripheral vision is maintained. There are two types of macular degeneration:

- Dry macular degeneration – associated with small, round, white yellow areas (drusens) in the macula. Dry macular degeneration accounts for 90% of all cases (Tortora and Derrickson, 2011a) There is no treatment available but progression is slow and thus sight loss is limited. Some lifestyle changes can be made to help reduce the seterioration and possible progression to wet macular degeneration, e.g. protecting the eyes from UV light, eating a healthy diet rich in antioxidants and stopping smoking.
- Wet macular degeneration (neurovascular) – caused by the development of abnormal blood vessels below the retina. All patients with wet macular degeneration will have had dry macular degeneration first. Current treatments are controversial and include dietary changes to include high levels of vitamins C and E, beta-carotene and zinc (Evans, 2009). A small number of patients may be suitable for photodynamic therapy (PDT) (Chakravarthy *et al.*, 2010), which involves the injection of a dye into the blood vessels; subsequent excitation of the dye by a 'cold' laser (which does not damage the retina) coagulates the targeted blood vessels. Increasingly drug therapies (antivascular endothelial growth factor) are being developed and are becoming more common in clinical use (Royal College of Opthalmologists, 2009).

Glaucoma

Glaucoma is a term relating to a series of disorders characterised by (Lewis *et al.*, 2010):

- increased intraocular pressure (IOP)
- optic nerve atrophy
- loss of peripheral vision – 'tunnel vision'.

Loss of vision is related to a loss of balance in the generation and reabsorption of aqueous humour; the subsequent rise in IOP leads to damage to the head of the optic nerve.

Treatment is dependent on the particular type of glaucoma:

- Open angle glaucoma – the mechanisms for the drainage of aqueous humour become blocked. The onset is subtle and without symptoms until the patient finally notices the loss of peripheral vision, by which time the visual loss is usually large (Walsh, 2007). Primary treatment is the reduction of IOP with eye drops. Laser treatment is effective in the short-term but surgery remains the main option for treatment.
- Acute closed angle glaucoma – the lens bulges forward and restricts aqueous humour drainage. The onset is rapid and the patient may report:

- headaches
- nausea and vomiting
- eye pain
- blurred vision.

This is an ocular emergency and requires immediate medical attention. The patient will require laser iridotomy (creation of a hole in the iris) as a matter of urgency.
Care includes:

- caring for the patient in a quiet, darkened, environment
- providing vomit bowls, tissues and mouth washes as required
- administering analgesia as prescribed
- cold compresses to the forehead to reduce pain
- administering of prescribed drugs, including an intravenous infusion of mannitol, antiemetics and eye drops
- reassurance and explanation.

Retinal detachment

Retinal detachment is the detachment of the neural layer from the rest of the retina. Patients may experience:

- flashing lights
- floaters – small dark particles in the vision caused by small haemorrhages
- loss of vision – related to the area of detachment.

Treatment is with surgery:

- Laser therapy or photocoagulation is used to seal tears or holes in the retina and prevent the further accumulation of subretinal fluid, which would otherwise make the detachment worse.
- Plombage (scleral buckling) – a small square of material is sutured onto the sclera over the site of the hole, thus pushing the retinal layers back together.
- Encirclement – a silicone band is placed around the eyeball. This is used where there is a large area of detachment or multiple holes.

Subretinal fluid is drained during all these procedures to allow the separated layers to come into contact again.
Patient care includes:

- Bed rest to prevent further detachment occurring before and after surgery.
- Patient may be required to rest in a position that causes the detachment to lie against the underlying layers and also encourage the subretinal fluid to be reabsorbed.
- Analgesia – patients will experience eye pain after surgery.
- Eye care – the eyelids and conjunctiva are usually swollen after surgery.

Retinopathy

The leading cause of retinopathy in the UK is diabetes mellitus (Pachaiappan et al., 2006). It can be divided into two types:

- Non-proliferative retinopathy – aneurysms of the capillaries of the eyes, retinal haemorrhages and hardened exudates of lipids.
- Proliferative retinopathy – the retina has become ischaemic and in response there is a development of new blood vessels in the eye; however, new blood vessels are fragile and have a tendency to bleed. These blood vessels also grow into the vitreous humour. Eventually, fibrous bands develop which pull on the retina and cause retinal detachment.

Treatment of retinopathy includes:

- Control of cholesterol levels.
- Advice on diet and glycaemic control.
- Laser therapy to the retina – dead retinal tissue does not encourage new blood vessel formation. Therefore, a laser beam is used to create multiple small areas of dead retinal tissue (scotomas), which will not have an effect on vision but will reduce the growth of new blood vessels.
- Vitrectomy – removal of the vitreous humour; this removes blood vessels and haemorrhages. Vitreous humour is not naturally replaced by the body; however, replacement with aqueous humour will occur.

Conclusion

Disorders of the senses can lead to the loss of the ability to maintain the activities of daily living and may even threaten life. When faced with these possibilities, the patient will often be anxious and frightened. In this situation, being cared for by a professional with knowledge of both the condition and the care required will help the patient to reduce these feelings. This chapter has introduced the reader to the physiology of the eye, ear, nose and throat and some of the conditions associated with these structures. Knowledge of the physiology and the associated conditions of these structures enables the healthcare professional to deliver care that is safe and effective. Whilst this chapter cannot hope to cover all the conditions associated with the special senses and the throat, it gives the reader a firm base from which to deliver competent and knowledgeable care and to develop their knowledge in these fascinating areas.

577

Test your knowledge

- What is the purpose of ear wax?
- Name the two types of humour in the eyes.
- What is 'swimmer's ear'?
- What is a quinsy?
- Give three reasons for a patient to have a tracheostomy.
- What are the two types of retinopathy?

Activities

Here are some activities and exercises to help test your learning. For the answers to these exercises, as well as further self-testing activities, visit our website at www.wiley.com/go/fundamentalsofappliedpathophysiology

Fill in the blanks

The eyeball (otherwise known as the _____) is made up of three layers. The _____ tunic is a tough outer layer that helps to protect the eyeball and is made up of the _____ and _____. The middle layer is the _____ tunic which contains the blood vessels that supply _____ to all the tunics of the eye. The _____ tunic is the _____ layer and is commonly known as the retina. This layer contains the _____ and _____ required for vision. Light that reaches the sensory tunic is focused by the _____ which is _____ and relaxed by the _____ muscles, depending on whether the eye is focusing on near or far objects. A major disorder of the lens of the eye is _____ which may cause a _____ in vision, misty vision, abnormal _____ or _____ (dazzling by bright lights).

Choose from:
Cataracts; Rods; Vascular; Cornea; Globe; Ciliary; Colour perception; Sclera; Nutrition; Fibrous; Sensory; Decrease; Glare; Contracted; Inner; Cones; Lens

Label the diagram

Using the list of words supplied, label the diagram.

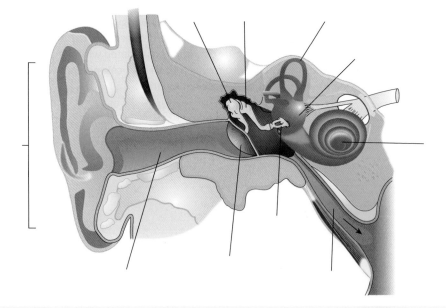

Malleus; Tympanic membrane; Eustachian tube; Vestibule; Cochlea; Pinna; External ear; Stapes; Semicircular canal; Incus

Word search

V	I	C	T	O	I	C	P	S	L	O	T	L	Y	I	O	S
E	E	I	A	E	V	Q	U	I	N	S	Y	T	S	I	A	I
R	A	L	U	C	R	I	C	I	M	E	S	I	R	I	C	T
T	L	I	D	U	O	I	S	I	R	A	S	I	N	A	R	D
I	T	A	S	A	I	R	T	U	L	C	R	U	A	S	A	I
G	T	R	E	T	I	N	O	P	A	T	H	Y	R	C	I	O
O	R	Y	E	G	Y	G	O	P	R	L	I	A	E	D	D	R
E	A	E	B	U	T	N	A	I	H	C	A	T	S	U	E	O
P	C	S	E	P	A	T	S	H	X	A	A	C	L	S	M	H
I	H	N	P	P	A	M	I	A	P	N	R	A	U	C	S	C
G	E	S	M	S	U	T	N	N	I	S	Y	Y	N	I	I	P
L	O	Y	U	S	U	I	R	B	N	H	Y	R	N	N	T	H
O	T	O	S	C	L	E	R	O	S	I	S	D	A	X	I	Y
T	O	N	Z	O	N	U	L	E	P	Y	T	P	U	L	T	P
T	M	E	P	A	T	I	E	L	A	H	M	U	A	I	O	A
I	Y	I	A	A	Y	G	C	O	A	Y	Y	Y	S	T	I	O
S	N	H	N	O	M	T	T	U	T	M	R	M	S	P	O	T

579

Tympanic	Pinna	Larynx
Tympanoplasty	Quinsy	Atrophy
Semicircular	Eustachiantube	Epiglottis
Otosclerosis	Trismus	Choroid
Malleus	Turbinate	Ciliary
Tinnitus	Visualacuity	Iris
Incus	Nares	Zonule
Dysphagia	Retinopathy	Otitismedia
Stapes	Oropharynx	Vertigo
Tracheotomy	Drusens	

Further resources

BMC Ear Nose and Throat Disorders

www.biomedcentral.com/bmcearnosethroatdisord/
This is an open source (free to read) journal focusing on ENT disorders. The website is also linked to all other BMC journals and so relevant articles form other BMC journals are also highlighted here.

Northern Ireland Cancer Network. E-learning Care of the Laryngectomee

www.cancerni.net/education/elearningcareofthelaryngectomee
This is a free multimedia course on the care of the laryngectomy patient.

Royal National Institute of Blind People

www.rnib.org.uk
This website is of interest to all health professionals. There is information on how to help patients with poor vision in any setting, resource pages on various conditions (some produced in conjunction with the Royal College of Ophthalmologists) and patient stories to help you understand the real impact of sight loss.

The National Association of Laryngectomee Clubs

www.laryngectomy.org.uk
This site has a useful glossary of terms related to laryngectomy and a wide range of leaflets for professionals and patients.

The Royal College of Ophthalmologists

www.rcophth.ac.uk
This website has a large electronic library both for professionals and the public. You will find many eye-related disorders explained here as well as information on eye health.

Sign Station

www.signstation.org
This is an interactive website that helps you to understand British Sign Language (BSL). It is free to register and registered users can access the BSL dictionary, view video scenarios on dealing with deaf people and take a free online course to learn the basics of BSL.

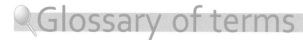
Glossary of terms

| Aneurysm: | a localised dilatation of the wall of a blood vessel, usually the aorta or the arteries at the base of the brain. |

Anticholinergic:	a drug that blocks the action of acetylcholine and thus inhibits the transmission or effect of parasympathetic nerve action.
Anti-emetic:	a drug that reduces nausea and vomiting.
Antihistamine:	a drug that inhibits the effect of histamines.
Antipyretic:	a drug that can reduce high temperatures (e.g. paracetamol, aspirin, ibuprofen).
Aspiration:	inhalation of a foreign body (such as food).
Atrophy:	wasting away; a diminution in the size of a cell, tissue or organ.
Aural:	related to the ear.
Cannula:	a flexible tube containing a stiff, pointed trocar. Once inserted into the body, the trocar is removed, allowing fluid to pass along the cannula.
Cartilage:	a type of connective tissue that contains collagen and elastic fibres. This strong tough material on the bone ends helps to distribute the load within the joint; the slippery surface allows smooth movement between the bones. Cartilage can withstand both tension and compression.
Cauterisation:	coagulation of tissues by heat or caustic substances.
Cilia:	small, hair-like processes on the outer surface of some cells; used to propel liquids.
Coagulation:	the process of transforming a liquid into a solid (especially blood) or the hardening of tissue by physical means.
Congenital:	present at birth, rather than acquired during life.
Connective tissue:	a primary tissue characterised by cells separated by a matrix; supports and binds other body tissue.
Distal:	away from the beginning.
Dysphagia:	difficulty in swallowing.
Epithelial cell:	a cell that covers the internal and external organs of the body.
Exudate:	escaping fluid that spills from a space; contains cellular debris and pus.
Facial palsy:	paralysis of some or all of the muscles of the face.
Fistula:	an abnormal passage from an internal organ to the surface of the skin or between two organs.

581

Foley catheter:	a rubber catheter with an inflatable balloon tip.
Glycaemic control:	the control of blood sugar levels.
Haemorrhage:	Bleeding.
Hereditary:	transmitted from parent to child.
Humidification:	increasing the water content of inhaled air.
Hypertension:	raised blood pressure.
Hypovolaemia:	low levels of fluid in the circulation.
Intracranial:	within the skull.
Intraocular pressure:	pressure within the eye.
Ischaemia:	a low oxygen state in a part of the body. Usually the result of obstruction to the blood supply to tissues.
Laxative:	a drug that promotes evacuation of the bowel.
Ligation:	tying off a blood vessel to stop or prevent bleeding.
Lipid:	an energy-rich organic compound that is soluble in organic substances such as alcohol and benzene.
Lymph node:	part of the lymphatic system, it contains many white cells to destroy bacteria that are trapped within the lymph node.
Malaise:	a feeling of body weakness.
Mucosa:	mucous membrane.
Mucous membrane:	thin sheet of tissue lining a part of the body that secretes mucus. Cover all the passageways leading into or out of the body (e.g. the mouth, nose, bronchi, urethra).
Mucus:	the secretions of mucous membranes.
Necrosis:	tissue death.
Needle aspiration:	the removal of fluid by a fine needle.
Neurological:	pertaining to the nervous system.
Olfactory:	pertaining to the sense of smell.
Opacity:	referring to the opaque quality of a substance.
Opaque:	does not allow the passage of light.
Palpation:	using the fingers or hands to examine by touch.

Pneumonia:	a condition characterised by acute inflammation of the lungs.
Polyp (plural polypi):	abnormal growth of tissue projecting from a mucous membrane.
Postnasal pack:	packing the upper nasopharynx with gauze or sponge to prevent the flow of blood into the nasopharynx. Also provides a firm base against which to pack the nasal cavity if required.
Pressure necrosis:	tissue death caused by prolonged or excessive pressure.
Prosthesis:	an artificial replacement for a missing part of the body.
Pulse oximetry:	non-invasive measurement of the oxygen content of the blood (SpO_2).
Purulent:	producing or containing pus.
Pus:	a thick green or cream fluid found at the site of a bacterial infection. It consists of millions of dead white blood cells of the immune system as well as dead bacteria.
Pyrexia:	elevated temperature associated with fever.
Regurgitation:	the return of swallowed food to the mouth.
Respiratory insufficiency:	inability to breathe due to weakness of the muscles of respiration.
Sac:	a pouch.
Secondary bacterial infection:	a bacterial infection following viral infection.
Sedation:	state of calm or sleepiness brought about by drugs.
Semirecumbent:	reclining position.
Stoma:	any opening; a mouth. Usually used to refer to a surgically created opening.
Suture:	stitch.
Syringing:	the procedure of introducing a fluid into a cavity to flush out debris or foreign bodies.
Tinnitus:	ringing noise in the ear.
Trocar:	a sharp pointed rod that fits inside a tube (cannula).
Vertigo:	dizziness.
Visual acuity:	detailed central vision.

References

Allen, D. and Vasavada, A. (2006). Cataract and surgery for cataract. *British Medical Journal.* 333: 128–132.

Bajaj, Y., Uppal, S., Bhatti, I. and Coatesworth, A.P. (2010). Otosclerosis 3: the surgical management of otosclerosis. *The International Journal of Clinical Practice.* 64(4): 505–510.

Benninger, M. (2008). Acute bacterial rhinosinusitis and otitis media: changes in pathogenicity following widespread use of pneumococcal conjugate vaccine. *Otolaryngology – Head Neck Surgery.* 183(3): 274–278.

Canaday, D.H. and Salata, R.A. (2008). Sinusitis and otitis. In: Tan, J.S., File, T.M., Salata, R.A. and Tan, M.J. (eds). *Expert Guide to Infectious Diseases*, 2nd edn. Philadelphia: American College of Physicians, pp. 387–400.

Chakravarthy, U., Evans, J. and Rosenfeld, P.J. (2010). Age related macular degeneration. *British Medical Journal.* 340: 526–530.

Clegg, A.J., Loveman, E., Gospodarevskaya, E. *et al.* (2010). The safety and effectiveness of different methods of earwax removal: a systematic review and economic evaluation. *Health Technology Assessment.* 14(28): 1–192.

Demarcantonio, M.A. and Han, J.K. (2011). Nasal polyps: Pathogenesis and treatment implications. *Otolaryngologic Clinics of North America.* 44(3): 685–695.

Evans, J.R. (2009). Antioxidant vitamin and mineral supplements for slowing the progression of age related macular degeneration. *Cochrane Library of Systematic Reviews.* Issue 2. Art No.: CD000254.

Fairhurst-Winstanley, W. (2007). Caring for the patient with a respiratory disorder. In: Walsh, M. and Crumbie, A. (eds). *Watson's Clinical Nursing and Related Sciences*, 7th edn. London. Elsevier, pp. 325–362.

Feber, T. (2006). Tracheostomy care for community nurses: Basic principles. *British Journal of Community Nursing*, 11(5): 186–193.

Gopen, Q. (2010). Pathology & clinical course: Inflammatory diseases of the middle ear. In: Gulya, A.J., Minar, L.B. and Poe, D.S. (eds). *Glassock-Shambaugh Surgery of the Ear*, 6th edn. Beijing, Peoples Medical Publishing House, pp. 425–436.

Guyton, A.C. and Hall, J. (2010). *Textbook of Medical Physiology*, 12th edn. Philadelphia: Elsevier Saunders.

Jenkins, G.W., Kemnitz, C.P. and Tortora, G.J. (2010). *Anatomy and Physiology. From Science to Life*, 2nd edn. International Student Edition. Hoboken, NJ: John Wiley & Sons.

Kaushik V., Malik T. and Saeed S.R. (2010). Interventions for acute otitis externa. *Cochrane Database of Systematic Reviews.* Issue 1. Art. No.: CD004740.

Kazi, R., Sayed, S.I. and Dwivedi, R.C. (2010). Post larygectomy speech and voice rehabilitation: past, present and future. *ANZ Journal of Surgery.* 80(11): 770–771.

Kumar, A and Wiet, R (2010). Aural complications of otitis media. In: Gulya, A.J., Minar, L.B. and Poe, D.S. (eds). *Glassock-Shambaugh Surgery of the Ear*, 6th edn. Beijing, Peoples Medical Publishing House, pp. 437–449.

Lewis, S.L., Dirksen, S.R., Heitkemper, M.M., Bucher, L. and Camera, I. (2010). *Medical – Surgical Nursing: Assessment and Management of Clinical Problems*, 8th edn. St. Louis: Mosby Elsevier.

Manes, R.P. (2010). Evaluating and managing the patient with nosebleeds. *Medical Clinics of North America.* 94(5): 903–912.

Marieb, E.N. and Hoehn, K. (2010). *Human Anatomy and Physiology*, 8th edn. San Francisco: Pearson Benjamin Cummings.

Masood, A., Moumoulidis, I. and Panesar, J. (2007). Acute rhinosinusitis in adults: an update on current management. *Postgraduate Medical Journal.* 83: 402–408.

McKerrow, W and Bradley, P.J. (2007). Sore throats. In: Ludman, H. and Bradley, P.J. (eds). *ABC of Ear Nose and Throat*. Oxford. Blackwell.

Pachaiappan, K.J., Patel, V., Morrissey, J. and Gadsby, R. (2006). Lipid management in type 1 diabetes. *Diabetic Medicine*, 23(Suppl 1): 11–14.

Pankhania, M., Judd, O. and Ward, A. (2011). Otorrhea. *British Medical Journal.* 342: d2299.

Riaz, Y., Mehta, J.S., Wormald, R. *et al.* (2006). Surgical interventions for age-related cataract. *Cochrane Database of Systematic Reviews.* Issue 4. Art. No.: CD001323.

Royal College of Ophthalmologists. (2009). *Age Related Macular Degeneration. Guidelines for Management*. London: Royal College of Ophthalmologists.

Sajjadi, H. and Paparella, M.M. (2008). Meniere's disease. *The Lancet*. 372(9636): 406–414.

Schlosser, R.J. (2009). Epistaxis. *New England Journal of Medicine*. 360: 784–789.

Schrauwen, I (2010) The etiology of otosclerosis: A combination of genes and environment. *The Laryngoscope*. 120(6): 1195–1202.

Scottish Intercollegiate Guidelines Network (SIGN) (2006). *Diagnosis and Management of Head and Neck Cancer. A National Clinical Guideline*. Edinburgh: SIGN.

Tortora, G.J. and Derrickson, B. (2011a). *Principles of Anatomy and Physiology. Volume 1. Organisation, Support and Movement, and Control of the Human Body*, 13th edn. International Student Version. Hoboken, NJ: John Wiley and Sons Inc.

Tortora, G.J. and Derrickson, B. (2011b). *Principles of Anatomy and Physiology. Volume 2.Maintenance and Continuity of the Human Body*, 13th edn. International Student Version. Hoboken, NJ: John Wiley and Sons Inc.

Walsh, M. (2007). Caring for the patient with a disorder of the senses. In: Walsh, M. and Crumbie, A. (eds). *Watson's Clinical Nursing and Related Sciences*, 7th edn. London: Elsevier, pp. 731–763.

Appendix A

Reference values in venous serum (adults)

Analysis	Reference range	
	SI units	**Non-SI units**
Albumin	36–47 g/L	3.6–4.7 g/100 mL
Alkaline phosphatase	40–125 U/L	–
Amylase	<100 U/L	–
Bilirubin (total)	2–17 μmol/L	0.12–1.0 mg/100 mL
Calcium	2.12–2.62 mmol/L	4.24–5.24 mEq/L or 8.50–10.50 mg/100 mL
Chloride	95–107 mmol/L	95–107 mEq/L
Cholesterol (total)	<5.5 mmol/L	–
HDL-cholesterol		
Male	0.5–1.6 mmol/L	19–62 mg/100 mL
Female	0.6–1.9 mmol/L	23–74 mg/100 mL
Copper	13–24 μmol/L	83–153 μg/100 mL

Fundamentals of Applied Pathophysiology: An Essential Guide for Nursing and Healthcare Students, Second Edition. Edited by Muralitharan Nair and Ian Peate.
© 2013 John Wiley & Sons, Ltd. Published 2013 by John Wiley & Sons, Ltd.

Analysis	Reference range	
	SI units	Non-SI units
Creatine kinase (total)		
Male	30–200 U/L	–
Female	30–150 U/L	–
Creatinine	55–120 µmol/L	0.62–1.36 mg/100 mL
Ferritin		
Male	17–300 µg/L	17–300 ng/mL
Female	14–150 µg/L	14–150 ng/mL
Glucose (fasting)	3.6–5.8 mmol/L	65–104 mg/100 mL
Glycated haemoglobin (HbA1)	5.0–6.5%	–
Immunoglobulin A	0.5–4.0 g/L	50–400 mg/100 mL
Immunoglobulin G	5.0–13.0 g/L	500–1300 mg/100 mL
Immunoglobulin M		
Male	0.3–2.2 g/L	30–220 mg/100 mL
Female	0.4–2.5 g/L	40–250 mg/100 mL
Iron		
Male	14–32 µmol/L	78–178 µg/100 mL
Female	10–28 µmol/L	56–156 µg/100 mL
Magnesium	0.75–1.0 mmol/L	1.5–2.0 mEq/L or 1.82–2.43 mg/100 mL
Osmolality	280–290 mmol/kg	280–290 mosm/L
Phosphate (fasting)	0.8–1.4 mmol/L	2.48–4.34 mg/100 mL
Potassium (plasma)	3.3–4.7 mmol/L	3.3–4.7 mEq/L
Potassium (serum)	3.6–5.1 mmol/L	3.6–5.1 mEq/L
Protein (total)	60–80 g/L	6–8 g/100 mL
Sodium	132–144 mmol/L	132–144 mEq/L
Total CO_2	24–30 mmol/L	24–30 mEq/L

Continued

Analysis	Reference range	
	SI units	Non-SI units
Transferrin	2.0–4.0 g/L	0.2–0.4 g/100 mL
Triglycerides (fasting)	0.6–1.7 mmol/L	53–150 mg/100 mL
Urate		
Male	0.12–0.42 mmol/L	2.0–7.0 mg/100 mL
Female	0.12–0.36 mmol/L	2.0–6.0 mg/100 mL
Urea	2.5–6.6 mmol/L	15–40 mg/100 mL
Zinc	11–22 µmol/L	72–144 µg/100 mL
Haematological values		
Bleeding time (Ivy)	Less than 8 minutes	–
Body fluid (total)	50% (obese) to 70% (lean) of body weight	–
Intracellular	30–40% of body weight	–
Extracellular	20–30% of body weight	–
Blood volume		
Male	75 ± 10 mL/kg	–
Female	70 ± 10 mL/kg	–
Coagulation screen		
Prothrombin time	8.0–10.5 seconds	–
Activated partial		
thromboplastin time	26–37 seconds	–
Erythrocyte sedimentation rate[a]		
Adult male	0–10 mm/h	–
Adult female	3–15 mm/h	–
Fibrinogen	1.5–4.0 g/L	0.15–0.4 g/100 mL
Folate		
Serum	1.5–20.6 µg/L	1.5–20.6 ng/mL
Red cell	95–570 µg/L	95–570 ng/mL

Analysis	Reference range	
	SI units	Non-SI units
Haemoglobin		
Male	130–180 g/L	13–18 g/100 mL
Female	115–165 g/L	11.5–16.5 g/100 mL
Leucocytes (adults)	$4.0\text{–}11.0 \times 10^9$/L	$4.0\text{–}11.0 \times 10^3$/mm^3
Differential white cell count		
Neutrophil granulocytes	$2.0\text{–}7.5 \times 10^9$/L	$2.0\text{–}7.5 \times 10^3$/mm^3
Lymphocytes	$1.5\text{–}4.0 \times 10^9$/L	$1.5\text{–}4.0 \times 10^3$/mm^3
Monocytes	$0.2\text{–}0.8 \times 10^9$/L	$0.2\text{–}0.8 \times 10^3$/mm^3
Eosinophil granulocytes	$0.04\text{–}0.4 \times 10^9$/L	$0.04\text{–}0.4 \times 10^3$/mm^3
Basophil granulocytes	$0.01\text{–}0.1 \times 10^9$/L	$0.01\text{–}0.1 \times 10^3$/mm^3
Packed cell volume (PCV) or haematocrit		
Male	0.40–0.54	–
Female	0.37–0.47	–
Platelets	$150\text{–}350 \times 10^9$/L	$150\text{–}350 \times 10^3$/mm^3
Red cell count		
Male	$4.5\text{–}6.5 \times 10^{12}$/L	$4.5\text{–}6.5 \times 10^6$/mm^3
Female	$3.8\text{–}5.8 \times 10^{12}$/L	$3.8\text{–}5.8 \times 10^6$/mm^3
Red cell lifespan (mean)	120 days	–
Red cell lifespan $T_2^{\frac{1}{2}}$ (^{51}Cr)	25–35 days	–
Reticulocytes (adults)	$25\text{–}85 \times 10^9$/L	$25\text{–}85 \times 10^3$/mm^3
Vitamin B$_{12}$	130–770 pg/mL	–

[a]Higher values in older patients are not necessarily abnormal.

Appendix B

List of units

cm	centimetre
mm	millimetre
L	litre
mL	millilitre
kg	kilogram
g	gram
mg	milligram
μg	microgram
ng	nanogram
pg	picogram
mol	mole
mmol	millimole
μmol	micromole
mEq	milliequivalent
mosm	milliosmole
mmHg	millimetres of mercury
kcal	kilocalorie

Fundamentals of Applied Pathophysiology: An Essential Guide for Nursing and Healthcare Students, Second Edition. Edited by Muralitharan Nair and Ian Peate.
© 2013 John Wiley & Sons, Ltd. Published 2013 by John Wiley & Sons, Ltd.

Index

Journals and bacteria are in *italics*. Page numbers for Illustrations and figures are in *italics*. Tables are in **bold**.

Fundamentals of Applied Pathophysiology: An Essential Guide for Nursing and Healthcare Students, Second Edition. Edited by Muralitharan Nair and Ian Peate.
© 2013 John Wiley & Sons, Ltd. Published 2013 by John Wiley & Sons, Ltd.